State of the Art Imaging of Osteoarthritis

Guest Editor

ALI GUERMAZI, MD

RHEUMATIC DISEASE CLINICS OF NORTH AMERICA

www.rheumatic.theclinics.com

August 2009 • Volume 35 • Number 3

SAUNDERS an imprint of ELSEVIER, Inc.

W.B. SAUNDERS COMPANY

A Division of Elsevier Inc.

1600 John F. Kennedy Blvd., Suite 1800 • Philadelphia, PA 19103-2899

http://www.theclinics.com

**RHEUMATIC DISEASE CLINICS OF NORTH AMERICA Volume 35, Number 3
August 2009 ISSN 0889-857X, ISBN 13: 978-1-4377-1750-1**

Editor: Rachel Glover
Developmental Editor: Donald Mumford

Rheumatic Disease Clinics of North America (ISSN 0889-857X) is published quarterly by Elsevier Inc., 360 Park Avenue South, New York, NY 10010-1710. Months of issue are February, May, August, and November. Business and editorial offices: 1600 John F. Kennedy Boulevard, Suite 1800, Philadelphia, PA 19103-2899. Periodicals postage paid at New York, NY and additional mailing offices. Subscription prices are USD 244.00 per year for US individuals, USD 414.00 per year for US institutions, USD 122.00 per year for US students and residents, USD 288.00 per year for Canadian individuals, USD 512.00 per year for Canadian institutions, USD 342.00 per year for international individuals, USD 512.00 per year for international institutions, and USD 171.00 per year for Canadian and foreign students/residents. To receive student/resident rate, orders must be accompanied by name of affiliated institution, date of term, and the *signature* of program/residency coordinator on institution letterhead. Orders will be billed at individual rate until proof of status received. Foreign air speed delivery is included in all *Clinics* subscription prices. All prices are subject to change without notice. **POSTMASTER:** Send address changes to *Rheumatic Disease Clinics of North America,* Elsevier Health Sciences Division, Subscription Customer Service, 3251 Riverport Lane, Maryland Heights, MO 63043. **Customer Service: 1-800-654-2452 (US and Canada). From outside of the US and Canada: 314-447-8871. Fax: 314-447-8029. For print support, e-mail: JournalsCustomerService-usa@elsevier.com. For online support, e-mail: Journals OnlineSupport-usa@elsevier.com.**

Reprints. For copies of 100 or more of articles in this publication, please contact the Commercial Reprints Department, Elsevier Inc., 360 Park Avenue South, New York, New York, 10010-1710; Tel.: (+1) 212-633-3813, Fax: (+1) 212-462-1935, and E-mail: reprints@elsevier.com.

Rheumatic Disease Clinics of North America is covered in *MEDLINE/PubMed (Index Medicus), Current Contents/Clinical Medicine, Science Citation Index, ISI/BIOMED,* and *EMBASE/Excerpta Medica.*

Printed and bound by CPI Group (UK) Ltd, Croydon, CR0 4YY

Transferred to Digital Print 2011

Contributors

GUEST EDITOR

ALI GUERMAZI, MD
Director, Quantitative Imaging Center, Associate Professor, Department of Radiology, Boston University School of Medicine, Boston, Massachusetts; President, Boston Imaging Core Lab (BICL), Boston, Massachusetts

AUTHORS

BERND BITTERSOHL, MD
Department of Orthopedic Surgery, University of Bern, Freiburgstrasse, Bern, Switzerland; Department of Orthopedic Surgery, University of Düsseldorf, Düsseldorf, Germany

ALAN BRETT, PhD
Optasia Medical, Manchester, United Kingdom

PHILIP G. CONAGHAN, MBBS, PhD, FRACP, FRCP
Professor of Musculoskeletal Diseases, NIHR Leeds Musculoskeletal Biomedical Research Unit and Section of Musculoskeletal Disease, Leeds Institute of Molecular Medicine, University of Leeds; Chapel Allerton Hospital, Leeds, United Kingdom

MICHEL D. CREMA, MD
Adjunct Assistant Professor, Department of Radiology, Quantitative Imaging Center, Boston University School of Medicine, Boston, Massachusetts; Boston Imaging Core Lab (BICL), Boston, Massachusetts; Institute of Diagnostic Imaging (IDI), Ribeirão Preto, SP, Brazil; Division of Radiology, Department of Internal Medicine, Ribeirão Preto School of Medicine, University of São Paulo, Ribeirão Preto, SP, Brazil

JEAN-LUC DRAPÉ, MD, PhD
Professor and Chairman of Radiology, Department of Radiology B, Cochin Hospital, Paris Descartes University, Paris, France

JEFF DURYEA, PhD
Brigham and Women's Hospital, Harvard Medical School, Boston, Massachusetts

FELIX ECKSTEIN, MD
Professor and Chairman, Institute of Anatomy & Musculoskeletal Research, Paracelsus Medical University, Salzburg, Austria; CEO, Chondrometrics GmbH, Ulrichshöglerstre, Ainring, Germany

MARTIN ENGLUND, MD, PhD
Musculoskeletal Sciences, Department of Orthopedics, Clinical Sciences Lund, Lund University, Lund, Sweden; Clinical Epidemiology Research & Training Unit, Boston University School of Medicine, Boston, Massachusetts

ANTOINE FEYDY, MD, PhD
Associate Professor of Radiology, Department of Radiology B, Cochin Hospital, Paris Descartes University, Paris, France

HENRI GUERINI, MD
Clinical Assistant Professor of Radiology, Department of Radiology B, Cochin Hospital, Paris Descartes University, Paris, France

ALI GUERMAZI, MD
Director, Quantitative Imaging Center, Associate Professor, Department of Radiology, Boston University School of Medicine, Boston, Massachusetts; President, Boston Imaging Core Lab (BICL), Boston, Massachusetts

MARIE-PIERRE HELLIO LE GRAVERAND, MD, DSc, PhD
Senior Director, Clinical Development and Medical Affairs, Inflammation, Specialty Care Business Unit, Pfizer Inc, New London, Connecticut

DAVID J. HUNTER, MBBS, FRACP, PhD
Chief of Research, Division of Research, Department of Orthopedics New England Baptist Hospital, Boston, Massachusetts

HELEN I. KEEN, MBBS, FRACP
Senior Lecturer, School of Medicine and Pharmacology, University of Western Australia, Perth, Australia

YOUNG-JO KIM, MD, PhD
Department of Orthopedic Surgery, Children's Hospital, Harvard Medical School, Boston, Massachusetts

L. STEFAN LOHMANDER, MD, PhD
Musculoskeletal Sciences, Department of Orthopedics, Clinical Sciences Lund, Lund University, Lund, Sweden

TALLAL C. MAMISCH, MD
Department of Orthopedic Surgery, University of Bern, Freiburgstrasse, Bern, Switzerland; Department of Radiology, Sonnenhof Clinics, Freiburgstrasse, Bern, Switzerland

MONICA D. MARRA, MD
Department of Radiology, Quantitative Imaging Center, Boston University School of Medicine, Boston, Massachusetts; Boston Imaging Core Lab (BICL), Boston, Massachusetts; Institute of Diagnostic Imaging (IDI), Ribeirão Preto, SP, Brazil

STEVE MAZZUCA, PhD
Indiana University School of Medicine, Indianapolis, Indiana

ETIENNE PLUOT, MD
Fellow of Radiology, Department of Radiology B, Cochin Hospital, Paris Descartes University, Paris, France

FRANK W. ROEMER, MD
Co-Director, Quantitative Imaging Center, Associate Professor, Department of Radiology, Boston University School of Medicine, Boston, Massachusetts; Attending Radiologist and Section Chief MRI, Stenglinstr, Augsburg, Germany; Director of Research, Boston Imaging Core Lab, Boston, Massachusetts

MARK SCHWEITZER, MD
Professor and Chair of Radiology, Department of Diagnostic Imaging, The Ottawa Hospital, University of Ottawa, General Campus, Ottawa, Canada

ADNAN SHEIKH, MD
Assistant Professor in Musculoskeletal Radiology, Department of Diagnostic Imaging, The Ottawa Hospital, University of Ottawa, General Campus, Ottawa, Canada

KLAUS A. SIEBENROCK, MD, PhD
Department of Orthopedic Surgery, University of Bern, Freiburgstrasse, Bern, Switzerland

STEFAN WERLEN, MD
Department of Radiology, Sonnenhof Clinics, Bern, Switzerland

DAVID R. WILSON, DPhil
Associate Professor, Department of Orthopaedics, University of British Columbia and Vancouver Coastal Health Research Institute, Vancouver, British Columbia, Canada

CHRISTOPH ZILKENS, MD
Department of Orthopedic Surgery, University of Düsseldorf, Düsseldorf, Germany; Department of Orthopedic Surgery, Children's Hospital, Harvard Medical School, Boston, Massachusetts

Contents

Preface   xiii

Ali Guermazi

Imaging Insights on the Epidemiology and Pathophysiology of Osteoarthritis   447

David J. Hunter

> This article highlights recent studies, particularly those with an emphasis on magnetic resonance imaging, that are providing unique insights into the relation between structures identified on imaging and the symptoms and genesis of osteoarthritis. These insights are changing the way disease prevalence is viewed and providing new insights into disease genesis. Furthermore, it is becoming increasingly apparent that the subchondral bone, periosteum, periarticular ligaments, periarticular muscle spasm, synovium, and joint capsule are all richly innervated and are the likely source of nociception in osteoarthritis. In addition, it is apparent that local tissue alterations in the bone and meniscus and alignment of the lower extremity are important in terms of disease genesis. The article is consistent with the literature in that much of the focus and understanding is knee-centric with less focus on the hip and hand.

Imaging the Role of Biomechanics in Osteoarthritis   465

David J. Hunter and David R. Wilson

> Osteoarthritis is widely believed to result from local mechanical factors acting within the context of systemic susceptibility. This narrative review delineates current understanding of the etiopathogenesis of osteoarthritis and more specifically examines the critical role of biomechanics in disease pathogenesis. There are several ways the mechanical forces across the joint can be measured, including some that rely heavily on imaging methods. These are described and methods to advance the field are proposed.

Radiographic Grading and Measurement of Joint Space Width in Osteoarthritis   485

Marie-Pierre Hellio Le Graverand, Steve Mazzuca, Jeff Duryea, and Alan Brett

> The progression of osteoarthritis is traditionally measured using radiographic joint space width (JSW). Numerous knee radiograph protocols have been developed with various levels of complexity and performance as it relates to detecting JSW loss (ie, joint space narrowing). Sensitivity to joint space narrowing is improved when radioanatomic alignment of the medial tibial plateau is achieved. Semiautomated software has been developed to improve the accuracy of JSW measurement over manual methods. JSW measurements include minimum JSW, mean JSW or joint space area, and JSW at fixed locations.

Usefulness of Ultrasound in Osteoarthritis   503

Helen I. Keen and Philip G. Conaghan

> Ultrasonography is a useful tool in understanding rheumatic conditions and in diagnosis and management. Much of the investigation into the

validity of ultrasonography and its clinical use has been undertaken in in-flammatory arthritides. Although ultrasonography has been applied to os-teoarthritis (OA) in clinical practice, there has been little investigation into the validity of ultrasonography in OA or its utility in clinical trials or routine clinical practice. This review outlines benefits and limitations of imaging OA with ultrasonography.

Magnetic Resonance Imaging-Based Semiquantitative and Quantitative Assessment in Osteoarthritis

521

Frank W. Roemer, Felix Eckstein, and Ali Guermazi

Whole organ magnetic resonance imaging (MRI)-based semiquantitative (SQ) assessment of knee osteoarthritis (OA), based on reliable scoring methods and expert reading, has become a powerful research tool in OA. SQ morphologic scoring has been applied to large observational cross-sectional and longitudinal epidemiologic studies as well as interventional clinical trials. SQ whole organ scoring analyzes all joint structures that are potentially relevant as surrogate outcome measures of OA and potential disease modification, including cartilage, subchondral bone, osteophytes, intra- and periarticular ligaments, menisci, synovial lining, cysts, and bursae. Resources needed for SQ scoring rely on the MRI protocol, image quality, experience of the expert readers, method of documentation, and the individual scoring system that will be applied. The first part of this article discusses the different available OA whole organ scoring systems, focusing on MRI of the knee, and also reviews alternative approaches. Rheumatologists are made aware of artifacts and differential diagnoses when applying any of the SQ scoring systems. The second part focuses on quantitative approaches in OA, particularly measurement of (subregional) cartilage loss. This approach allows one to determine minute changes that occur relatively homogeneously across cartilage structures and that are not apparent to the naked eye. To this end, the cartilage surfaces need to be segmented by trained users using specialized software. Measurements of knee cartilage loss based on water-excitation spoiled gradient recalled echo acquisition in the steady state, fast low-angle shot, or double-echo steady-state imaging sequences reported a 1% to 2% decrease in cartilage thickness annually, and a high degree of spatial heterogeneity of cartilage thickness changes in femorotibial subregions between subjects. Risk factors identified by quantitative measurement technology included a high body mass index, meniscal extrusion and meniscal tears, knee malalignment, advanced radiographic OA grade, bone marrow alterations, and focal cartilage lesions.

Magnetic Resonance Imaging Assessment of Subchondral Bone and Soft Tissues in Knee Osteoarthritis

557

Michel D. Crema, Frank W. Roemer, Monica D. Marra, and Ali Guermazi

Knee osteoarthritis (OA) has to be considered a whole joint disease. Magnetic resonance imaging (MRI) allows superior assessment of all joint tissues that may be involved in OA, such as the subchondral bone, synovium, ligaments, and periarticular soft tissues. Reliable MRI-based scoring systems are available to assess and quantify these structures and associated pathology. Cross-sectional and longitudinal evaluation has enabled practitioners to understand their relevance in explaining pain and structural progression.

The Meniscus in Knee Osteoarthritis   579

Martin Englund, Ali Guermazi, and L. Stefan Lohmander

The meniscus is a critical tissue in the healthy knee joint because of its shock absorption and load distribution properties. Meniscal damage is a frequent finding on MRI of the osteoarthritis (OA) knee. The damage appears as horizontal, flap, or complex tears; meniscal maceration; or destruction. Asymptomatic meniscal lesions are common incidental findings on knee MRI of the middle-aged or older person. This challenges the health professional in choosing the best treatment. A meniscal tear can lead to knee OA, but knee OA can also lead to a spontaneous meniscal tear. A degenerative meniscal lesion often suggests early-stage knee OA. Surgical resection of nonobstructive degenerate lesions may merely remove evidence of the disorder while the OA and associated symptoms proceed.

Hip MRI and Its Implications for Surgery in Osteoarthritis Patients   591

Tallal C. Mamisch, Christoph Zilkens, Klaus A. Siebenrock, Bernd Bittersohl, Young-Jo Kim, and Stefan Werlen

Osteoarthritis (OA) of the hip joint stems from a combination of intrinsic factors, such as joint anatomy, and extrinsic factors, such as injuries, diseases, and load. Possible risk factors for OA are instability and impingement. Different surgical techniques, such as osteotomies of the pelvis and femur, surgical dislocation, and hip arthroscopy, are being performed to delay or halt OA. Success of salvage procedures of the hip depends on the existing cartilage and joint damage before surgery. The likelihood of therapy failure rises with advanced OA. For imaging of intra-articular hip pathology, MRI represents the best technique because it enables clinicians to directly visualize cartilage, it provides superior soft tissue contrast, and it offers the prospect of multidimensional imaging. However, opinions differ on the diagnostic efficacy of MRI and on the question of which MRI technique is most appropriate. This article gives an overview of the standard MRI techniques for diagnosis of hip OA and their implications for surgery.

Role of Imaging in Spine, Hand, and Wrist Osteoarthritis   605

Antoine Feydy, Etienne Pluot, Henri Guerini, and Jean-Luc Drapé

Osteoarthritis (OA) of the wrist is mainly secondary to traumatic ligamentous or bone injuries. Involvement of the radiocarpal joint occurs early on in the disease, whereas the mediocarpal joint is involved at a later stage. Metabolic diseases may also involve the wrist and affect specific joints such as the scapho-trapezio-trapezoid joint. Although OA of the wrist is routinely diagnosed on plain films, a thorough assessment of cartilage injuries on computed tomographic arthrography, magnetic resonance imaging (MRI), or MR arthrography remains necessary before any surgical procedure. OA of the fingers is frequently encountered in postmenopausal women. Distal interphalangeal joints and trapezio-metacarpal joint are the most frequently involved joints. Whereas the clinical diagnosis of OA of the wrist and hand is straightforward, the therapeutic management of symptomatic forms remains unclear, with no clear guidelines. OA of the spine is related to degenerative changes of the spine involving the disc space, vertebral endplates, the facet joints, or the supportive and surrounding soft tissues. The sequelae of disc degeneration are among the leading causes of functional incapacity in both sexes, and are a common source of chronic disability in the working years. Disc degeneration involves structural disruption and cell-mediated changes in composition. Radiography remains usually the first-line imaging method. MRI is ideally suited for delineating the presence, extent, and complications of degenerative spinal disease. Other imaging modalities such as computed tomography, dynamic radiography, myelography, and discography may provide complementary information in selected cases, especially before an imaging-guided percutaneous treatment or spinal surgery. The presence of degenerative changes on imaging examinations is by no means an indicator of symptoms, and there is a high prevalence of lesions in asymptomatic individuals. This article focuses on imaging of OA of the wrist and hand, as well as lumbar spine OA, with an emphasis on current MRI grading systems available for the assessment of discovertebral lesions.

Pre- and Postoperative Assessment in Joint Preserving and Replacing Surgery   651

Adnan Sheikh and Mark Schweitzer

Advances in imaging technology have increased its suitability for diagnosing musculoskeletal disease. Modification of imaging techniques and improved image quality have led to increased use of computed tomography and magnetic resonance imaging in the assessment of postoperative complications. This article discusses the indications, pre- and postoperative imaging findings, and postoperative complications of knee and hip arthroplasty, articular cartilage repair, and high tibial osteotomy.

Index   675

FORTHCOMING ISSUES

November 2009
Quantitative Assessment
of Musculoskeletal Conditions
in Standard Clinical Care
Theodore Pincus and
Yusuf Yazici, *Guest Editors*

February 2010
Systemic Lupus Erythematosus
Ellen Ginzler, MD, *Guest Editor*

RECENT ISSUES

May 2009
Fibromyalgia
Philip J. Mease, MD, *Guest Editor*

February 2009
Infections and Rheumatic Diseases
Luis R. Espinoza, MD, *Guest Editor*

November 2008
Sjögren's Syndrome
Steven E. Carsons, MD, *Guest Editor*

RELATED INTEREST
Radiologic Clinics of North America
Volume 47, Issue 3
Musculoskeletal Radiology: Past, Present, and Future
Carolyn M. Sofka, MD, *Guest Editor*

THE CLINICS ARE NOW AVAILABLE ONLINE!
Access your subscription at:
www.theclinics.com

Preface–Osteoarthritis: From the Simple X-ray to Compositional MRI: What Have We Learned?

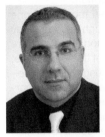

Ali Guermazi, MD
Guest Editor

Osteoarthritis (OA) is an extraordinarily prevalent disease. Approximately 50 million Americans and 800 million people worldwide have reported having OA and approximately 20 million Americans arthritis-associated activity limitations.[1] OA of the knee, which is the joint most well investigated, affects an estimated 6% of adults and is a leading cause of disability among adults in the United States. The economic burden of arthritis is estimated to be approximately $120 billion, which is equivalent to 1.2% of the gross domestic product.[2] OA, however, remains an enigmatic disease. At the meeting of the Osteoarthritis Research Society International held in Montreal, Canada, September 10–13, 2009, it was reported that 10% of the population has asymptomatic OA, 58% of persons with knee OA have no radiographic findings, and 80% of persons who have had an anterior cruciate ligament develop OA. Today, knowledge of the pathophysiology and natural history of OA is so limited that most of the patients and even physicians believe that there is little we can do to treat or prevent the disease other than trying to alleviate the inflammatory symptoms when they occur. In the meantime, several epidemiologic studies were or are currently under way to help understand the relationship between structure and function and how best to intervene in this disease process. Imaging is playing a major role in these studies and providing insights in understanding of this complex disease. In this issue of *Rheumatic Disease Clinics of North America*, world-renowned researchers and clinicians report on the latest advances in understanding of the disease using imaging.

Dr Hunter presents insights on epidemiology of the disease and how to tackle its risk factors. Drs Hunter and Wilson describe the importance of alignment and mechanics in pathophysiology of OA and in the treatment of the disease.

Rheum Dis Clin N Am 35 (2009) xiii–xiv
doi:10.1016/j.rdc.2009.09.003
0889-857X/09/$ – see front matter © 2009 Elsevier Inc. All rights reserved.

rheumatic.theclinics.com

Dr Le Graverand and colleagues report on the utility of radiographs in OA and Drs Keen and Conaghan on ultrasound use in OA. Dr Roemer and colleagues and Dr Crema and colleagues report on the place of MRI in semiquantitative and quantitative assessment of knee OA. Dr Englund and colleagues report on the place of meniscus in the genesis and progression of knee OA. Because OA is usually a multijoint disease, Dr Mamisch and colleagues and Dr Feydy and colleagues report on OA of other joints, including hip, spine, hand, and wrist. Finally, Drs Sheikh and Schweitzer report on the role of imaging in pre- and postoperative assessment in joint preserving and replacing surgery, when preservative therapy is no longer an option.

Today, it is obvious that the disease has a complex etiology, as more than one pathway exists to explain the pathophysiology of the disease. Although several study working groups are focusing on better defining OA using imaging modalities that are more sensitive than radiography, there is a common theme to many of these activities: whether or not to image pre-OA or in early OA. Ultimately,when waiting for the development of radiographic changes, the potential for reversibility is small, and the opportunity for interventions to modify structural changes may be lost. The ability to modify the structural changes of OA is the holy grail of many researchers (and, soon, also clinicians) who are engaged in OA management. We have witnessed the recent revolution in the management of other chronic musculoskeletal diseases, including osteoporosis and rheumatoid arthritis, and know that as each day passes we are closer to similar major progress in the way OA is managed. At the forefront of the ultimate ability to modify structural changes is the ability to detect early disease and measure structural changes in a responsive manner. MRI is a promising tool not only in understanding the pathophysiology of the disease but also in disclosing the painful structure and monitoring the different structural changes, especially bone marrow lesions and cartilage. Moreover, compositional MRI, although still in its early stage, may play a role in the future in showing premorphologic changes as a biomarker of preclinical disease. Only then will treatment of OA or, even better, its prevention, be possible.

I hope this issue will bring insights to the readership of *Rheumatic Disease Clinics of North America* to better understand OA and also encourage more researchers to join this excellent opportunity in elucidating this enigmatic disease.

Ali Guermazi, MD
Department of Radiology
Section of Musculoskeletal
Quantitative Imaging Center
Boston University School of Medicine
820 Harrison Avenue
FGH Building, 3rd Floor
Boston, MA 02118, USA

E-mail address:
ali.guermazi@bmc.org

REFERENCES

1. Centers for Disease Control and Prevention. Prevalence of doctor-diagnosed arthritis and arthritis-attributable activity limitation—United States, 2003–2005. MMWR Morb Mortal Wkly Rep 2006;55:1089–92.
2. Centers for Disease Control and Prevention. National and state medical expenditures and lost earnings attributable to arthritis and other rheumatic conditions—United States, 2003. MMWR Morb Mortal Wkly Rep 2007;56:4–7.

Imaging Insights on the Epidemiology and Pathophysiology of Osteoarthritis

David J. Hunter, MBBS, FRACP, PhD

KEYWORDS

• Epidemiology • Pathophysiology • Osteoarthritis • MRI • Pain

Symptomatic osteoarthritis (OA) causes substantial physical and psychosocial disability.[1] Interestingly, the risk for disability (defined as needing help walking or climbing stairs) attributable to knee OA is as great as that attributable to cardiovascular disease and greater than that caused by any other medical condition in the elderly.[1] Estimates suggest that the public health consequences will deteriorate as the prevalence of knee OA is projected to double by the year 2020, due in part to increases in obesity and longevity.

The synovial joint is an organ, and OA represents failure of that organ. The disease process can be initiated by abnormalities arising in any of its constituent tissues.[2] At a molecular level, the disease occurs when the dynamic equilibrium between the breakdown and repair of the synovial joint tissues is overwhelmed.[3] During disease development, inflammatory changes occur secondary to particulate and soluble breakdown products of cartilage and bone. OA is commonly misnamed "degenerative joint disease," as the cells of the cartilage and bone are normal and, if the inciting breakdown mechanism is reduced, can restore the damaged tissue to normal.

This article briefly describes the epidemiology and pathophysiology of OA. It also delineates what knowledge imaging has brought to these scientific areas in recent years. The predominant symptoms in most patients presenting with OA are pain and functional limitation. Over recent years, several imaging-based studies have narrowed the discord between knowledge about structural findings on imaging and symptoms. In addition, several new risk factors that portend to more rapid structural progression have been identified using novel imaging methods. Much of the research

A version of this article originally appeared in the 47:4 issue of Radiologic Clinics of North America.

Division of Research, Department of Orthopedics, New England Baptist Hospital, 125 Parker Hill Avenue, Boston, MA 02120, USA
E-mail address: djhunter@caregroup.harvard.edu

Rheum Dis Clin N Am 35 (2009) 447–463
doi:10.1016/j.rdc.2009.08.001
0889-857X/09/$ – see front matter © 2009 Elsevier Inc. All rights reserved.

and understanding of OA are centered on the knee (as opposed to the hip or hand), and as such this article reflects this imbalance.

EPIDEMIOLOGY

In epidemiologic investigation, OA typically is defined using conventional radiographs, and less frequently self-report. The reported prevalence of OA varies according to the method used to evaluate it. The characteristic radiographic features used to define and classify OA severity are osteophytes (osteocartilaginous growths), subchondral sclerosis, and joint space narrowing (**Fig. 1**).

Both the presence and severity of OA traditionally are classified using the Kellgren and Lawrence (K&L) grading system,[4] a system that depends heavily on the osteophytes for disease definition (**Table 1**). This system suffers from additional limitations including mixing distinct constructs (eg, osteophytes, joint space narrowing, subchondral sclerosis, subchondral bone shape changes, and cysts) into one scale. Further, the scale is not linear; thus, the use of K&L grade as a measure of disease progression is best avoided.

Understanding the radiographic method of disease definition becomes important when one considers that osteophytes, typically the first features identified on radiographs, are not necessarily a deleterious finding and may represent an effort on the part of the joint to promote stability. They are important, however, if they represent a source of symptoms, and yet most of the epidemiologic research in OA is based on the presence of self-reported OA or radiographic osteophytes and not on symptomatic OA, defined as the concomitant presence of pain and radiographic features. It is the presence of symptomatic OA that is important clinically, not simply the radiographic identification of an osteophyte or self-reported OA (where misclassification is

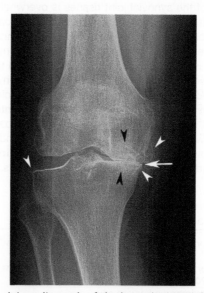

Fig. 1. A weight-bearing plain radiograph of the knee depicting the characteristic features seen in OA: medial tibiofemoral joint space narrowing (*arrow*), marginal femoral and tibial osteophytosis (*white arrowhead*), and medial tibial and femoral subchondral sclerosis (*black arrowheads*).

Table 1	
The Kellgren and Lawrence grading system	
Grade 0	Normal
Grade 1	Doubtful narrowing of joint space and possible osteophytic lipping
Grade 2	Definite osteophytes and possible narrowing of joint space
Grade 3	Moderate multiple osteophytes, definite narrowing of joint space and some sclerosis, and possible deformity of bone ends
Grade 4	Large osteophytes, marked narrowing of joint space, severe sclerosis, and definite deformity of bone ends

From Kellgren JH, Lawrence JS. Atlas of standard radiographs. Oxford (UK): Blackwell Scientific; 1963. P. 2; with permission.

even more problematic than the commonly used radiographic OA definition). In addition, by the time a person has disease sufficient to produce the characteristic changes of OA on conventional radiographs, marked structural damage is already present using other methods capable of identifying early disease.[5–10]

During a 1-year period, 25% of people over 55 years old have a persistent episode of knee pain, of whom about one in six consult their general practitioner about it.[11] In this British sample, symptomatic knee OA defined as pain on most days and radiographic features consistent with OA occurred in approximately 12% of those aged over 55 years.[11] From US estimates, about 6% of adults aged over 30 years[12] and 13% of people aged 60 years and over[13] had symptomatic knee OA.

Although OA is common in the knee, it is even more prevalent in the hands, especially the distal (DIP) and proximal (PIP) interphalangeal joints and the base of the thumb (carpometacarpal [CMC]). When symptomatic, especially so for the base of thumb joint, hand OA is associated with functional impairment.[14,15] OA of the thumb CMC joint is a common condition that can lead to substantial pain, instability, deformity, and loss of motion.[16] Over the age of 70 years, approximately 5% of women and 3% of men have symptomatic OA affecting this joint with impairment of hand function.[14]

The prevalence of hip OA is about 9% in white populations.[17] In contrast, studies in Asian, black, and East Indian populations indicate a very low prevalence of hip OA.[18] The prevalence of symptomatic hip OA is approximately 4%.[13] It has been suggested that the lower rates detected among certain ethnic populations may be due to lower rates of congenital or developmental abnormalities and, in some cultures, the common use of squatting postures, which force the hip through extreme ranges of motion.[19]

Risk Factors for OA

OA perhaps is understood best as resulting from excessive mechanical stress applied in the context of systemic susceptibility (**Fig. 2**). Susceptibility to OA may be increased in part by genetic inheritance (a positive family history increases risk), age, ethnicity, diet, and female gender.[20]

In people vulnerable to the development of knee OA, local mechanical factors such as abnormal joint congruity, malalignment (varus or valgus deformity), muscle weakness, or alterations in the structural integrity of the joint environment such as meniscal damage, bone marrow lesions (BMLs), or ligament rupture can facilitate the progression of OA. Loading also can be affected by obesity and joint injury (either acutely as in a sporting injury or after repetitive overuse such as occupational exposure), both of which can increase the likelihood of development or progression of OA.

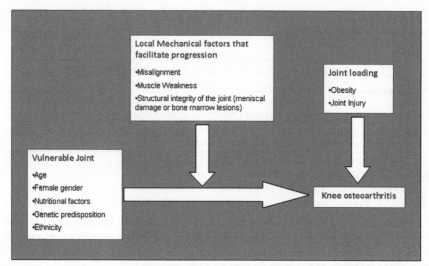

Fig. 2. Schemata demonstrating the risk factors for OA onset and progression.

INSIGHTS FROM IMAGING ON EPIDEMIOLOGY

Bearing in mind that radiographs are notoriously insensitive to the earliest pathologic features of OA, the absence of positive radiographic findings should not be interpreted as confirming the complete absence of symptomatic disease. Conversely, the presence of positive radiographic findings does not guarantee that an osteoarthritic joint is also the active source of the patient's current knee or hip symptoms where other sources of pain including periarticular sources such as pes anserine bursitis at the knee and trochanteric bursitis at the hip often contribute.[21] According to the American College of Rheumatology (ACR) criteria for classification of hand OA (unlike the hip and knee, where radiographs enhance the sensitivity and specificity), radiographs are less sensitive and specific than physical examination in the diagnosis of symptomatic hand OA.[22] The usefulness of radiographs relates more importantly to the exclusion of other diagnostic possibilities rather than confirmation of osteoarthritic disease.[23] Thus in clinical practice, the diagnosis of OA should be made on the basis of history and physical examination and the role of radiography is to rule out other conditions.

Recent imaging studies have provided new insights into disease genesis. This section will focus on these as they pertain to the hip and hand, with the remainder of the article providing a larger focus on the knee.

Hip OA is a major cause of disability in the United States,[24] and the major reason for the approximately 200,000 hip replacements performed annually.[25] Recent evidence highlights the importance of local mechanical factors, including acetabular dysplasia, which may account for up to 40% of hip OA.[26,27]

OA of the thumb CMC joint is a common condition that can lead to substantial pain, instability, deformity, and loss of motion.[16] The agility of the thumb is afforded mainly by the mobility of the trapeziometacarpal joint or so-called base of thumb joint.[28–30] Eaton and Littler[28] proposed that instability of the trapeziometacarpal joint combined with strenuous use could lead to OA. The author recently confirmed this suspicion and demonstrated that radial subluxation predisposes to subsequent OA of the trapeziometacarpal joint in men.[31]

A recent study using high-resolution magnetic resonance imaging (MRI) and surface coils adapted for clinical scanners, with an in-plane resolution of 80 to 100 mm identified early phenotypic features of hand OA where enthesophytic changes were prominent.[32] The most striking abnormalities were in the collateral ligaments (abnormalities ranging from thickening to frank disruption) and capsules of the PIP and DIP joints, rather than in the articular cartilage or subchondral bone.

PATHOPHYSIOLOGY OF OA

Early investigators tended to regard OA as an isolated disease of articular cartilage. Although cartilage loss is a prominent feature of OA, contemporary models recognize that the entire synovial joint organ is affected by OA. OA can be viewed as the clinical and pathologic outcome of a range of disorders that results in structural and functional failure of the synovial joint organ with loss and erosion of articular cartilage, subchondral bone alteration, meniscal degeneration, a synovial inflammatory response, and bone and cartilage overgrowth (osteophytes).[33] Joint failure may cause pain, physical disability, and psychological distress,[1] although many people with structural changes consistent with OA are asymptomatic.[21] The reasons why there is this disconnect between radiographic severity and the level of reported pain and disability is largely unknown, although recent imaging studies are beginning to shed light on this.

INSIGHTS FROM IMAGING ON SYMPTOM GENESIS

The structural determinants of pain and mechanical dysfunction in OA are not well understood, but they are believed to involve multiple interactive pathways that are best framed in a biopsychosocial framework (posits that biologic, psychological, and social factors all play a significant role in pain in OA).[34,35] Local to the joint, there are several tissues that contain nociceptive fibers, and these are the likely sources of pain in OA. The subchondral bone, periosteum, periarticular ligaments, periarticular muscle, synovium, and joint capsule are all richly innervated and are the likely source of nociception in OA.

In population studies, there is a significant discordance between radiographically diagnosed OA and knee pain.[21] Although radiographic evidence of joint damage predisposes to joint pain, it is clear that the relation of the severity of joint damage to the severity of the pain is not strong. Using other imaging modalities such as MRI, however, numerous structural alterations evident on MRI, such as subchondral BMLs,[36,37] subarticular bone attrition,[38] synovitis, and effusion[39,40] have been related to knee pain. It remains unclear which of these local tissue factors predominate, as until recently, these analyses did not account for the fact that much of the structural change is collinear (a person who has more severe disease will have worse structural change in multiple tissues including the bone and synovium).Additionally, the studies were not adjusting for other tissue changes. A recent analysis confirmed most beliefs that it is likely that changes in the subchondral bone and synovial activation/effusion predominate.[41] The different tissues within the joint and their respective contribution to symptoms are discussed.

Hyaline Articular Cartilage

Articular cartilage is both aneural and avascular. As such, cartilage is incapable of directly generating pain, inflammation, stiffness, or any of the symptoms that patients with OA typically describe.[42] This said, some studies have suggested a relation between cartilage morphometry and lesions and the symptoms of OA.[43] The studies that have demonstrated a relation of cartilage damage to pain traditionally have investigated the role of cartilage in predisposing to symptoms in isolation from other tissues and as such are fundamentally flawed. It is important to note that this disease of the whole joint concurrently affects other tissues that contain nociceptors. The relation of cartilage to symptoms in OA is likely through secondary mechanisms such as:

Exposing the underlying subchondral bone nociceptors

Vascular congestion of subchondral bone leading to increased intraosseous pressure

Synovitis secondary to articular cartilage damage with activation of synovial membrane nociceptors

Subchondral Bone

Periarticular bone changes associated with OA can be segregated into distinct patterns based on their anatomic location and pathogenic mechanisms. These alterations include progressive increase in subchondral plate thickness, alterations in the architecture of subchondral trabecular bone, formation of new bone at the joint margins (osteophytes), development of subchondral bone cysts, and advancement of the tidemark associated with vascular invasion of the calcified cartilage.

Of these lesions, that which has the most supportive evidence for a role in symptom genesis is the bone marrow lesion (**Fig. 3**). Lesions in the bone marrow play an integral if not pivotal role in the symptoms that emanate from knee OA and its structural progression.[36] BMLs were found in 272 of 351 (77.5%) people with painful knees, compared with 15 of 50 (30%) people with no knee pain ($P<.001$). Large lesions were present almost exclusively in people with knee pain (35.9% versus 2%; $P<.001$). After adjustment for severity of radiographic disease, effusion, age, and sex, all lesions, and in particular large lesions, remained associated with the occurrence of knee pain. More recently, their relation to pain severity[37] and incident pain[44] also was demonstrated. There are conflicting data, albeit from smaller studies with different methods, suggesting no relation of BMLs to pain[45,46]; however the balance of data would support a strong relation of BMLs to pain.

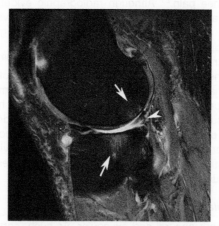

Fig. 3. Sagittal fat-suppressed intermediate-weighted MRI depicts diffuse ill-defined hyperintensities (*arrows*) abutting the subchondral plate in the weight-bearing lateral tibia and femur characteristic of bone marrow lesions. There is also an extensive osteophytosis and cartilage defect of the lateral tibial plateau and femoral condyle and bone attrition of the tibial plateau. There is an oblique tear of the partially macerated posterior horn of the lateral meniscus (*arrowhead*).

Other potential causes of pain from a boney origin in OA include periostitis associated with osteophyte formation,[47] subchondral microfractures,[48] bone attrition.[38] and bone angina caused by decreased blood flow and elevated intraosseous pressure.[49] One likely source that remains relatively underexplored is that of intraosseous hypertension. The pathophysiology remains unclear, although phlebographic studies in OA indicate impaired vascular clearance from bone and raised intraosseous pressure in the bone marrow near the painful joint.[49–52] What may cause pain subsequently is unknown. Increased trabecular bone pressure, ischemia, and inflammation are all possible stimuli.

Synovitis and Effusion

The synovial reaction in OA includes synovial hyperplasia, fibrosis, thickening of synovial capsule, activated synoviocytes, and in some cases lymphocytic infiltrate (B- and T-cells as well as plasma cells).[53] The site of infiltration of the synovium is of obvious relevance, as one of the most densely innervated structures of the joint is the white adipose tissue of the fat pad, which also shows evidence of inflammation and can act as a rich source of inflammatory adipokines.[54] Synovial causes of pain include irritation of sensory nerve endings within the synovium from osteophytes and synovial inflammation that is caused, at least in part, by the release of prostaglandins, leukotrienes, proteinases, neuropeptides, and cytokines.[35,55]

Synovitis and effusion are frequently present in OA and relate to pain and other clinical outcomes (**Fig. 4**).[39] Synovial thickening around the infrapatellar fat pad using noncontrast MRI has been shown on biopsy to represent mild chronic synovitis.[56] A semiquantitative measure of synovitis from the infrapatellar fat pad is associated with pain severity, and similarly, change in synovitis is associated with change in pain severity.[40] Of the three locations for synovitis in this study, changes in the infrapatellar fat pad were related most strongly to pain change (4.2 mm increase in pain per unit increase in synovitis).

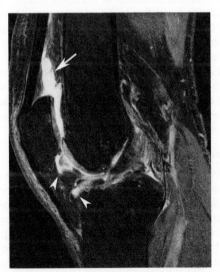

Fig. 4. Sagittal fat-suppressed intermediate-weighted MRI shows knee joint effusion (*arrow*) and infrapatellar synovitis (*arrowhead*). On this noncontrast MRI, the magnitude of synovitis is difficult to determine.

In an important caveat to this analysis, a recent study compared nonenhanced fat-suppressed proton density-weighted MRI with fat-suppressed contrast-enhanced (CE) T1-weighted MRI for semiquantitative assessment of peripatellar synovitis in OA.[57] These data suggested that signal alterations in Hoffa's fat pad on nonenhanced MRI do not always represent synovitis as seen on CE T1-weighted MRI but are a rather nonspecific albeit sensitive finding. This study concluded that semiquantitative scoring of peripatellar synovitis in OA ideally should be performed using CE T1-weighted MRI and should include scoring of synovial thickness.

Meniscus

The meniscus has many functions in the knee, including load bearing, shock absorption, stability enhancement, and lubrication.[58,59] The menisci transmit anywhere from 45% to 60% of the compressive loads in the knee.[58] If the meniscus does not cover the articular surface that it is designed to protect because of change in position, or if a tear leaves it unable to resist axial loading, it will not perform this role. The absence of a functioning meniscus increases peak and average contact stresses in the medial compartment of the knee in a range of 40% to 700%.[60–62]

Knee OA after meniscectomy/meniscal repair traditionally is considered a result of the joint injury that leads to the meniscectomy in the first instance and the increased cartilage contact stress caused by the loss of meniscal tissue.[63–65] Meniscectomy often is accompanied by the onset of OA because of the high focal stresses imposed on articular cartilage and subchondral bone subsequent to excision of the meniscus. The studies that have explored the relationship between the meniscus and risk of disease progression in OA provide a clear indication of the risk inherent with damage to this vital tissue.[66–68] Each aspect of meniscal abnormality (whether change in position or damage) (**Fig. 5**) had a major effect on risk of cartilage loss in OA.

Thus, the intact and functional meniscus is clearly important to preserve joint integrity and prevent further joint damage. In contrast, the meniscus plays a much smaller role in symptom genesis. An unfortunate consequence of the frequent use of MRI in clinical practice is the frequent detection of meniscal tears.[69] Degenerative lesions, described as horizontal cleavages, flap (oblique), or complex tears or meniscal maceration or destruction are associated with older age and are almost universal in people with OA.[69] In asymptomatic subjects with a mean age of 65 years, a tear was found in 67% using MRI, whereas in patients with symptomatic knee OA, a meniscal tear was found in 91% of patients.[70] In the interests of preserving menisci, an important cautionary note; meniscal tears are nearly universal in people with knee OA and are unlikely to be a cause of increased symptoms.[70,71] The penchant to remove menisci is to be avoided, unless there are symptoms of locking or extension blockade, at which point surgical treatment often becomes necessary.[72]

The Role of Other Tissues

Periarticular muscles influence joint loading, and impairments in muscle function have been observed in people with OA.[73] Various studies have investigated the role of muscle strength on joint integrity, and some have explored the impact on physical functioning. Sharma and colleagues[74] conducted a 3-year longitudinal cohort study investigating factors contributing to poor physical functioning in 257 patients with knee OA. They found that in addition to factors such as age, reduced absolute quadriceps and hamstrings strength and poor proprioceptive acuity increased the likelihood of poor physical functioning as measured by the time to perform five repetitions of rising and sitting in a chair. In addition to their exploration in observational studies, there is ample evidence from clinical trials demonstrating that muscle

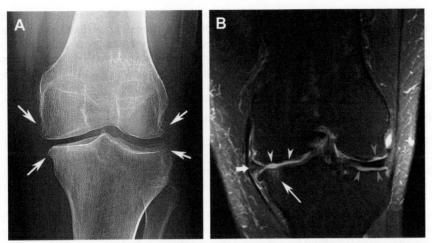

Fig. 5. Anteroposterior left knee radiograph (*A*) shows diffuse marginal osteophytosis of the tibia and femur (*arrows*). There is a mild-to-moderate medial tibiofemoral joint space narrowing. Coronal fat-suppressed proton density-weighted MRI performed the same day shows subchondral bone marrow lesion (*arrow*) at the medial tibial plateau just subjacent to a focal full thickness cartilage defect. (*B*) There are multiple partial thickness defects of the medial femoral condyle cartilage (*yellow arrowheads*). Surprisingly, there are more extensive focal full-thickness cartilage defects (*green arrowhead*) at the lateral femoral condyle and almost complete denudation (*red arrowheads*) subchondral bone at the lateral tibia, as opposed to a radiographically normal-appearing lateral tibiofemoral joint space width. Indeed, most of the joint space narrowing of the medial tibiofemoral joint is secondary to a partially macerated and extruded medial meniscus (*thick arrow*). There is attrition of the medial and lateral tibial plateaus and marginal osteophytosis.

strengthening exercises result in improvements in pain, physical function, and quality of life in people with knee OA.[75,76]

Obesity is the single most important risk factor for developing severe OA of the knee and more so than other potentially damaging factors including heredity.[77] Even if it usually is accepted that mechanical loading contributes to joint destruction in overweight patients, recent advances in the understanding of adipose tissue pathophysiology add further insights in understanding the relationship between obesity and OA. Indeed, the positive association between overweight or obesity and OA is observed not only for knee joints but also for nonweight-bearing joints such as hands.[78,79] Furthermore, if weight loss may prevent the onset of OA, the loss of body fat is related more closely to symptomatic benefit than is the loss of body weight.[80] Local fat depots may play an important role in disease and symptoms genesis. Among these tissues, the synovium and infrapatellar fat pad appear to produce large amounts of adipokines.[81] Until recently, the fat pad, which is an extrasynovial but an intra-articular tissue, had been neglected. This adipose tissue, however, is able to release growth factors, cytokines, and adipokines.[54] Because obese individuals have higher concentrations of inflammatory markers, inflammation may contribute to functional limitation and disease progression in those with OA.[82] Besides direct effects on the joint, inflammatory mediators can affect muscle function and lower the pain threshold.

Another source of joint pain in OA may be from the nerves themselves. Following joint injury in which there is ligamentous rupture, the nerves that reinnervate the healing soft tissues contain an overabundance of algesic chemicals such as substance P and calcitonin gene-related peptide. An interesting observation of these new nerves is that their overall morphology is abnormal, with fibers appearing punctate and disorganized.[83,84] Because these phenomena are consistent with the innervation profiles described in nerve injury models, the author speculates that injured joints may develop neuropathic pain after trauma. Indeed, treatment of inflamed joints with the neuropathic pain analgesic gabapentin can relieve arthritis pain.[85]

INSIGHTS FROM IMAGING ON DISEASE PATHOGENESIS

Traditionally, measurement of OA structural change has been performed using radiographs. Standardized techniques for measuring joint space width (JSW) in the medial tibiofemoral compartment, using standardized radiographic protocols, have become accepted for quantifying changes in knee OA.[86] Because of inherent limitations in conventional radiograph technology, further research and development have investigated other techniques that may improve the assessment of disease, its early development, and its progression. Foremost among these is MRI, a noninvasive three-dimensional method for assessing joint morphology that may supplant the widespread use of conventional radiographs in clinical trials.[87] Although MRI has enormous potential, recent studies provide a note of caution for its immediate ability to supersede the weight-bearing radiograph. The responsiveness of different measures of cartilage morphometry may not be as great as early data suggested.[6,88,89]

Because of limitations in the responsiveness of both radiographic and MRI measures of progression, efforts are being made to stratify those with the highest risk of progression. Several studies have suggested that baseline clinical, biomarker, and imaging features are predictive of progression of cartilage loss in the medial compartment of the knee and could be used to provide greater study power by selecting a population at greater risk for more rapid progression. Risk factors include increased body mass index (BMI),[90] an increased level of type II collagen C-terminal degradation products detected in the urine (uCTX-II),[91] the presence of varus malalignment at the tibiofemoral joint,[92,93] the presence on MRI of subchondral BMLs,[94] or meniscal abnormalities.[68] What follows is a discussion of constructs identified on imaging studies that provide insights on factors that predispose to disease progression.

Alignment

Mechanical factors are the dominant risk factors for structural progression. Varus and valgus malalignment have been shown to increase the risk of subsequent medial and lateral knee OA radiographic progression, respectively.[92] Varus malalignment has been shown to lead to a fourfold amplification of focal medial knee OA progression, while valgus malalignment has been shown to predispose to a two- to fivefold increase in lateral OA progression.[92,95] In an MRI-based study, varus malalignment predicted medial tibial cartilage volume and thickness loss, and tibial and femoral denuded bone increase, after adjusting for other local factors (meniscal damage and extrusion and laxity).[93] Understanding the role alignment plays in OA progression is important, because it modulates the effect of standard risk factors for knee OA progression, including obesity,[96] quadriceps strength,[97] laxity,[97] and stage of disease.[92,95]

Meniscal Damage

Biswal and colleagues[66] studied 43 subjects and demonstrated that the 26 subjects who had sustained meniscal tears had a higher average rate of progression of cartilage loss (22%) than seen in those who had intact menisci (14.9%) ($P \leq .018$).

Berthiaume and colleagues[67] investigated the relation between knee meniscus structural damage and cartilage degradation in 32 subjects and found similar effects. The author demonstrated a strong association of meniscal position and meniscal damage and cartilage loss,[68] with the highest quartile of medial meniscal damage having an odds ratio of medial progression of 6.3 (range 3.1 to 12.6). Each aspect of meniscal abnormality (whether change in position or damage) had a major effect on risk of cartilage loss.

BMLs

BMLs also have been found to be associated with compartment-specific OA cartilage progression measured semiquantitatively.[94,98] Medial tibiofemoral compartment BMLs occurred mostly in those with varus malalignment, and lateral tibiofemoral lesions occurred in those with valgus limbs. Of 75 knees with medial lesions, 25 (36.0%) showed medial progression versus only 12 of 148 knees (8.1%) without lesions (odds ratio [OR] for progression, 6.5; 95% confidence interval [CI] 3.0,14.0). Sixty-nine percent of knees destined to progress medially had medial lesions. Lateral lesions conferred a similar marked risk of lateral progression. These increased risks were attenuated by 30% to 50% after adjusting for limb alignment. This demonstrates that BMLs are potent risk factors for predicting progression in knee OA, and their relation to progression is explained, in part, by their association with limb alignment.

Stage of Disease

A recent longitudinal analysis demonstrated that by selecting people with K&L grade 3 (pre-existent JSN) at baseline, this group demonstrated the greatest change in JSW over 12 months.[99] A recent study selected participants with the presence of a full-thickness cartilage defect (denuded area), and demonstrated that cartilage loss in that plate was improved markedly. Before stratification, the highest standardized response mean (SRM) for any region was 0.35,[89] and after stratification and selection of those with a denuded area, this improved to 0.62.

Other Risk Factors or Profiling Indices

Synovitis is frequently present in OA and may correlate with pain and other clinical outcomes.[39,40] Although synovitis may play a role in mediating symptoms, its role in predisposing to further structural progression appears limited,[40] so using this as a method for identifying those at high risk of progression is not optimal.

Among those with established knee OA, an estimated 20% to 35% have an incidental anterior cruciate ligament (ACL) tear identified by MRI.[100] The effect of an incidental complete ACL tear on the risk for cartilage loss appears to be mediated by concurrent meniscal pathology,[101] so using this as a method for identifying those at high risk of progression is not optimal.

SUMMARY

Recent studies, particularly those with an emphasis on MRI, are providing unique insights into the relation between structure identified on imaging and symptom and disease genesis. The traditional predominant focus of imaging studies and preclinical investigation is on hyaline cartilage. However, the subchondral bone, periosteum, periarticular ligaments, periarticular muscles, synovium, and joint capsule are all richly innervated and are the likely source of nociception in OA. In addition, local tissue alterations in the bone, meniscus, and alignment of the lower extremity are important in terms of disease genesis.

Although imaging studies have provided many insights, much remains unknown and uncertain. Imaging developments in OA are an important rate-limiting step to further therapeutic development. If and when structure-modifying agents are available, their efficacy will need to be determined using appropriate structure constructs. Some of these fundamental questions include:

What structural changes on MRI are consistent with the diagnosis of OA?
How does one define early disease on MRI?
What metrics of structural change (on either conventional radiograph or MRI) are
    most useful at different stages of disease and for clinical trial application?
What are the optimal platforms and sequences for specific structural features?

Hopefully over the years to come answers to these questions will be developed, and the field will move forward with these advances.

REFERENCES

1. Guccione AA, Felson DT, Anderson JJ, et al. The effects of specific medical conditions on the functional limitations of elders in the Framingham Study. Am J Public Health 1994;84:351–8.
2. Brandt KD, Dieppe P, Radin EL. Etiopathogenesis of osteoarthritis. Rheum Dis Clin North Am 2008;34:531–59.
3. Eyre DR. Collagens and cartilage matrix homeostasis. Clin Orthop Relat Res 2004;(427 Suppl):S118–22.
4. Kellgren JH, Lawrence JS. Atlas of standard radiographs. Oxford: Blackwell Scientific; 1963.
5. Pessis E, Drape JL, Ravaud P, et al. Assessment of progression in knee osteoarthritis: results of a 1-year study comparing arthroscopy and MRI. Osteoarthritis Cartilage 2003;11:361–9.
6. Eckstein F, Burstein D, Link TM. Quantitative MRI of cartilage and bone: degenerative changes in osteoarthritis. NMR Biomed 2006;19:822–54.
7. Karachalios T, Zibis A, Papanagiotou P, et al. MR imaging findings in early osteoarthritis of the knee. Eur J Radiol 2004;50:225–30.
8. Hunter DJ, Patil V, Niu JB, et al. The etiology of knee pain in the community. Arthritis Rheum 2004;50:1885.
9. Reichenbach S, Guermazi A, Niu J, et al. Prevalence of bone attrition on knee radiographs and MRI in a community-based cohort. Osteoarthr Cartilage 2008;16:1005–10.
10. Amin S, LaValley MP, Guermazi A, et al. The relationship between cartilage loss on magnetic resonance imaging and radiographic progression in men and women with knee osteoarthritis. Arthritis Rheum 2005;52:3152–9.
11. Peat G, McCarney R, Croft P. Knee pain and osteoarthritis in older adults: a review of community burden and current use of primary health care. Ann Rheum Dis 2001;60:91–7.
12. Hunter D, Felson D. Osteoarthritis. BMJ 2006;332:639–42.
13. Lawrence RC, Helmick CG, Arnett FC, et al. Estimates of the prevalence of arthritis and selected musculoskeletal disorders in the United States. Arthritis Rheum 1998;41:778–99.
14. Zhang Y, Niu J, Kelly-Hayes M, et al. Prevalence of symptomatic hand osteoarthritis and its impact on functional status among the elderly: The Framingham Study. Am J Epidemiol 2002;156:1021–7.

15. Cunningham LS, Kelsey JL. Epidemiology of musculoskeletal impairments and associated disability. Am J Public Health 1984;74:574–9.
16. Armstrong AL, Hunter JB, Davis TR. The prevalence of degenerative arthritis of the base of the thumb in postmenopausal women. J Hand Surg Br 1994;19: 340–1.
17. Felson DT, Zhang Y. An update on the epidemiology of knee and hip osteoarthritis with a view to prevention. Arthritis Rheum 1998;41:1343–55.
18. Nevitt MC, Xu L, Zhang Y, et al. Very low prevalence of hip osteoarthritis among Chinese elderly in Beijing, China, compared with whites in the United States: the Beijing Osteoarthritis Study. Arthritis Rheum 2002;46:1773–9.
19. Zhang Y, Hunter DJ, Nevitt MC, et al. Association of squatting with increased prevalence of radiographic tibiofemoral knee osteoarthritis: the Beijing Osteoarthritis Study. Arthritis Rheum 2004;50:1187–92.
20. Felson DT. An update on the pathogenesis and epidemiology of osteoarthritis. Radiol Clin North Am 2004;42:1–9.
21. Hannan MT, Felson DT, Pincus T. Analysis of the discordance between radiographic changes and knee pain in osteoarthritis of the knee. J Rheumatol 2000;27:1513–7.
22. Altman RD. Classification of disease: osteoarthritis. Semin Arthritis Rheum 1991; 20:40–7.
23. Cibere J. Do we need radiographs to diagnose osteoarthritis? Best Pract Res Clin Rheumatol 2006;20:27–38.
24. Centers for Disease Control and Prevention (CDC). Prevalence of self-reported arthritis or chronic joint symptoms among adults–United States, 2001. MMWR Morb Mortal Wkly Rep 2002;51:948–50.
25. Fortin PR, Clarke AE, Joseph L, et al. Outcomes of total hip and knee replacement: preoperative functional status predicts outcomes at six months after surgery. Arthritis Rheum 1999;42:1722–8.
26. Harris WH. Etiology of osteoarthritis of the hip. Clin Orthop Relat Res 1986;213: 20–33.
27. Solomon L. Patterns of osteoarthritis of the hip. J Bone Joint Surg Br 1976;58: 176–83.
28. Eaton RG, Littler JW. Ligament reconstruction for the painful thumb carpometacarpal joint. J Bone Joint Surg Am 1973;55:1655–66.
29. Cooke KS, Singson RD, Glickel SZ, et al. Degenerative changes of the trapeziometacarpal joint: radiologic assessment. Skeletal Radiol 1995;24(7):523–7.
30. Glickel SZ. Clinical assessment of the thumb trapeziometacarpal joint. Hand Clin 2001;17(2):185–95.
31. Hunter DJ, Zhang Y, Sokolove J, et al. Trapeziometacarpal subluxation predisposes to incident trapeziometacarpal osteoarthritis (OA): the Framingham Study. Osteoarthritis Cartilage 2005;13:953–7.
32. Tan AL, Grainger AJ, Tanner SF, et al. High-resolution magnetic resonance imaging for the assessment of hand osteoarthritis. Arthritis Rheum 2005;52: 2355–65.
33. Nuki G. Osteoarthritis: a problem of joint failure. Z Rheumatol 1999;58:142–7.
34. Dieppe PA, Lohmander LS. Pathogenesis and management of pain in osteoarthritis. Lancet 2005;365:965–73.
35. Hunter DJ, McDougall JJ, Keefe FJ. The symptoms of osteoarthritis and the genesis of pain. Rheum Dis Clin North Am 2008;34:623–43.
36. Felson DT, Chaisson CE, Hill CL, et al. The association of bone marrow lesions with pain in knee osteoarthritis. Ann Intern Med 2001;134:541–9.

37. Hunter D, Gale D, Grainger G, et al. The reliability of a new scoring system for knee osteoarthritis MRI and the validity of bone marrow lesion assessment: BLOKS (Boston Leeds Osteoarthritis Knee Score). Ann Rheum Dis 2008;67:206–11.

38. Torres L, Dunlop DD, Peterfy C, et al. The relationship between specific tissue lesions and pain severity in persons with knee osteoarthritis. Osteoarthritis Cartilage 2006;14:1033–40.

39. Hill CL, Gale DG, Chaisson CE, et al. Knee effusions, popliteal cysts, and synovial thickening: association with knee pain in osteoarthritis. J Rheumatol 2001; 28:1330–7.

40. Hill CL, Hunter DJ, Niu J, et al. Synovitis detected on magnetic resonance imaging and its relation to pain and cartilage loss in knee osteoarthritis. Ann Rheum Dis 2007;66:1599–603.

41. Lo G, McAlindon T, Niu J, et al. Strong association of bone marrow lesions and effusion with pain in osteoarthritis. Arthritis Rheum 2008;56(9):S790.

42. Felson D. The sources of pain in knee osteoarthritis. Curr Opin Rheumatol 2005; 17:624–8.

43. Hunter DJ, March L, Sambrook PN. The association of cartilage volume with knee pain. Osteoarthritis Cartilage 2003;11:725–9.

44. Felson DT, Niu J, Guermazi A, et al. Correlation of the development of knee pain with enlarging bone marrow lesions on magnetic resonance imaging. Arthritis Rheum 2007;56:2986–92.

45. Link TM, Steinbach LS, Ghosh S, et al. Osteoarthritis: MR imaging findings in different stages of disease and correlation with clinical findings. Radiology 2003;226:373–81.

46. Kornaat PR, Bloem JL, Ceulemans RY, et al. Osteoarthritis of the knee: association between clinical features and MR imaging findings. Radiology 2006;239:811–7.

47. Cicuttini FM, Baker J, Hart DJ, et al. Association of pain with radiological changes in different compartments and views of the knee joint. Osteoarthritis Cartilage 1996;4:143–7.

48. Burr DB. The importance of subchondral bone in the progression of osteoarthritis. J Rheumatol Suppl 2004;70:77–80.

49. Simkin P. Bone pain and pressure in osteoarthritic joints. Novartis Found Symp 2004;260:179–86.

50. Arnoldi CC, Lemperg K, Linderholm H. Intraosseous hypertension and pain in the knee. J Bone Joint Surg Br 1975;57:360–3.

51. Arnoldi CC, Djurhuus JC, Heerfordt J, et al. Intraosseous phlebography, intraosseous pressure measurements and 99mTC-polyphosphate scintigraphy in patients with various painful conditions in the hip and knee. Acta Orthop Scand 1980;51:19–28.

52. Arnoldi CC. Vascular aspects of degenerative joint disorders. A synthesis. Acta Orthop Scand Suppl 1994;261:1–82.

53. Roach HI, Aigner T, Soder S, et al. Pathobiology of osteoarthritis: pathomechanisms and potential therapeutic targets. Curr Drug Targets 2007;8:271–82.

54. Ushiyama T, Chano T, Inoue K, et al. Cytokine production in the infrapatellar fat pad: another source of cytokines in knee synovial fluids. Ann Rheum Dis 2003; 62:108–12.

55. McDougall J. Arthritis and pain. Neurogenic origin of joint pain. Arthritis Res Ther 2006;8:220.

56. Fernandez-Madrid F, Karvonen RL, Teitge RA, et al. Synovial thickening detected by MR imaging in osteoarthritis of the knee confirmed by biopsy as synovitis. Magn Reson Imaging 1995;13:177–83.

57. Roemer FW, Guermazi A, Zhang Y, et al. Hoffa's fat pad: evaluation on unenhanced MR Images as a measure of patellofemoral synovitis in osteoarthritis. AJR Am J Roentgenol 2009;192:1696–700.
58. Seedhom BB, Dowson D, Wright V. Proceedings: functions of the menisci. A preliminary study. Ann Rheum Dis 1974;33:111.
59. Verstraete KL, Verdonk R, Lootens T, et al. Current status and imaging of allograft meniscal transplantation. Eur J Radiol 1997;26:16–22.
60. Baratz ME, Fu FH, Mengato R. Meniscal tears: the effect of meniscectomy and of repair on intra-articular contact areas and stress in the human knee. A preliminary report. Am J Sports Med 1986;14(4):270–5.
61. Fukubayashi T, Kurosawa H. The contact area and pressure distribution pattern of the knee. A study of normal and osteoarthrotic knee joints. Acta Orthop Scand 1980;51(6):871–9.
62. Kurosawa H, Fukubayashi T, Nakajima H. Load-bearing mode of the knee joint: physical behavior of the knee joint with or without menisci. Clin Orthop Relat Res 1980;(149):283–90.
63. Tapper EM, Hoover NW. Late results after meniscectomy. J Bone Joint Surg Am 1969;51:517–26.
64. Johnson RJ, Kettelkamp DB, Clark W, et al. Factors effecting late results after meniscectomy. J Bone Joint Surg Am 1974;56:719–29.
65. Englund M, Roos EM, Lohmander LS. Impact of type of meniscal tear on radiographic and symptomatic knee osteoarthritis: a sixteen-year follow-up of meniscectomy with matched controls. Arthritis Rheum 2003;48:2178–87.
66. Biswal S, Hastie T, Andriacchi TP, et al. Risk factors for progressive cartilage loss in the knee: a longitudinal magnetic resonance imaging study in forty-three patients. Arthritis Rheum 2002;46:2884–92.
67. Berthiaume MJ, Raynauld JP, Martel-Pelletier J, et al. Meniscal tear and extrusion are strongly associated with progression of symptomatic knee osteoarthritis as assessed by quantitative magnetic resonance imaging. Ann Rheum Dis 2005;64:556–63.
68. Hunter DJ, Zhang YQ, Niu JB, et al. The association of meniscal pathologic changes with cartilage loss in symptomatic knee osteoarthritis. Arthritis Rheum 2006;54:795–801.
69. Englund M, Guermazi A, Gale D, et al. Incidental meniscal findings on knee MRI in middle-aged and elderly persons. N Engl J Med 2008;359:1108–15.
70. Bhattacharyya T, Gale D, Dewire P, et al. The clinical importance of meniscal tears demonstrated by magnetic resonance imaging in osteoarthritis of the knee. J Bone Joint Surg Am 2003;85-A:4–9.
71. Englund M, Niu J, Guermazi A, et al. Effect of meniscal damage on the development of frequent knee pain, aching, or stiffness. Arthritis Rheum 2007;56:4048–54.
72. Englund M, Lohmander LS. Risk factors for symptomatic knee osteoarthritis fifteen to twenty-two years after meniscectomy. Arthritis Rheum 2004;50:2811–9.
73. Hurley MV. The role of muscle weakness in the pathogenesis of osteoarthritis. Rheum Dis Clin North Am 1999;25:283–98.
74. Sharma L, Cahue S, Song J, et al. Physical functioning over three years in knee osteoarthritis: role of psychosocial, local mechanical, and neuromuscular factors. Arthritis Rheum 2003;48:3359–70.
75. Roddy E, Zhang W, Doherty M, et al. Aerobic walking or strengthening exercise for osteoarthritis of the knee? A systematic review. Ann Rheum Dis 2005;64:544–8.

76. Roddy E, Zhang W, Doherty M, et al. Evidence-based recommendations for the role of exercise in the management of osteoarthritis of the hip or knee—the MOVE consensus. Rheumatology 2005;44:67–73.

77. Coggon D, Reading I, Croft P, et al. Knee osteoarthritis and obesity. Int J Obes Relat Metab Disord 2001;25:622–7.

78. Cicuttini FM, Baker JR, Spector TD. The association of obesity with osteoarthritis of the hand and knee in women: a twin study. J Rheumatol 1996;23:1221–6.

79. Sayer AA, Poole J, Cox V, et al. Weight from birth to 53 years: a longitudinal study of the influence on clinical hand osteoarthritis. Arthritis Rheum 2003;48: 1030–3.

80. Toda Y, Toda T, Takemura S, et al. Change in body fat, but not body weight or metabolic correlates of obesity, is related to symptomatic relief of obese patients with knee osteoarthritis after a weight control program. J Rheumatol 1998;25: 2181–6.

81. Presle N, Pottie P, Dumond H, et al. Differential distribution of adipokines between serum and synovial fluid in patients with osteoarthritis. Contribution of joint tissues to their articular production. Osteoarthritis Cartilage 2006;14:690–5.

82. Spector TD, Hart DJ, Nandra D, et al. Low-level increases in serum C-reactive protein are present in early osteoarthritis of the knee and predict progressive disease. Arthritis Rheum 1997;40:723–7.

83. McDougall JJ, Bray RC, Sharkey KA. Morphological and immunohistochemical examination of nerves in normal and injured collateral ligaments of rat, rabbit, and human knee joints. Anat Rec 1997;248:29–39.

84. McDougall JJ, Yeung G, Leonard CA, et al. A role for calcitonin gene-related peptide in rabbit knee joint ligament healing. Can J Physiol Pharmacol 2000; 78:535–40.

85. Hanesch U, Pawlak M, McDougall JJ, et al. Gabapentin reduces the mechano-sensitivity of fine afferent nerve fibres in normal and inflamed rat knee joints. Pain 2003;104:363–6.

86. Guermazi A, Burstein D, Conaghan P, et al. Imaging in osteoarthritis. Rheum Dis Clin North Am 2008;34:645–87.

87. Eckstein F, Mosher T, Hunter D. Imaging of knee osteoarthritis: data beyond the beauty. Curr Opin Rheumatol 2007;19:435–43.

88. Hunter D, Conaghan P, Peterfy C, et al. Responsiveness, effect size, and small-est detectable difference of magnetic resonance imaging in knee osteoarthritis. Osteoarthritis Cartilage 2006;14(Suppl 1):112–5.

89. Hunter DJ, Niu J, Zhang Y, et al. Change in cartilage morphometry: a sample of the progression cohort of the Osteoarthritis Initiative. Ann Rheum Dis 2009;68: 349–56.

90. Felson DT. Obesity and osteoarthritis of the knee. Bull Rheum Dis 1992;41:6–7.

91. Garnero P, Ayral X, Rousseau JC, et al. Uncoupling of type II collagen synthesis and degradation predicts progression of joint damage in patients with knee osteoarthritis. Arthritis Rheum 2002;46:2613–24.

92. Sharma L, Song J, Felson DT, et al. The role of knee alignment in disease progression and functional decline in knee osteoarthritis. [erratum appears in JAMA 2001;286(7):792]. JAMA 2001;286:188–95.

93. Sharma L, Eckstein F, Song J, et al. Relationship of meniscal damage, meniscal extrusion, malalignment, and joint laxity to subsequent cartilage loss in osteoar-thritic knees. Arthritis Rheum 2008;58:1716–26.

94. Felson DT, McLaughlin S, Goggins J, et al. Bone marrow edema and its relation to progression of knee osteoarthritis. Ann Intern Med 2003;139:330–6.

95. Cerejo R, Dunlop DD, Cahue S, et al. The influence of alignment on risk of knee osteoarthritis progression according to baseline stage of disease. Arthritis Rheum 2002;46:2632–6.
96. Sharma L, Lou C, Cahue S, et al. The mechanism of the effect of obesity in knee osteoarthritis: the mediating role of malalignment. Arthritis Rheum 2000;43: 568–75.
97. Sharma L, Dunlop DD, Cahue S, et al. Quadriceps strength and osteoarthritis progression in malaligned and lax knees. Ann Intern Med 2003;138:613–9.
98. Hunter D, Zhang Y, Niu J, et al. Increase in bone marrow lesions is associated with cartilage loss: a longitudinal MRI study in knee osteoarthritis. Arthritis Rheum 2006;54:1529–35.
99. Hellio Le Graverand MP, Vignon E, Brandt KD, et al. Head-to-head comparison of the Lyon-Schuss and fixed flexion radiographic techniques. Long-term repro-ducibility in normal knees and sensitivity to change in osteoarthritic knees. Ann Rheum Dis 2008;67:1562–6.
100. Hill CL, Seo GS, Gale D, et al. Cruciate ligament integrity in osteoarthritis of the knee. Arthritis Rheum 2005;52:794–9.
101. Amin S, Guermazi A, LaValley M, et al. Complete anterior cruciate ligament tear and the risk for cartilage loss and progression of symptoms in men and women with knee osteoarthritis. Osteoarthritis Cartilage 2008;16:897–902.

Imaging the Role of Biomechanics in Osteoarthritis

David J. Hunter, MBBS, FRACP, PhD[a],*, David R. Wilson, DPhil[b]

KEYWORDS

• Alignment • Biomechanics • Osteoarthritis
• Imaging • Joint loading

Osteoarthritis (OA) affects an estimated 21 million Americans,[1,2] and recent estimates suggest that symptomatic knee OA occurs in 13% of persons aged 60 and over.[1,3] The risk of mobility disability (defined as needing help walking or climbing stairs) attributable to knee OA alone is greater than that due to any other medical condition in people aged 65 and over.[4,5] Although this prevalence is high, it is expected to increase even further with the increasing prevalence of obesity and the aging of the community.[6]

The etiopathogenesis of OA is widely believed the result of local mechanical factors acting within the context of systemic susceptibility. Several studies have highlighted the importance of mechanical factors in the etiopathogenesis of this disease.[7–12] Knee alignment and the stance-phase adduction moment[13] are key determinants of the disproportionate medial transmission of load.[14]

This narrative review focuses on the influence of biomechanics on the causes of OA and on the imaging methods that may be used to quantify these forces. Although it is recognized that joint mechanics are critical to disease pathogenesis, and there are some tools that enable modeling joint mechanics, there is desperate need of further advanced imaging methods to allow critical evaluation of the forces within the joint under more physiologic loading conditions and evaluation of the impact of targeted therapeutics on them. This review focuses on which mechanical parameters are of greatest interest and some steps that may facilitate movement toward measuring them using medical imaging methods.

A version of this article originally appeared in the 47:4 issue of Radiologic Clinics of North America.
[a] Division of Research, New England Baptist Hospital, 125 Parker Hill Avenue, Boston, MA 02120, USA
[b] Department of Orthopaedics, University of British Columbia and Vancouver Coastal Health Research Institute, Vancouver, BC, Canada
* Corresponding author.
E-mail address: djhunter@caregroup.harvard.edu (D.J. Hunter).

ETIOPATHOGENESIS OF OSTEOARTHRITIS

OA is a significant public health challenge, ranked as the leading cause of disability in elders.[4] Recent estimates suggest that symptomatic knee OA occurs in 6% of adults 30 years of age and older[15] and 13% of persons age 60 and over.[3] The prevalence of OA is expected to increase as the United States population ages and the prevalence of obesity rises. By 2020, the number of people with OA may double.[6,16]

OA occurs in joints when the dynamic equilibrium between the breakdown and repair of joint tissues becomes unbalanced.[17] This progressive joint failure may cause pain and disability,[5] although many persons with structural changes consistent with OA are asymptomatic.[18] OA can occur in any synovial joint in the body but is most common in the knees, hips, and hands.

THE ROLE OF MECHANICS IN THE CAUSE OF KNEE OSTEOARTHRITIS

OA is perhaps best understood as resulting from excessive mechanical stress applied in the context of systemic susceptibility. Susceptibility to OA may be increased in part by genetic inheritance (a positive family history increases risk), age, ethnicity, nutritional factors, and female gender.[19]

The susceptibility to OA can also, in theory, be influenced by the mechanical environment. For example, the greater prevalence for OA in women than men may partly be explained on the basis of the female knee being more mechanically vulnerable to OA. Quadriceps strength in men is greater than in women and this difference may play a role in reducing postural sway and improving joint stability.[20] The higher fat mass and lower muscle mass in women may explain some of the gender difference in OA susceptibility, although this is conjectural and needs to be formally tested.[21] Other gender differences that have an impact on joint loading include pelvic dimensions, knee morphology, Q angle, and neuromuscular strength.[22] For instance, disproportionate loading of the lateral compartment in women likely arises from differences in knee stability and stiffness that is lower in women as a result of lower neuromuscular strength and higher ligamentous laxity.[22–24]

Local mechanical factors, such as adduction moment, malalignment, and quadriceps strength, potentially make the knee joint vulnerable to the development and progression of OA.[25] Local mechanical factors also mediate the impact of more systemic factors, such as obesity, on the knee.[26]

The human knee is a complex joint with considerable forces on the articular surfaces during weight bearing. The knee has three joint compartments: the patellofemoral and the medial and lateral tibiofemoral joints. The medial compartment is subjected to more stress than the lateral compartment, which may account, in part, for why OA affects the medial tibiofemoral compartment more often than the lateral compartment in men and women (75% of knee OA affects the medial compartment as opposed to 25% affecting the lateral compartment).[27]

In theory, any shift from a neutral or collinear alignment of the hip, knee, and ankle affects load distribution at the knee.[28] The load-bearing mechanical axis is traditionally represented on radiographs by a line drawn from the center of the femoral head to the center of the ankle talus. In neutrally aligned limbs, this line passes through a midpoint between the tibial spines. The medial compartment bears a resultant 60% to 70% of the force across the neutrally aligned knee during weight bearing[13] and, because it is subjected to more load than the lateral compartment, may play a role in the predisposition to medial tibiofemoral compartment progression in OA.[27] In a varus knee, this axis passes medial to the knee and has a moment arm about the center of the knee, which further increases force across the medial compartment. In contrast, in a valgus knee, the load-bearing axis passes lateral to the knee, and there is an associated increase in force across the lateral compartment.[28] The neutral full-limb (mechanical) alignment in those without OA is approximately 1° varus; as a result, by convention, neutral is typically categorized as 0° to 2° varus.[29]

The acquisition and measurement of the mechanical axis of the knee is technically difficult and requires a full-limb radiograph, which is considered the gold standard method for assessing knee alignment (**Fig. 1**). More recently, some studies have assessed anatomic alignment on short-film radiographs centered at the knee (**Fig. 2**).[30] These measures on the short film do not capture proximal and distal

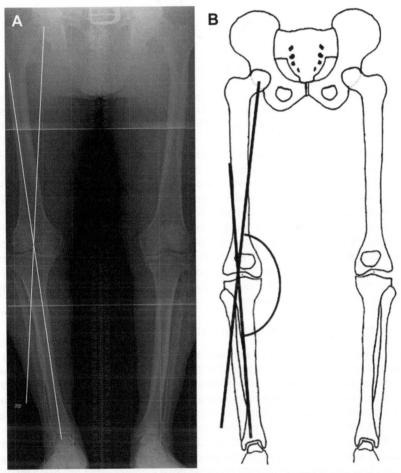

Fig. 1. Long limb film (*A*) and schematic (*B*) of varus malaligned right knee. Hip-knee-ankle alignment contributes to the load distribution across the knee articular surface by proportionately dividing load between the medial and lateral compartments. The load-bearing mechanical axis is traditionally represented on radiographs by a line drawn from the center of the femoral head to the center of the ankle talus. In a varus knee, this axis passes medial to the knee and a moment arm is created, which further increases force across the medial compartment.

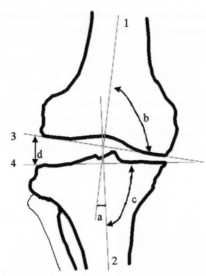

Fig. 2. Measures of alignment depicted on a short film of a typical varus knee. 1. Femoral anatomic axis line. 2. Tibial anatomic axis line. 3. Condylar line. 4. Tibial plateau line. a. Anatomic axis angle. b. Condylar angle. c. Tibial plateau angle. d. Condylar plateau angle.

anatomy but do avoid unwanted pelvic radiation, high cost, and specialized equipment. A study by Kraus and colleagues[30] demonstrated strong correlation between data obtained from full-limb measures of the mechanical axis and short-film measures of the anatomic axis. In this study, the anatomic axis was offset a mean 4.21° valgus from the mechanical axis (3.5° in women and 6.4° in men). The high correlation in this study suggests that the more easily obtainable, standard knee films can be substituted for the more cumbersome full-length radiographs during the radiographic assessment of knee alignment.[31] Although these measures may strongly correlate, there are differences, and optimal exploration of the relationship between knee alignment (mechanical axis) and OA should be pursued using measures of mechanical axis, which may afford greater precision.

EFFECT OF TIBIOFEMORAL MALALIGNMENT ON DISEASE PROGRESSION

Varus and valgus malalignment have been shown to increase the risk of subsequent medial and lateral (respectively) knee OA radiographic progression.[32] That is, in the presence of existing knee OA, abnormal alignment is associated with accelerated structural deterioration in the compartment subjected to abnormally increased compressive stress. Varus malalignment has been shown to lead to a fourfold amplification of focal medial knee OA progression, whereas valgus malalignment has been shown to predispose to a two- to fivefold increase in lateral OA progression.[32,33] In an MRI-based study, varus malalignment predicted medial tibial cartilage volume and thickness loss and tibial and femoral denuded bone increase, after adjusting for other local factors (meniscal damage and extrusion, laxity).[34]

Malalignment has consequences beyond the direct effects on cartilage, including alteration in other knee-related tissues, such as bone marrow lesions, which further propagate OA disease.[35,36] These changes in the cartilage and other local tissues about the knee lead to further malalignment, and it is this vicious cycle that is the major determinant of the rate of structural progression in knee OA. Understanding the role alignment plays in OA etiopathogenesis is important because it modulates the effect of standard risk factors for knee OA progression, including obesity,[37] quadriceps strength,[38] laxity,[38] and stage of disease.[32,33]

IMPACT OF DYNAMIC MOMENTS ON DISEASE PROGRESSION

Malalignment provides only a static impression of the mechanical forces transmitted by a joint in one plane. Appropriately determining these forces in more than one plane requires 3-D analysis. During the stance phase of gait, the force acting at the foot during gait passes medial to the center of the knee joint in a normally aligned leg. The perpendicular distance from the line of action of this force to the center of the knee joint is the lever arm of this force about the joint center. This force combined with this lever arm produces a moment that tends to adduct the knee joint.[13] This moment can be substantial and provides a major contribution to the total loading across the knee joint, which is usually labeled the adduction (or external varus) moment at the knee.

The mean maximum magnitude of the adduction moment during normal gait is approximately 3.3% body weight times height[14] and is greater than either of the moments tending to flex or extend the knee. Studies of patients with medial knee OA show that they have, on average, a higher adduction moment (4.2% body weight × height) than those without OA.[14,39] This translates to a higher maximum reaction force on the medial compartment by 25% over normal values in those with medial knee OA.[40,41]

Progressive varus alignment of the lower limb by medial joint space narrowing increases the perpendicular distance of the ground reaction force vector from the center of the knee joint and, as a result, is associated with an increase in the magnitude of the peak knee adduction moment (which occurs even if there is no increase in the magnitude of the ground reaction force).[40,41] Only 50% of knee adduction moment variability in subjects with medial tibiofemoral OA is accounted for by the mechanical axis of the lower limb, however, emphasizing the need for dynamic evaluation of the knee joint loading environment.[41] The adduction moment might also be affected by habitual postures during locomotion or by more distal malalignments, such as tibial or calcaneal varum.

Higher maximum adduction moments at the knee are related to OA disease severity and to a higher rate of progression of knee OA.[40,42] Of the risk factors associated with disease progression, the adduction moment is potentially the most potent that has been identified.[40] In addition to the effects this has on joint space, it also seems strongly associated with remodeling in the subchondral bone as measured by bone mineral density.[39]

THE RELATIONSHIP BETWEEN MECHANICS AND KNEE SYMPTOMS

A full understanding of the risk factors for pain and other symptoms in knee OA requires consideration of a range of biopsychosocial factors.[43] The symptoms of knee OA are typically described as mechanical (ie, they occur with physical activity). Subjects with the same degree of structural damage, however, experience widely different levels of pain, a phenomenon that is poorly understood. Differences in joint forces and joint stress during functional activities may assist in explaining the dissociation between radiographic structural findings and pain. Malalignment has been previously shown to be a predictor for functional decline in knee OA and may play a role in the "mechanical" nature of OA-related pain.[32]

Knee OA may lead to adaptive strategies in gait to reduce the loading in an otherwise vulnerable joint.[41,44] These strategies include adopting a toe-out gait or slower walking speed. They can be reinforced or learned by appropriate rehabilitation and offer a potential for another conservative approach to knee OA therapy.

In addition to strategies used by patients, prescribed medication may alter knee loading. Commensurate with reductions in pain, nonsteroidal anti-inflammatory drugs (NSAIDs) also offer improvements in a person's walking speed.[45] Some of the increase in joint loading may be a direct consequence of faster walking speeds after the use of the NSAIDs, but previous analyses have also demonstrated increase in both the adduction moment and quadriceps moment in persons who experienced pain relief with piroxicam.[46] Of particular concern is that that anti-inflammatory or analgesic therapy may be associated with an increase in joint forces. Whether or not this is the mechanism that explains the potential for increased structural damage associated with NSAID use remains unclear.[47]

RELATION OF JOINT MECHANICS TO PATELLOFEMORAL OSTEOARTHRITIS

The patellofemoral (PF) joint transmits relatively high forces through relatively small contact areas. The PF joint reaction force (JRF) increases with increasing knee flexion. The JRF during walking (10°–15° of flexion) is approximately 50% of bodyweight. Walking up stairs (60°), the JRF is 3.3 times bodyweight. During squats (130°), the JRF is 7.8 times bodyweight.[48] It is, therefore, not surprising that the patella is involved in more than half of cases of symptomatic knee OA, with combined tibiofemoral and PF OA found in 41% of subjects and isolated PF disease found in 11% of subjects.[49]

Contemporary surgical and conservative treatment of PF OA is based, to a large extent, on Ficat's hypothesis that pain and cartilage degeneration occur when abnormal kinematics (lateral patellar tilt) produce excessive pressure on the lateral patellar facet.[50,51] Several studies have demonstrated that the radiographically assessed relation of the patella relative to the femur plays a critical role in determining the rate of disease progression and predisposing to symptoms in persons with PF OA.[52–55] Patellar alignment measures are associated with markers of PF OA[53]: medial displacement and tilt of the patella is associated with medial PF compartment OA progression and lateral displacement is associated with lateral PF compartment OA progression. The few studies that have explored PF OA show that the lateral PF compartment is affected more frequently than the medial.[56–58]

RELATION OF JOINT MECHANICS TO HIP OSTEOARTHRITIS

There is strong evidence that mechanical and structural changes around the hip are major etiologic factors in the development of OA.[59,60] Childhood diseases, such as Legg-Perthes disease and slipped capital femoral epiphysis, predispose the hip to OA at a young age.[61–64] Acetabular dysplasia is a major precursor of OA.[59,65] Patients with acetabular dysplasia, overload of the acetabular rim is the pathomechanism that ultimately leads to OA.[66] These structural deformities can be corrected with a range of operative strategies, including pelvic and femoral osteotomies, in an effort to improve patient symptoms and delay OA progression.[67] It was originally assumed that 50% of hip OA was idiopathic (not associated with any obvious deformity).[68] More recent studies have found that 90% or more of hip OA cases can be attributed to anatomic abnormalities (discussed later).[59,60,69]

One of the most provocative new hypotheses in orthopedics is that femoroacetabular impingement (FAI) accounts for most cases of idiopathic hip OA.[70] This hypothesis has gained prominence over the past 5 years because of its many implications for prevention and treatment of OA. FAI describes repetitive abutment between the proximal femur and the acetabular rim, due to abnormal hip morphology or excessive hip motion, in patients with no childhood history of hip pathology.[71,72] Patients, typically young (20s and 30s),[73] active adults, generally present with groin pain.[71] FAI is estimated to affect 10% to 15% of the general population,[74] suggesting that not all cases lead to OA.

The diagnosis of FAI is currently based on a history of groin pain, decreased range of motion on clinical examination, impingement test (pain elicited by combined flexion to 90°, adduction, and internal rotation), and radiographic evidence.[71] Several recent reviews have described the clinical examination process for FAI in detail with considerations for other potential overlapping diagnoses.[71,75,76] A detailed systematic examination can identify the origin of pain in the hip and groin area.[77] Conventional radiographs are often used to assess the lack of femoral offset that characterizes FAI, but they may miss abnormalities.[78] MRI can quantify the femoral neck "bump" in FAI.[79] A study using CT showed the value of 3-D reconstruction of the hip in understanding the morphologic deformities in cases of FAI.[80]

Recent evidence has demonstrated links between cartilage degeneration and the clinical symptoms and morphologic characteristics of FAI, but many questions about the association between FAI and cartilage degeneration remain. Two mechanisms by which the cartilage and labrum are affected by FAI have been described.[70,79,81,82] Cam impingement is a result of a nonspherical femoral head abutting against the acetabular rim in flexion and internal rotation (**Fig. 3**A). The abutment creates shear forces resulting in damage to the anterosuperior acetabular cartilage. Pincer impingement occurs as a result of linear contact between the femoral head-neck junction and the acetabular rim (**Fig. 3**B). Repeated abutment leads to degeneration of the labrum and circumferential cartilage damage. In a study of 149 hips with mild or no radiographic OA, patients with radiologic features of cam impingement (26 hips) had damage to the anterosuperior acetabular cartilage, whereas patients with radiologic features of pincer impingement (16 hips) had a narrow strip of circumferential cartilage damage.[83] Most patients had features of both mechanisms and showed a combination of these patterns of damage.

ROLE OF IMAGING IN ASSESSMENT OF JOINT BIOMECHANICS
What to Measure and Why it Cannot be Done?

There are several hypotheses about the links between mechanics and OA, and these hypotheses define the mechanical quantities of primary interest to researchers.

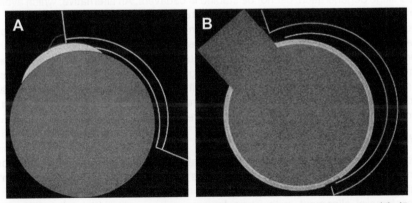

Fig. 3. Schematic illustrations of cam impingement (*A*) and pincer impingement (*B*). (*From* Ganz R, Parvizi J, Beck M, et al. Femoroacetabular impingement: a cause for osteoarthritis of the hip. Clin Orthop Relat Res 2003;417:112–20; with permission.)

Unfortunately, the most interesting quantities are among the most difficult to measure. Force on the joint surfaces is a key quantity in many hypotheses, but it can only be measured directly by implanting a measurement device into the joint, which is too interventional (in the case of the natural joint) for most in vivo studies of humans. Force distribution on the cartilage surface is also widely believed important—a moderate force transmitted through a small contact area may produce local stresses that cause cartilage damage whereas the same force transmitted through a large contact area produces no cartilage injury. Although there are sensors available to measure force distribution,[84] they must also be implanted, which carries the same limitations in vivo as direct measurements of force. Loading rate has been postulated to play a role in OA.[85] Assessing loading rate requires rapid measurements of force (typically every 100th of a second or faster), which is more challenging than static force measurements. There is also substantial interest in how force is transmitted through joint structures, such as cartilage and bone (stress). Measuring stress in simple machines and structures is a challenge, and stress has not been measured in joints in vivo. Some approaches are emerging for measuring strain or deformation of the joint tissues in response to stress,[86] but the relationship between stress and strain is more complex in joint tissues than in, for instance, steel, which makes it difficult to use strain measurements to predict stress. Kinematics (joint movement) are easier to measure and several methods for accurately quantifying joint kinematics in vivo have been developed in recent years. Kinematics describe how the bones that make up the joint move relative to each other, which can reflect where load is transmitted through the surfaces and the lines of action of structures that transmit forces. Kinematics may also have a more direct influence on OA because relative velocity in the joint has been implicated in OA progression.[87]

Ex Vivo Studies and Joint Models

Current understanding of joint mechanics is founded on ex vivo studies, which are inappropriate for linking mechanics with clinical symptoms. In ex vivo studies, kinematics and contact mechanics have been measured in cadaver specimens loaded in mechanical rigs.[88–95] Although studies of this type have helped understanding of the biomechanics of healthy joints, their central limitation for studying OA is that morphologic adaptations due to the disease process or the healing process and mechanical links to clinical symptoms, such as pain, and ongoing processes, such as cartilage degeneration, cannot be studied in cadavers. An alternative, which avoids some of the limitations of mechanical measurements that can be made in vivo, is to predict joint mechanics using mathematic models. Models incorporating sophisticated descriptions of joint structures have been developed and validated[96–101] and used to answer specific clinically motivated questions.[102–105] Two primary limitations of mathematic models are (1) many simplifying assumptions must be made about the properties of the joint, which limits their validity and applicability, and (2) like ex vivo studies, they are inappropriate for studying links with ongoing in vivo symptoms and processes, unless these changes are measured and incorporated into the model.

Radiographic Measures of Alignment

Most of the measures used clinically to quantify joint mechanics assess joint alignment. For example, tibiofemoral alignment is often quantified with the femorotibial angle or hip-knee-ankle angle.[106] A range of measures has emerged for quantifying patellofemoral alignment, with particular emphasis on medial-lateral position and patellar tilt. A central limitation of this approach is that the measures describe the joint (whose primary function is to move) at only one static position. In addition, although it is intuitive that these alignment measures are related to how load is transmitted in the joint, for most measures it is unclear how any given change in alignment measure would change force distribution in the joint. A further limitation is that the accuracy and repeatability of these measures is affected by their 2-D nature. 2-D radiographic measurements are prone to errors due to magnification and subject positioning. MRI and CT collect 3-D information about joint anatomy, which has been used in such applications as quantifying femoral neck deformities that are thought associated with hip OA.[79] In many cases, however, the 3-D data are still reduced to a 2-D measurement, which does not describe 3-D deformities adequately. This limitation is true for many measures, including patellar tilt, Q angle, anatomic alignment of the tibiofemoral joint, and the hip center-edge-angle.

Gait Analysis

Gait analysis (often more generally referred to as motion analysis) is a modality for estimating joint mechanics in activity. In motion analysis, movement of the joint segments is tracked with an optical, magnetic, or optoelectronic system and loads applied to the body (such as ground reaction forces) are measured. Mechanical analysis can then be used to assess the resultant forces and moments at the joints. It is essential to note that the resultant forces and moments at the joints, which are output by the majority of commercial motion analysis systems, are entirely different from the contact forces in the joint. Determining contact forces requires the resultant forces and moments determined from motion analysis and further analysis using joint models.[107] The advantage of gait analysis is that movement is relatively unconstrained by the measurement system and, therefore, a large range of activities can be analyzed. One key limitation of gait analysis is that joint movement is typically measured with markers fixed to the skin, which move substantially relative to the bones and can, therefore, introduce substantial error. Large groups of skin-mounted markers have reduced error due to skin movement.[108] A second key limitation is that the models and analysis required for determination of joint contact loads require many simplifications and assumptions, limiting the accuracy with which these can be measured. Typically, only general rather than subject-specific models are used. This limits the usefulness of these methods when pathologic joints are involved.

In Vivo Radiographic Measurement of Kinematics

Some of the limitations of motion analysis have been addressed with radiographic-based methods of measuring motion, including biplanar radiography and fluoroscopy. 3-D knee kinematics have been measured during activity in vivo using fluoroscopy and subsequent image processing. This has been done in joints after arthroplasty[109] and in natural joints.[110] A limitation of this approach is that measurement errors are large out of the imaging plane. The most accurate measurements of kinematics are made with biplanar radiography, which has been used to study kinematics in several joints.[111,112] Although many biplanar radiography studies are done with a series of static positions, recent work using high-speed biplanar radiography has made accurate measurements of kinematics during dynamic activity possible.[113] Because these measurements are so accurate, combining kinematics with known joint geometry yields predictions of joint contact interactions.[114] One key limitation of these approaches is that markers (typically small tantalum spheres) need to be implanted into the bones, an invasive procedure. The second key limitation is that these approaches expose patients to ionizing radiation, which always carries some risk and limits the number of repeat assessments that can be made.

MRI Measurements of Kinematics

Several different approaches are described that use MRI to assess joint kinematics. They are distinguished from each other by whether or not they measure 2-D or 3-D movement, whether or not kinematics are measured when the joint is actively loaded, and whether or not the movement is measured continuously. Some 2-D measurements of patellar tracking have been made in loaded flexion.[115,116] 2-D studies of the PF joint have shown that patterns of patellar tracking are different in loaded flexion as opposed to unloaded flexion but found that patterns measured in very slow flexion are not different from those measured in rapid flexion.[116] The primary limitation of 2-D studies is that they neglect at least half of the movement: completely describing any joint's movement requires six quantities of movement (typically three rotations and three translations). Planar studies can measure a maximum of three quantities. One 3-D kinematic approach includes cine phase–contrast MRI[117–122] and fast phase–contrast MRI,[123] in which velocity information is extracted from MRI and used to measure 3-D tracking of the joint. Applications have focused on the knee. Although promising, these techniques have some limitations; most notably, subjects must flex their knees through many cycles, limiting the magnitude of load that can be applied and the applicability of the technique in symptomatic subjects. Subject interexamination variability ranges from 0.8° to 2.4° for fast phase–contrast MRI and 1.3° to 6.1° for cine phase–contrast MRI.[123] Another approach involves imaging the joint statically at several positions of loaded flexion. Although some variations of this method[124,125] have not quantified its accuracy in real knees, the accuracy and repeatability of other variations have been measured.[126–128] A limitation of this approach is that movement is not measured during continuous flexion. One of the limitations of all of these MRI-based approaches is that kinematics are measured when participants are supine in the confined cylindric bore of an MRI scanner. Some recent work has explored using open configuration MRI scanners with a vertical gap, in which participants can stand and load their weight-bearing joints while being scanned.[129] Although this configuration provides a superior simulation of active weight bearing to that simulated in closed-bore scanners, open scanners have lower field strengths than standard closed-bore scanners, which limits the image quality that can be obtained.

MRI Measurements of Contact Area

Several methods for assessing cartilage contact area from MRI in vivo are described, although most methods have not yet been validated extensively. Contact area can be used to infer force distribution and some measurement approaches describe where contact occurs in the joint, which may also be relevant in OA. Although MRI has been used to measure contact area in animals, the applicability of measurements in cats[130] and dogs[131] to humans is difficult due to differences in geometry. In one study in humans, knees of healthy volunteers were imaged in a 1.5-T MRI scanner at several angles of flexion while they pressed against a weighted foot pedal to simulate standing load.[125] Area was assessed by constructing B-spline curves along the contact boundary of the PF joint in each slice and integrating across all of the slices to calculate area. A similar method has also been applied to standing volunteers in a 0.5-T open MRI scanner.[132,133] Most studies have focused on the PF joint—although contact areas in the elbow have been studied,[134] there is little work on the hip, shoulder, wrist, or the tibiofemoral joint (due in part to the presence of the meniscus).

THE WAY FORWARD

The OA scientific community has been taking tools available to us in imaging and using them to try to image the joint. The most obvious impact has been in the reliance on plain radiography to delineate the presence and severity of disease for OA. This is also true, however, for much of the effort thus far in MRI, where the attention has been on applying MRI metrics used for other disease areas to OA. These are characteristically static images obtained in what are often not physiologically functional positions.

In addition, many of the tissues of the joint are unlike those of other organ systems in several inherent ways. For example, many MRI contrast mechanisms are dependent on the cellular/interstitial volume ratios; articular cartilage is almost acellular and, therefore, these contrast mechanisms may not be applicable to the study of cartilage. Furthermore, in most other systems, the function of the organ is that of cellular function (ie, cellular contraction, filtering, and electrical transmission); however, in the joint, the function of the tissues is biomechanical and is generally provided by the characteristics of the extracellular matrix itself (although the cells are responsible for producing that matrix). As a result, many of the indices and contrast mechanisms that are used for other body systems may not provide the information or contrast needed to study OA.

Although it is clear that malalignment is critical in determining disease progression, less is known of factors that contribute to alignment. Certain local factors within the joint, such as the tibiofemoral congruence (through bone and cartilage disease), anterior cruciate ligament integrity, and meniscal degeneration and position, seem to play a role in determining alignment. These same factors govern load distribution across the articular cartilage of a given joint.[135] Further elucidation of the factors that influence alignment may contribute to knowledge about OA pathophysiology and provide insight into therapeutic options.

Clinicians managing knee OA should make efforts, where possible, to influence modifiable risk factors. At present, there are several therapeutic options that can modify joint forces, including braces, wedges, and osteotomies for the knee and surgical correction of hip deformity associated with FAI syndrome. Through altering joint mechanics, the rate of disease progression may be altered. There is substantial opportunity for further therapeutic development in this area, which at present needs imaging methods to quantify the impact these therapeutic advances have on joint mechanics.

Clearly biomechanics (by whatever measure or construct that is used to quantify them) plays a critical role in the etiopathogenesis of OA. Unfortunately, the most interesting quantities are among the most difficult to measure. Although force, stress, and loading rate figure most prominently in mechanical hypotheses about OA, the methods to measure them in vivo are limited.

In order to improve understanding of the relation between biomechanics and OA and develop, test, and disseminate therapies aimed at modifying biomechanics, the methods of acquisition currently available need to be improved. This will require a discourse between imaging manufacturers, imaging scientists, biomechanists, and OA clinical researchers to forge this new path.

SUMMARY

The pathogenesis of OA seems to be the result of a complex interplay between mechanical, cellular, and biochemical forces. Of these factors, mechanical forces are paramount. Extensive investigation of femorotibial alignment has demonstrated its pivotal role in knee OA progression. Understanding of the pivotal role of mechanical loading under physiologic and functional loading conditions is more limited in part because of limitations in measurement technology. Greater attention to the role of mechanical factors in OA etiopathogenesis is required to find ways of reducing the public health impact of this condition. Therapies directed at unloading or reducing the forces in the knee are not used as frequently as they should be; there is substantial opportunity for further therapeutic development in this area; and factors for this, in particular those that pertain to limitations in imaging methods to measure the impact of these interventions, need to be explored.

REFERENCES

1. Centers for Disease Control and Prevention (CDC). Prevalence and impact of chronic joint symptoms—seven states, 1996. MMWR Morb Mortal Wkly Rep 1998;47:345–51.
2. Lawrence RC, Helmick CG, Arnett FC, et al. Estimates of the prevalence of arthritis and selected musculoskeletal disorders in the United States [comments]. Arthritis Rheum 1998;41:778–99.
3. Dunlop DD, Manheim LM, Song J, et al. Arthritis prevalence and activity limitations in older adults. Arthritis Rheum 2001;44:212–21.
4. Centers for Disease Control and Prevention (CDC). Prevalence of disabilities and associated health conditions among adults—United States, 1999 [erratum appears in MMWR Morb Mortal Wkly Rep 2001 Mar 2;50(8):149]. MMWR Morb Mortal Wkly Rep 2001;50:120–5.
5. Guccione AA, Felson DT, Anderson JJ, et al. The effects of specific medical conditions on the functional limitations of elders in the Framingham Study. Am J Public Health 1994;84:351–8.
6. Centers for Disease Control and Prevention (CDC). Arthritis prevalence and activity limitations—United States, 1990. MMWR Morb Mortal Wkly Rep 1994; 43:433–8.
7. Kerin A, Patwari P, Kuettner K, et al. Molecular basis of osteoarthritis: biomechanical aspects [review] [72 refs]. Cell Mol Life Sci 2002;59:27–35.
8. Jackson BD, Wluka AE, Teichtahl AJ, et al. Reviewing knee osteoarthritis—a biomechanical perspective [review] [38 refs]. J Sci Med Sport 2004;7:347–57.
9. Teichtahl A, Wluka A, Cicuttini FM. Abnormal biomechanics: a precursor or result of knee osteoarthritis? [review] [20 refs]. Br J Sports Med 2003;37:289–90.
10. Carter DR, Beaupre GS, Wong M, et al. The mechanobiology of articular cartilage development and degeneration. [review] [54 refs]. Clin Orthop Relat Res 2004;S69–77.
11. Shakoor N, Moisio K. A biomechanical approach to musculoskeletal disease [review] [85 refs]. Best Pract Res Clin Rheumatol 2004;18:173–86.
12. Andriacchi TP, Mundermann A, Smith RL, et al. A framework for the in vivo pathomechanics of osteoarthritis at the knee [review] [101 refs]. Ann Biomed Eng 2004;32:447–57.
13. Andriacchi TP. Dynamics of knee malalignment [review] [28 refs]. Orthop Clin North Am 1994;25:395–403.
14. Schipplein OD, Andriacchi TP. Interaction between active and passive knee stabilizers during level walking. J Orthop Res 1991;9:113–9.
15. Felson DT, Lawrence RC, Dieppe PA, et al. Osteoarthritis: new insights. Part 1: the disease and its risk factors [review] [120 refs]. Ann Intern Med 2000;133: 635–46.

16. Badley E, DesMeules M. Arthritis in Canada: an ongoing challenge 2003; Ottawa, Health Canada [report].
17. Eyre DR. Collagens and cartilage matrix homeostasis [review] [37 refs]. Clin Orthop Relat Res 2004;S118–22.
18. Hannan MT, Felson DT, Pincus T. Analysis of the discordance between radiographic changes and knee pain in osteoarthritis of the knee. J Rheumatol 2000;27:1513–7.
19. Felson DT. An update on the pathogenesis and epidemiology of osteoarthritis [review] [39 refs]. Radiol Clin North Am 2004;42:1–9.
20. Hassan BS, Doherty SA, Mockett S, et al. Effect of pain reduction on postural sway, proprioception, and quadriceps strength in subjects with knee osteoarthritis. Ann Rheum Dis 2002;61:422–8.
21. Madsen OR, Brot C, Petersen MM, et al. Body composition and muscle strength in women scheduled for a knee or hip replacement. A comparative study of two groups of osteoarthritic women [erratum appears in Clin Rheumatol 1997 Nov;16(6):640]. Clin Rheumatol 1997;16:39–44.
22. Huston LJ, Greenfield ML, Wojtys EM. Anterior cruciate ligament injuries in the female athlete. Potential risk factors [review] [98 refs]. Clin Orthop Relat Res 2000;50–63.
23. Hewett TE. Neuromuscular and hormonal factors associated with knee injuries in female athletes. Strategies for intervention [review] [60 refs]. Sports Med 2000; 29:313–27.
24. Shelbourne KD, Davis TJ, Klootwyk TE. The relationship between intercondylar notch width of the femur and the incidence of anterior cruciate ligament tears. A prospective study. Am J Sports Med 1998;26:402–8.
25. Felson DT. Risk factors for osteoarthritis: understanding joint vulnerability [review] [32 refs]. Clin Orthop Relat Res 2004;S16–21.
26. Felson DT, Goggins J, Niu J, et al. The effect of body weight on progression of knee osteoarthritis is dependent on alignment. Arthritis Rheum 2004;50:3904–9.
27. Ledingham J, Regan M, Jones A, et al. Radiographic patterns and associations of osteoarthritis of the knee in patients referred to hospital. Ann Rheum Dis 1993; 52:520–6.
28. Tetsworth K, Paley D. Malalignment and degenerative arthropathy [review] [44 refs]. Orthop Clin North Am 1994;25:367–77.
29. Cooke TD, Sled EA, Scudamore RA. Frontal plane knee alignment: a call for standardized measurement. J Rheumatol 2007;34:1796–801.
30. Kraus VB, Vail TP, Worrell T, et al. A comparative assessment of alignment angle of the knee by radiographic and physical examination methods. Arthritis Rheum 2005;52:1730–5.
31. Hinman RS, May RL, Crossley KM, et al. Is there an alternative to the full-leg radiograph for determining knee joint alignment in osteoarthritis? Arthritis Rheum 2006;55:306–13.
32. Sharma L, Song J, Felson DT, et al. The role of knee alignment in disease progression and functional decline in knee osteoarthritis [erratum appears in JAMA 2001 Aug 15;286(7):792]. JAMA 2001;286:188–95.
33. Cerejo R, Dunlop DD, Cahue S, et al. The influence of alignment on risk of knee osteoarthritis progression according to baseline stage of disease. Arthritis Rheum 2002;46:2632–6.
34. Sharma L, Eckstein F, Song J, et al. Relationship of meniscal damage, meniscal extrusion, malalignment, and joint laxity to subsequent cartilage loss in osteoarthritic knees. Arthritis Rheum 2008;58:1716–26.

35. Felson DT, McLaughlin S, Goggins J, et al. Bone marrow edema and its relation to progression of knee osteoarthritis. Ann Intern Med 2003;139:330–6.
36. Hunter D, Zhang Y, Niu J, et al. Increase in bone marrow lesions is associated with cartilage loss: a longitudinal MRI study in Knee Osteoarthritis. Arthritis Rheum 2006;54:1529–35.
37. Sharma L, Lou C, Cahue S, et al. The mechanism of the effect of obesity in knee osteoarthritis: the mediating role of malalignment. Arthritis Rheum 2000;43: 568–75.
38. Sharma L, Dunlop DD, Cahue S, et al. Quadriceps strength and osteoarthritis progression in malaligned and lax knees [comment][summary for patients in Ann Intern Med. 2003 Apr 15;138(8):I1; PMID: 12693914]. Ann Intern Med 2003;138:613–9.
39. Wada M, Maezawa Y, Baba H, et al. Relationships among bone mineral densities, static alignment and dynamic load in patients with medial compartment knee osteoarthritis. Rheumatology 2001;40:499–505.
40. Miyazaki T, Wada M, Kawahara H, et al. Dynamic load at baseline can predict radiographic disease progression in medial compartment knee osteoarthritis. Ann Rheum Dis 2002;61:617–22.
41. Hurwitz DE, Ryals AB, Case JP, et al. The knee adduction moment during gait in subjects with knee osteoarthritis is more closely correlated with static alignment than radiographic disease severity, toe out angle and pain. J Orthop Res 2002; 20:101–7.
42. Sharma L, Hurwitz DE, Thonar EJ, et al. Knee adduction moment, serum hyaluronan level, and disease severity in medial tibiofemoral osteoarthritis. Arthritis Rheum 1998;41:1233–40.
43. Dieppe PA, Lohmander LS. Pathogenesis and management of pain in osteoarthritis [review] [100 refs]. Lancet 2005;365:965–73.
44. Mundermann A, Dyrby CO, Hurwitz DE, et al. Potential strategies to reduce medial compartment loading in patients with knee osteoarthritis of varying severity: reduced walking speed [erratum appears in Arthritis Rheum. 2004 Dec;50(12):4073]. Arthritis Rheum 2004;50:1172–8.
45. Blin O, Pailhous J, Lafforgue P, et al. Quantitative analysis of walking in patients with knee osteoarthritis: a method of assessing the effectiveness of non-steroidal anti-inflammatory treatment. Ann Rheum Dis 1990;49:990–3.
46. Schnitzer TJ, Popovich JM, Andersson GB, et al. Effect of piroxicam on gait in patients with osteoarthritis of the knee. Arthritis Rheum 1993;36:1207–13.
47. Huskisson EC, Berry H, Gishen P, et al. Effects of antiinflammatory drugs on the progression of osteoarthritis of the knee. LINK Study Group. Longitudinal investigation of nonsteroidal antiinflammatory drugs in knee osteoarthritis. J Rheumatol 1995;22:1941–6.
48. Grelsamer RP, Weinstein CH. Applied biomechanics of the patella [review] [39 refs]. Clin Orthop Relat Res 2001;9–14.
49. McAlindon T, Zhang Y, Hannan M, et al. Are risk factors for patellofemoral and tibiofemoral knee osteoarthritis different? J Rheumatol 1996;23:332–7.
50. Ficat RP, Hungerford DS. Disorders of the patello-femoral joint. Baltimore (MD): The Williams and Wilkins Co; 1977.
51. Ficat P. [The syndrome of lateral hyperpressure of the patella]. [in French]. Acta Orthop Belg 1978;44:65–76.
52. Kalichman L, Zhu Y, Zhang Y, et al. The association between patella alignment and knee pain and function: an MRI study in persons with symptomatic knee osteoarthritis. Osteoarthritis Cartilage 2007;15:1235–40.

53. Kalichman L, Zhang YQ, Niu JB, et al. The association between patellar alignment on magnetic resonance imaging and radiographic manifestations of knee osteoarthritis. Arthritis Res Ther 2007;9:R26.
54. Hunter DJ, Zhang YQ, Niu JB, et al. Patella malalignment, pain and patellofemoral progression: the Health ABC Study. Osteoarthritis Cartilage 2007;15:1120–7.
55. Niu J, Zhang YQ, Nevitt M, et al. Patellar malalignment and knee pain among subjects with no radiographic knee osteoarthritis: the Beijing Osteoarthritis Study. Arthritis Rheum 2005;52:1191.
56. Elahi S, Cahue S, Felson DT, et al. The association between varus-valgus alignment and patellofemoral osteoarthritis. Arthritis Rheum 2000;43:1874–80.
57. Harrison MM, Cooke TD, Fisher SB, et al. Patterns of knee arthrosis and patellar subluxation. Clin Orthop Relat Res 1994;56–63.
58. Iwano T, Kurosawa H, Tokuyama H, et al. Roentgenographic and clinical findings of patellofemoral osteoarthrosis. With special reference to its relationship to femorotibial osteoarthrosis and etiologic factors. Clin Orthop Relat Res 1990;190–7.
59. Harris WH. Etiology of osteoarthritis of the hip. Clin Orthop Relat Res 1986;20–33.
60. Tanzer M, Noiseux N. Osseous abnormalities and early osteoarthritis: the role of hip impingement [review] [26 refs]. Clin Orthop Relat Res 2004;170–7.
61. Goodman DA, Feighan JE, Smith AD, et al. Subclinical slipped capital femoral epiphysis. Relationship to osteoarthrosis of the hip [comment][erratum appears in J Bone Joint Surg Am 1999 Apr;81(4):592]. J Bone Joint Surg Am 1997;79:1489–97.
62. Leunig M, Werlen S, Ungersbock A, et al. Evaluation of the acetabular labrum by MR arthrography [erratum appears in J Bone Joint Surg Br 1997 Jul;79(4):693]. J Bone Joint Surg Br 1997;79:230–4.
63. Rab GT. The geometry of slipped capital femoral epiphysis: implications for movement, impingement, and corrective osteotomy. J Pediatr Orthop 1999;19:419–24.
64. Snow SW, Keret D, Scarangella S, et al. Anterior impingement of the femoral head: a late phenomenon of Legg-Calve-Perthes' disease. J Pediatr Orthop 1993;13:286–9.
65. Cooperman DR, Wallensten R, Stulberg SD. Acetabular dysplasia in the adult. Clin Orthop Relat Res 1983;79–85.
66. Klaue K, Durnin CW, Ganz R. The acetabular rim syndrome. A clinical presentation of dysplasia of the hip [review] [62 refs]. J Bone Joint Surg Br 1991;73:423–9.
67. Millis MB, Kim YJ. Rationale of osteotomy and related procedures for hip preservation: a review [review] [59 refs]. Clin Orthop Relat Res 2002;108–21.
68. Lloyd-Roberts GC. Osteoarthritis. J Bone Joint Surg Br 1955;37:8–47.
69. Solomon L. Patterns of osteoarthritis of the hip. J Bone Joint Surg Br 1976;58:176–83.
70. Ganz R, Parvizi J, Beck M, et al. Femoroacetabular impingement: a cause for osteoarthritis of the hip [review] [30 refs]. Clin Orthop Relat Res 2003;112–20.
71. Crawford JR, Villar RN. Current concepts in the management of femoroacetabular impingement [review] [37 refs]. J Bone Joint Surg Br 2005;87:1459–62.
72. Lavigne M, Parvizi J, Beck M, et al. Anterior femoroacetabular impingement: part I. Techniques of joint preserving surgery [review] [27 refs]. Clin Orthop Relat Res 2004;61–6.

73. Sampson TG. Arthroscopic treatment of femoroacetabular impingement: a proposed technique with clinical experience. Instr Course Lect 2006;55: 337–46.

74. Leunig M, Beck M, Dora C, et al. [Femoroacetabular impingement: trigger for the development of coxarthrosis] [review] [54 refs] [in German]. Orthopade 2006;35:77–84.

75. Beall DP, Sweet CF, Martin HD, et al. Imaging findings of femoroacetabular impingement syndrome [review] [21 refs]. Skeletal Radiol 2005;34:691–701.

76. Guanche CA, Bare AA. Arthroscopic treatment of femoroacetabular impingement. Arthroscopy 2006;22:95–106.

77. Holmich P, Dienst M. [Differential diagnosis of hip and groin pain. Symptoms and technique for physical examination] [review] [6 refs] [in German]. Orthopade 2006;35:10–5.

78. Meyer DC, Beck M, Ellis T, et al. Comparison of six radiographic projections to assess femoral head/neck asphericity. Clin Orthop Relat Res 2006;445:181–5.

79. Ito K, Minka MA, Leunig M, et al. Femoroacetabular impingement and the cam-effect. A MRI-based quantitative anatomical study of the femoral head-neck offset. J Bone Joint Surg Br 2001;83:171–6.

80. Beaule PE, Zaragoza E, Motamedi K, et al. Three-dimensional computed tomography of the hip in the assessment of femoroacetabular impingement. J Orthop Res 2005;23:1286–92.

81. Leunig M, Casillas MM, Hamlet M, et al. Slipped capital femoral epiphysis: early mechanical damage to the acetabular cartilage by a prominent femoral metaphysis. Acta Orthop Scand 2000;71:370–5.

82. Leunig M, Beck M, Woo A, et al. Acetabular rim degeneration: a constant finding in the aged hip. Clin Orthop Relat Res 2003;201–7.

83. Beck M, Kalhor M, Leunig M, et al. Hip morphology influences the pattern of damage to the acetabular cartilage: femoroacetabular impingement as a cause of early osteoarthritis of the hip. J Bone Joint Surg Br 2005;87:1012–8.

84. Wilson DR, Apreleva MV, Eichler MJ, et al. Accuracy and repeatability of a pressure measurement system in the patellofemoral joint. J Biomech 2003;36: 1909–15.

85. Radin EL, Ehrlich MG, Chernack R, et al. Effect of repetitive impulsive loading on the knee joints of rabbits. Clin Orthop Relat Res 1978;288–93.

86. Song Y, Greve JM, Carter DR, et al. Articular cartilage MR imaging and thickness mapping of a loaded knee joint before and after meniscectomy. Osteoarthritis Cartilage 2006;14:728–37.

87. Andherst W, Tashman S. The association between velocity of the center of closest proximity on subchondral bones and osteoarthritis progression. J Orthop Res 2009;27:71–7.

88. Ahmed AM, Burke DL, Yu A. In-vitro measurement of static pressure distribution in synovial joints–Part II: retropatellar surface. J Biomech Eng 1983;105:226–36.

89. Ahmed AM, Duncan NA, Tanzer M. In vitro measurement of the tracking pattern of the human patella. J Biomech Eng 1999;121:222–8.

90. Ahmed AM, Duncan NA. Correlation of patellar tracking pattern with trochlear and retropatellar surface topographies. J Biomech Eng 2000;122:652–60.

91. Huberti HH, Hayes WC. Patellofemoral contact pressures. The influence of q-angle and tendofemoral contact. J Bone Joint Surg Am 1984;66:715–24.

92. Huberti HH, Hayes WC. Contact pressures in chondromalacia patellae and the effects of capsular reconstructive procedures. J Orthop Res 1988;6: 499–508.

93. Ateshian GA, Kwak SD, Soslowsky LJ, et al. A stereophotogrammetric method for determining in situ contact areas in diarthrodial joints, and a comparison with other methods. J Biomech 1994;27:111–24.

94. Brown TD, Shaw DT. In vitro contact stress distributions in the natural human hip. J Biomech 1983;16:373–84.

95. Apreleva M, Hasselman CT, Debski RE, et al. A dynamic analysis of glenohumeral motion after simulated capsulolabral injury. A cadaver model. J Bone Joint Surg Am 1998;80:474–80.

96. Blankevoort L, Kuiper JH, Huiskes R, et al. Articular contact in a three-dimensional model of the knee. J Biomech 1991;24:1019–31.

97. Blankevoort L, Huiskes R. Validation of a three-dimensional model of the knee. J Biomech 1996;29:955–61.

98. Elias JJ, Wilson DR, Adamson R, et al. Evaluation of a computational model used to predict the patellofemoral contact pressure distribution. J Biomech 2004;37:295–302.

99. Wismans J, Veldpaus F, Janssen J, et al. A three-dimensional mathematical model of the knee-joint. J Biomech 1980;13:677–85.

100. van der Helm FC. A finite element musculoskeletal model of the shoulder mechanism. J Biomech 1994;27:551–69.

101. Brown TD, DiGioia AM III. A contact-coupled finite element analysis of the natural adult hip. J Biomech 1984;17:437–48.

102. Ahmad CS, Kwak SD, Ateshian GA, et al. Effects of patellar tendon adhesion to the anterior tibia on knee mechanics [comment]. Am J Sports Med 1998;26:715–24.

103. Kwak SD, Ahmad CS, Gardner TR, et al. Hamstrings and iliotibial band forces affect knee kinematics and contact pattern. J Orthop Res 2000;18:101–8.

104. Cohen ZA, Roglic H, Grelsamer RP, et al. Patellofemoral stresses during open and closed kinetic chain exercises. An analysis using computer simulation. Am J Sports Med 2001;29:480–7.

105. Cohen ZA, Henry JH, McCarthy DM, et al. Computer simulations of patellofemoral joint surgery. Patient-specific models for tuberosity transfer. Am J Sports Med 2003;31:87–98.

106. Kanamiya T, Naito M, Hara M, et al. The influences of biomechanical factors on cartilage regeneration after high tibial osteotomy for knees with medial compartment osteoarthritis: clinical and arthroscopic observations. Arthroscopy 2002;18:725–9.

107. Morrison JB. The mechanics of the knee joint in relation to normal walking. J Biomech 1970;3:51–61.

108. Andriacchi TP, Alexander EJ, Toney MK, et al. A point cluster method for in vivo motion analysis: applied to a study of knee kinematics. J Biomech Eng 1998;120:743–9.

109. Delport HP, Banks SA, De SJ, et al. A kinematic comparison of fixed- and mobile-bearing knee replacements. J Bone Joint Surg Br 2006;88:1016–21.

110. Komistek RD, Dennis DA, Mahfouz M. In vivo fluoroscopic analysis of the normal human knee. Clin Orthop Relat Res 2003;69–81.

111. Karrholm J, Brandsson S, Freeman MA. Tibiofemoral movement 4: changes of axial tibial rotation caused by forced rotation at the weight-bearing knee studied by RSA. J Bone Joint Surg Br 2000;82:1201–3.

112. Fleming BC, Peura GD, Abate JA, et al. Accuracy and repeatability of Roentgen stereophotogrammetric analysis (RSA) for measuring knee laxity in longitudinal studies. J Biomech 2001;34:1355–9.

113. You BM, Siy P, Anderst W, et al. In vivo measurement of 3-D skeletal kinematics from sequences of biplane radiographs: application to knee kinematics. IEEE Trans Med Imaging 2001;20:514–25.

114. Anderst WJ, Tashman S. A method to estimate in vivo dynamic articular surface interaction. J Biomech 2003;36:1291–9.

115. Powers CM, Ward SR, Fredericson M, et al. Patellofemoral kinematics during weight-bearing and non-weight-bearing knee extension in persons with lateral subluxation of the patella: a preliminary study. J Orthop Sports Phys Ther 2003;33:677–85.

116. Muhle C, Brossmann J, Heller M. Kinematic CT and MR imaging of the patello-femoral joint [review] [47 refs]. Eur Radiol 1999;9:508–18.

117. Sheehan FT, Zajac FE, Drace JE. Using cine phase contrast magnetic reso-nance imaging to non-invasively study in vivo knee dynamics. J Biomech 1998;31:21–6.

118. Sheehan FT, Zajac FE, Drace JE. In vivo tracking of the human patella using cine phase contrast magnetic resonance imaging. J Biomech Eng 1999;121:650–6.

119. Sheehan FT, Drace JE. Quantitative MR measures of three-dimensional patellar kinematics as a research and diagnostic tool. Med Sci Sports Exerc 1999;31: 1399–405.

120. Barrance PJ, Williams GN, Novotny JE, et al. A method for measurement of joint kinematics in vivo by registration of 3-D geometric models with cine phase contrast magnetic resonance imaging data. J Biomech Eng 2005;127:829–37.

121. Barrance PJ, Williams GN, Snyder-Mackler L, et al. Altered knee kinematics in ACL-deficient non-copers: a comparison using dynamic MRI. J Orthop Res 2006;24:132–40.

122. Barrance PJ, Williams GN, Snyder-Mackler L, et al. Do ACL-injured copers exhibit differences in knee kinematics? an MRI study. Clin Orthop Relat Res 2007;454:74–80.

123. Rebmann AJ, Sheehan FT. Precise 3D skeletal kinematics using fast phase contrast magnetic resonance imaging. J Magn Reson Imaging 2003;17:206–13.

124. Patel VV, Hall K, Ries M, et al. A three-dimensional MRI analysis of knee kine-matics. J Orthop Res 2004;22:283–92.

125. Patel VV, Hall K, Ries M, et al. Magnetic resonance imaging of patellofemoral kinematics with weight-bearing. J Bone Joint Surg Am 2003;85:2419–24.

126. Fellows RA, Hill NA, Macintyre NJ, et al. Repeatability of a novel technique for in vivo measurement of three-dimensional patellar tracking using magnetic reso-nance imaging. J Magn Reson Imaging 2005;22:145–53.

127. Fellows RA, Hill NA, Gill HS, et al. Magnetic resonance imaging for in vivo assessment of three-dimensional patellar tracking. J Biomech 2005;38: 1643–52.

128. Lerner AL, Tamez-Pena JG, Houck JR, et al. The use of sequential MR image sets for determining tibiofemoral motion: reliability of coordinate systems and accuracy of motion tracking algorithm. J Biomech Eng 2003;125:246–53.

129. McWalter E, Wilson D, Kacher D, et al. Three dimensional patellar kinematics in weightbearing flexion [abstract]. World Congress of Biomechanics 2006:135 Munich. August.

130. Ronsky JL, Herzog W, Brown TD, et al. In vivo quantification of the cat patello-femoral joint contact stresses and areas. J Biomech 1995;28:977–83.

131. Tashman S, Anderst W. In-vivo measurement of dynamic joint motion using high speed biplane radiography and CT: application to canine ACL deficiency. J Bio-mech Eng 2003;125:238–45.

132. Gold GE, Besier TF, Draper CE, et al. Weight-bearing MRI of patellofemoral joint cartilage contact area. J Magn Reson Imaging 2004;20:526–30.
133. Besier TF, Draper CE, Gold GE, et al. Patellofemoral joint contact area increases with knee flexion and weight-bearing. J Orthop Res 2005;23:345–50.
134. Goto A, Moritomo H, Murase T, et al. In vivo elbow biomechanical analysis during flexion: three-dimensional motion analysis using magnetic resonance imaging. J Shoulder Elbow Surg 2004;13:441–7.
135. Hunter DJ, Zhang Y, Niu J, et al. Structural factors associated with malalignment in knee osteoarthritis: the Boston osteoarthritis knee study [comment]. J Rheumatol 2005;32:2192–9.

Radiographic Grading and Measurement of Joint Space Width in Osteoarthritis

Marie-Pierre Hellio Le Graverand, MD, DSc, PhD[a],*, Steve Mazzuca, PhD[b],
Jeff Duryea, PhD[c], Alan Brett, PhD[d]

KEYWORDS

- Radiograph • Joint space width
- Joint space narrowing • Osteoarthritis
- Medial tibial plateau alignment

Osteoarthritis (OA) is the most common and costly form of arthritis. The disease is a slowly, progressive, ultimately degenerative disorder confined to movable joints. OA occurs when the equilibrium between breakdown and repair of the joint tissues becomes unbalanced. Clinically, OA is mainly characterized by joint pain and functional limitation; however, many subjects with definite structural changes consistent with OA are asymptomatic.

OA remains a condition that is poorly understood, and for which only symptom-modifying drugs are available. In contrast, no disease-modifying OA drugs that alter the structural progression of OA are currently approved. Disease-modifying OA drug development is constrained by its heterogeneous clinical manifestations, the unclear relationship between structural progression and clinical end points, and the need for long-term follow-up to observe changes in structure. Accurate and highly reproducible measurement of the rate of progression is a prerequisite for assessing structural change both for clinical trials and subsequently for patients in clinical practice.

A version of this article originally appeared in the 47:4 issue of Radiologic Clinics of North America.

[a] Clinical Development and Medical Affairs, Inflammation, Specialty Care Business Unit, Pfizer Inc, 50 Pequot Avenue, New London, CT 06320, USA
[b] Indiana University School of Medicine, Department of Medicine, Rheumatology Division, Long Hospital, Room 545,1110 W. Michigan Street, Indianapolis, IN 46202–5100, USA
[c] Radiology Brigham and Women's Hospital, Harvard Medical School, 75 Francis Street, Boston, MA 02115, USA
[d] Optasia Medical Ltd, Haw Bank House, High Street, Cheadle SK8 1AL, UK
* Corresponding author.
E-mail address: helliomp@pfizer.com (M-P. Hellio Le Graverand).

Rheum Dis Clin N Am 35 (2009) 485–502
doi:10.1016/j.rdc.2009.08.005
0889-857X/09/$ – see front matter © 2009 Published by Elsevier Inc.

rheumatic.theclinics.com

Traditionally, measurement of OA structural change has been performed using radiographs. Conventional radiography is the simplest and least expensive method for imaging joints affected by OA. Radiography is used in clinical practice in patients to establish the diagnosis of OA and to monitor the progression of the disease. Radiographs clearly visualize bony features including marginal osteophytes, subchondral sclerosis, and subchondral cysts that are associated with OA and provide an estimate of cartilage thickness and meniscal integrity by the interbone distance or joint space width (JSW). The radiographic definition of OA mainly relies on the evaluation of both osteophytes and joint space narrowing (JSN) (ie, the loss of JSW). Because osteophytes are considered specific to OA, develop at an earlier stage than JSN, are more correlated with knee pain, and are easier to ascertain than other radiographic features, they represent the widely applied criterion to define the presence of OA.[1–3] Assessment of OA severity, however, mainly relies on JSN and subchondral bone lesions. In addition, progression of JSN is the most commonly used criterion for the assessment of OA progression and the complete loss of JSW characterized by bone-on-bone contact is one of the factors considered in the decision for joint replacement.

The severity of OA can be estimated using semiquantitative scoring systems. Published atlases provide images that represent specific grades.[4,5] Several grading scales incorporating combinations of features also have been developed including the most widely used Kellgren and Lawrence grade classification.[6] The Kellgren and Lawrence grade scoring system suffers from limitations based on the invalid assumptions that changes in radiographic features (eg, osteophytes, JSN) are linear over the course of the disease and that the relationship between these features is constant. In contrast, the Osteoarthritis Research Society International Atlas Classification grades separately the tibiofemoral JSN and osteophytes in each compartment of the knee.[4]

Current clinical research tends to focus on knee OA because of the prevalence of the disease in this joint. This article focuses on the assessment of OA in the femorotibial compartment of the knee. Traditionally, the progression of knee OA in clinical trials has been assessed by measuring changes in JSW between the medial femoral condyle and medial tibial plateau on plain radiographs,[7] because the medial femorotibial compartment is the most common site of involvement in knee OA. Both a reduction in cartilage thickness and meniscal integrity are inferred from a reduction in JSW.[7–9]

RADIOANATOMIC ALIGNMENT OF THE TIBIOFEMORAL JOINT

The sine qua non for accurate measurement of radiographic JSW is a reproducible image of the joint space. A reproducible radiographic image of the tibiofemoral joint space requires adherence to exacting standards of positioning of the knee, which include specifications for flexion and rotation of the joint, and for angulation of the x-ray beam.[10] In most individuals, the anatomy of the knee is such that full extension of the joint (as is required for a conventional weight-bearing extended knee radiograph) tilts the tibial plateau to an angle that is skewed (ie, not parallel) to a horizontally directed x-ray beam (**Fig. 1**).[11] Skewed radioanatomic alignment of the tibial plateau in an anteroposterior (AP) or posteroanterior (PA) knee radiograph is apparent in the displacement of the anterior and posterior margins of the medial plateau (**Fig. 2**). Reproducibility of positioning notwithstanding, when the alignment of the plateau is notably skewed, the floor of the joint space can become indistinct, and a key reference point for the measurement of minimum JSW (minJSW) (ie, the shortest distance between femoral condyle and tibial plateau) is less reliably ascertained.

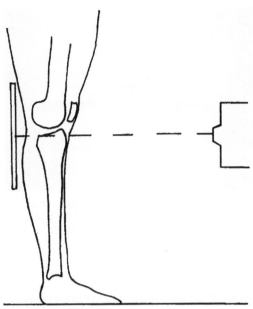

Fig. 1. Schematic drawing showing the positioning for the conventional extended knee radiograph. For most subjects, full knee extension tilts the tibial plateau to an angle that is skewed to a horizontal x-ray beam.

Buckland-Wright and colleagues[12] demonstrated that individualized flexion of the knee to achieve superimposition (± 1 mm) of the anterior and posterior margins of the medial tibial plateau (**Fig. 3**) confirmed under fluoroscopy before image acquisition resulted in measurements of medial tibiofemoral JSW in repeat AP radiographs that were significantly more reproducible than those obtained from concurrent extended knee radiographs. Subsequently, so-called "parallel radioanatomic alignment" of

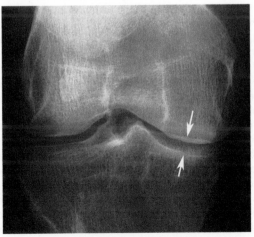

Fig. 2. Skewed radioanatomic alignment of the medial tibial plateau alignment, apparent in the displacement of anterior and posterior margins of the plateau (*arrows*).

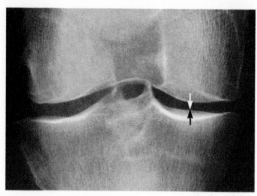

Fig. 3. Parallel radioanatomic alignment of the medial tibial plateau, apparent in superimposition of the anterior and posterior margins of the plateau (*arrows*). A maximum intermargin distance of 1–1.5 mm or less is generally taken as evidence of satisfactory parallel alignment.

the medial tibial plateau, which affords a distinct reference point for measurement of tibiofemoral JSW, has been a goal of developers of alternative protocols for standardized knee radiography.

PROTOCOLS FOR STANDARDIZED RADIOGRAPHIC EXAMINATION OF THE KNEE

For 40 years the extended knee radiograph (ie, a bilateral weight-bearing AP view of both knees in full extension) has been the conventional plain radiograph used to image the tibiofemoral joint.[13,14] It was the procedure used to acquire reference images for contemporary pictorial atlases of the radiographic severity of tibiofemoral OA[4,6,15] and remains an accepted radiographic technique for characterizing the bony changes of OA (eg, osteophytosis, subchondral sclerosis). Although the diagnostic use of the extended knee radiograph is established, this technique is severely limited as a means by which to visualize reproducibly the radiographic joint space.[16] This limitation stems from numerous technical shortcomings of the examination with respect to variability in the positioning of the knee in serial examinations. For example, longitudinal changes in weight-bearing (eg, because of weight gain or loss) may affect the extent of voluntary knee extension. Changes in the distance between the knee and x-ray cassette may alter the degree of radiographic magnification in the image. Although these sources of variation in knee position are likely to contribute random measurement error to estimates of tibiofemoral JSW, changes in knee pain from examination to examination (as may occur in a clinical trial of a purported disease-modifying OA drug) may introduce systematic measurement error. This was demonstrated by Mazzuca and colleagues,[17] who detected significant increases in tibiofemoral JSW in extended knee radiographs taken 7 to 14 days apart of OA patients who had undergone relief of an induced flare of knee OA pain. These sources of error seriously limit the use of the extended knee radiograph to detect true JSN.[6]

Over the past 15 years, several alternative protocols have been developed for standardized positioning of the knee for a radiographic examination of the tibiofemoral joint. Common to all of the techniques is a standard for knee flexion, rather than extension, that provides contact between the tibia and the posterior aspect of the femoral condyle (ie, the region in which cartilage damage in OA is often most prominent).[18] The

Table 1
Comparison of technical specifications for alternative protocols for standardized knee radiography

	Buckland-Wright Semiflexed[12]	Lyon Schuss[21]	Semiflexed Metatarsophalangeal[24]	Fixed Flexion[28]
Fluoroscopically assisted	Yes	Yes	No	No
Orientation of knee	Anteroposterior	Posteroanterior	Posteroanterior	Posteroanterior
Degree of flexion	Variable (7–10 degrees)	Fixed (20–35 degrees)	Fixed (7–10 degrees)	Fixed (20–35 degrees)
Standard for knee flexion	Flex to superimpose the anterior and posterior margins of the medial tibial plateau	Schuss position[a]	Coplanar alignment of the patella, first metatarsophalangeal joint, and x-ray cassette	Schuss position[a]
Standard for foot rotation	Rotate to center the tibial spines beneath the femoral notch	10 degrees	15 degrees	10 degrees
Standard for x-ray beam angulation	Horizontal	Adjust to bring the medial tibial plateau on sharpest focus	Horizontal	10 degrees caudal
Adjustment for radiographic magnification	Required	Optional	Optional	Optional

[a] Coplanar alignment of the front surface of the x-ray cassette with the hip, patella, and tip of the great toe.

protocols differ, however, with respect to the degree of flexion required, angulation of the x-ray beam, and the parameter that is adjusted to meet the examination's positioning standards (**Table 1**). A key distinction among current positioning protocols is the use (or not) of fluoroscopy to confirm satisfactory radioanatomic positioning of the medial tibial plateau (ie, parallel or near-parallel alignment with the central x-ray beam) before acquisition of the radiograph.

Fluoroscopically Assisted Protocols

Semiflexed AP view

Buckland-Wright and colleagues[12] described the semiflexed AP knee examination using fluoroscopy to guide knee flexion and rotation to achieve reproducible anatomic markers of parallel alignment of the medial tibial plateau relative to a horizontal x-ray beam. Under fluoroscopy, small degrees of flexion (7–10 degrees) are evaluated in terms of the resulting distance between anterior and posterior margins of the medial tibial plateau (**Fig. 4**A). When semiflexion affords an intermargin distance (IMD) less than or equal to 1 mm, the foot is rotated internally or externally as needed to center the tibial spines beneath the femoral notch.

Horizontality of the beam prevents parallax distortion of the joint space. Semiflexion of the AP knee draws the joint away from the x-ray film, however, and introduces

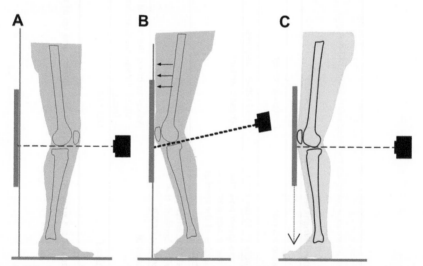

Fig. 4. Schematic drawings showing the positioning of the subject for the semiflexed AP view (*A*), Lyon-schuss (LS) or fixed-flexion (FF) posteroanterior views (*B*), and the metatarsophalangeal (MTP) PA view (*C*). In both the LS and FF protocols the x-ray beam is centered on the joint line. The FF protocol uses a fixed 10-degree caudal x-ray beam and positions the thighs, patellae, and pelvis flush with the film cassette and coplanar with the tips of the great toes, resulting in fixed knee angulation of approximately 20-degree flexion. In the LS protocol, positioning is identical to that for an FF view. The angle of the x-ray beam is not fixed, however, but is adjusted for each examination to align the MTP with the x-ray beam. Alignment is achieved by using fluoroscopy to superimpose the anterior and posterior margins of the medial tibial plateau. In the modified LS, an initial acquisition is performed at a 10-degree caudal angulation of the x-ray beam. If the medial tibial plateau alignment in the initial image is skewed, repeat examinations with a 1-unit caudal or cranial increment in the beam angle (1–2 degrees) is obtained for parallel alignment of the medial tibial plateau with the x-ray beam.

radiographic magnification, a potential obstacle to accurate JSW measurement. The semiflexed AP protocol requires use of a foot map to reproduce the joint-to-film distance and a magnification marker (ie, a small steel ball of known diameter affixed to the skin over the head of the fibula) to permit correction of JSW estimates for longitudinal variations in radiographic magnification, which may be as great as 35%.[12] Although magnification correction poses several challenges to accurate measurement of tibiofemoral JSW,[8] the semiflexed AP view has been shown to afford estimates of JSW that are more precise than those obtained from the conventional extended knee view[12,20] and less subject to the confounding effects of longitudinal changes in knee pain.[17]

Lyon schuss view

Vignon and colleagues[21] have developed an alternative protocol that used PA schuss position of the subject (ie, placement of the anterior aspect of the hip, the patella, and tip of the great toe against the x-ray cassette or surface of the vertical x-ray table). Lyon schuss positioning requires a greater degree of flexion than that seen in semiflexed AP views (see **Table 1**). Coplanar alignment of the hip, patella, and great toe fixes the degree of flexion for repeat examinations (20–35 degrees, depending on the relative lengths of the tibia and foot). This is an element of positioning that is not guaranteed to be reproduced with the semiflexed AP protocol. To compensate for the effect of knee flexion on the orientation of the medial tibial plateau, relative to the horizontal plane, fluoroscopy is used to adjust the angle of the x-ray beam caudally to bring the tibial plateau into sharpest focus (see **Fig. 4**B).

Early data derived from the Lyon schuss radiograph confirmed that it afforded reproducibility of measurement of medial tibiofemoral JSW superior to that of the conventional extended knee view.[21] A recent modification of the Lyon schuss protocol has incorporated use of the SynaFlexer (Synarc, San Francisco, California), an acrylic positioning frame in which subjects stand and position themselves to fix knee flexion and external foot rotation in schuss position. Recent applications of the protocol have also adopted the IMD as the standard for evaluating radioanatomic alignment of the medial tibial plateau.[19,22,23]

Non-fluoroscopically Assisted Protocols

Semiflexed metatarsophalangeal view

To develop a more exportable, non–fluoroscopically assisted alternative to their semiflexed AP view, Buckland-Wright and colleagues[24] have disseminated procedures for the semiflexed metatarsophalangeal (MTP) view. The MTP protocol provides a PA radiograph of both knees with the subject standing so that the MTP joints of both great toes are directly beneath the front surface of the x-ray cassette with knees flexed slightly until the patellae are in contact with the cassette, directly above the MTP joints (see **Table 1**). Positioning for the MTP view resembles that for the semiflexed view with respect to knee flexion and foot rotation. JSW measurements from the MTP view do not require correction for radioanatomic magnification. Use of a foot map is advised, however, to facilitate reproducibility of foot rotation (15 degrees) and placement of first MTP joints beneath the front of the x-ray cassette (see **Fig. 4**C).

The reproducibility of the semiflexed MTP view has been demonstrated with respect to measurements of tibiofemoral JSW and radioanatomic alignment of the medial tibial plateau in examinations repeated on the same day.[24,25] Several cross-sectional and longitudinal analyses of the performance of the MTP protocol have noted, however, that as many as 70% of MTP radiographs exhibit skewed alignment of the medial tibial plateau.[26,27] Moreover, alignment in MTP views is notably less reproducible over time than it is in the short term, resulting in lesser sensitivity to JSN than concurrent semiflexed AP radiographs.[26]

Fixed-flexion view

Peterfy and colleagues[28] have developed an empirically derived set of positioning standards for standardized knee radiography. Based on fluoroscopically guided measurements of beam angulation that produced parallel radioanatomic alignment of the medial tibial plateau in samples of normal and OA knees in schuss position (9 ± 3.6 degrees), they designed positioning standards for the PA fixed-flexion view. As with the Lyon schuss technique, both knees are in contact with the cassette and coplanar with the hips, patellae, and tips of the great toes (see **Table 1**). Whereas the beam angle in the Lyon schuss view is varied with each examination to align the beam with the medial tibial plateau, however, the fixed-flexion view requires that the x-ray beam be directed 10 degrees caudally. Positioning of the knee and foot for the fixed-flexion view is facilitated by use of the SynaFlexer positioning frame.

Like other standardization protocols, the fixed-flexion PA view permits highly precise measurements of JSW.[28] Because of biologic variability in the anatomy of the tibial plateau, however, the fixed-flexion technique often produces a radiograph with skewed radioanatomic alignment of the medial tibial plateau.[26] This has led investigators to explore a modification of the fixed-flexion protocol that entails ascertainment of the quality of alignment produced by 10 degrees caudal angulation and reacquisition of the radiograph with small adjustments of the angle (cranially or caudally) until satisfactory alignment is achieved.[22,29]

Sensitivity to JSN

The developers of the standardized knee radiography protocols described previously have each offered evidence to indicate that their protocol affords measurements of tibiofemoral JSW that are more precise and reproducible than those obtainable from the conventional extended knee radiograph.[12,21,24–28] Although measurement precision is an important theoretical determinant of sensitivity to the detection of change (eg, thinning of articular cartilage), it is not a sufficient basis to conclude that one standardized technique is more advisable than another for use in longitudinal studies of OA progression. Such choices are best made on the basis of direct comparisons of alternative protocols in the same subjects.

Head-to-head comparisons of alternative positioning protocols are rare in the OA literature. One such study compared the semiflexed AP view with its non–fluoroscopically assisted counterpart (MTP view) in examinations of 52 OA knees performed 14 months apart.[26] Serial MTP views suggested a small average increase in mean minJSW over 14 months that was not significantly greater than zero (mean ± SD = +0.09 ± 0.66 mm). In contrast, concurrent semiflexed AP examinations showed a marginally significant decrease in mean minJSW (−0.09 ± 0.31 mm; $P = .10$) in the same knees. Also important was the observation that the SD of JSN in serial Lyon schuss views was less than half the magnitude of that in measurements from MTP views. This suggests a notably smaller level of random measurement error in JSW estimates from semiflexed AP radiographs than from MTP views. The relative insensitivity of the MTP view to JSN in OA knees was attributed, at least in part, to longitudinal changes in the radioanatomic position of the medial plateau despite adherence to positioning standards for the examination. IMDs measured in repeat baseline MTP radiographs were very highly correlated (+0.88), whereas IMDs in the MTP views taken 14 months apart were only moderately correlated (+0.45).[26]

A recent study compared the Lyon schuss view with its non–fluoroscopically assisted counterpart (fixed-flexion view) in examinations of 62 OA and 99 non-OA knees taken 12 months apart.[19] In radiographically normal knees, mean minJSW did not change over 12 months in either view. In the OA knees, mean change in medial minJSW was −0.22 ± 0.43 mm in Lyon schuss views and +0.01 ± 0.46 mm in fixed-flexion views (P = .0002 and P = .92, respectively). At both time points the mean IMD in Lyon schuss views was only half as large as that in fixed-flexion views (approximately 0.9 ± 0.5 mm versus 1.9 ± 1.2 mm; $P<.0001$).[19]

Investigators from the same study have also evaluated the performance of a non–fluoroscopically guided variation on the Lyon schuss radiograph, in which an initial PA radiograph of the knee in schuss position was acquired with 10-degree caudal angulation (ie, as in the fixed-flexion view).[22] If the IMD in the initial radiograph exhibited skewed alignment, the examination was repeated up to three more times. Each iteration of the examination occurred with a small (1–2 degree) adjustment of beam angulation until parallel MTP alignment was achieved. The performance of original and modified Lyon schuss radiographs was compared with that of standard fixed-flexion radiographs in serial examinations of 74 OA knees performed 12 months apart. Compared with fixed-flexion, modified Lyon schuss radiographs afforded a smaller mean IMD at baseline (0.89 versus 2.06 mm; P = .002); more reproducible alignment over 12 months (mean IMD change = 0.49 versus 0.91 mm; P = .007); and more rapid JSN (mean change in minJSW = −0.25 versus −0.02 mm/y; P = .005). These differences paralleled those observed between original Lyon schuss and fixed-flexion procedures with respect to baseline alignment (0.96 versus 1.94 mm; $P<.001$); reproducibility of alignment (0.49 versus 1 mm; $P<.001$); and sensitivity to JSN (−0.16 versus 0.01 mm/y; P = .007).[22]

Although these comparisons indicate clearly that sensitivity to radiographic JSN is enhanced by fluoroscopically assisted joint positioning or beam angulation, it should be acknowledged that the non–fluoroscopically assisted methods described can detect disease progression in knee OA. A report from the Health, Aging and Body Composition Study offered evidence that the fixed-flexion radiograph exhibits noteworthy sensitivity to JSN in OA knees over a 3-year interval (mean JSN ± SD = 0.43 ± 0.66 mm).[30] Sensitivity of this view to JSN over shorter intervals is uncertain. The semiflexed MTP view was the source of primary outcome data for the Glucosamine/Chondroitin Arthritis Intervention Trial. A recent report suggests that the MTP view detected loss of JSW over 2 years in treatment and control groups of the Glucosamine/Chondroitin Arthritis Intervention Trial (eg, mean JSN in the placebo group = 0.166 mm); however, the failure of the trial to detect significant differences between treatment groups with respect to JSN was attributed, in part, by the authors to "increased variability of measurement."[31]

TIBIOFEMORAL JSW AND PROGRESSION OF OA
Manual Methods

Before the development of the automated and semiautomated methods of the early 1990s, JSW measurement was conducted using purely manual methods in which both the site of measurement within the compartment and the locations of the landmarks for measurement were judged purely by eye. Various methods have been used to obtain measurements from a radiograph laid on a light box including applying a ruler to the radiograph and reading the distance directly from the ruler; direct measurement from the radiograph using a magnifying lens with an internal measurement scale; direct measurement using a set of dial calipers; and a method developed by Lequesne,[32] which involved applying a set of simple calipers to the distance to be measured before transferring its points to a ruler[33] to measure the distance between them. A modified version of the last of these methods was introduced by Laoussadi and Menkes[34] in which the points were transferred to a sheet of paper to make prick-marks, the distance between which could then be measured using a 1/10 mm graduated magnifying glass. In this modified form, the method has become a standard for performing manual measurements from radiographs, often referred to as chondrometry or "Lequesne's method."

Although these manual methods benefit from simplicity of equipment and application, and from the fact that the same method could be used to measure any linear distance, they are time-consuming, subjective, and very labor-intensive, even for trained staff.

Semiautomated and Automated Methods

The purpose of the development of automated and semiautomated techniques for use in clinical trials was to develop more rapid, objective, and precise measurements of JSW. Software algorithms have been used to evaluate digital radiographic images for well over two decades. Initially, much of this work was in such fields as mammography and the purpose of the software was to provide a computer-aided diagnosis of potentially malignant structures.[35] The goal of image processing software applied to knee radiography for OA assessment is generally to provide quantitative measures of structural changes over time rather than a one-time diagnosis. Most of the work has been aimed at quantifying radiographic JSW to replace semiquantitative scoring, or the need for a reader to make measurements manually. **Fig. 5** shows an example of a cropped image of the knee, where the image analysis software has delineated both margins of the joint and determined the location of minJSW in the medial tibiofemoral compartment.

An early study by Dacre and colleagues[36] examined radiographic images of the knee using a video capture of the films illuminated by a light box. This technique produced 512 × 512 pixels images that were presented on a screen along with a mouse tool that the reader could use to trace the joint margins and allow for the measurement of the JSW and area at selected locations along the joint. The study

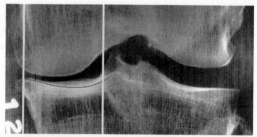

Fig. 5. Illustration of the delineation of the tibiofemoral joint space and identification of minimum joint space width (minJSW) by semiautomated measurement software. The vertical yellow lines are delineated by the operator to define the regions of interest where minJSW is to be measured. These regions are drawn to limit measurement to weight-bearing areas and to avoid bony changes (ie, osteophytes) at the extreme margins of the joint space that may bias measurement. Within each region, the software delineates the femoral and tibial margins of the joint space (*red lines*) and identifies the shortest distance between each pair of margins (*blue line*).

demonstrated improved reproducibility compared with manual readings and a good correlation to qualitative scoring. A subsequent paper by this group[37] used a more direct capture method to convert the image into a digital file that was stored on the local computer for further analysis. For this second study the researchers used automated edge detection software algorithms provided by a commercial software package to delineate the joint margins and make the measurements of JSW. Conrozier and Vignon[38] also demonstrated an improved reproducibility of a digital assessment over manual methods. The study used a modified digital caliper and the viewing of images on a back-lighted table to make measurements of radiographic JSW.

Lynch and colleagues[39] described a study using a new custom-designed software algorithm[40] written in the C programming language by the researchers in their laboratory. The software functioned by delineating both margins of the knee joint aided by the placement of seed points on the image by the reader. The software was validated by measuring the reproducibility on duplicate films, digitized using a 1280 × 1024 pixel CCD camera, of in vivo subjects and postmortem knees. An improved reproducibility of the minJSW compared with the manual technique was demonstrated. A subsequent publication confirmed these results on macro radiographs of the knee.[12]

Duryea and colleagues[41] described a different "rule-based" custom-written software algorithm used to delineate the joints of the knee and make a measurement of minJSW. The method is "trainable," meaning that the core algorithm can be optimized for different data sets by applying the software to a representative subset of the data in a study. Validation of the software was made using duplicate films digitized with a commercial radiographic film digitizer. Comparisons with a manual reading using a graduated hand-held lens demonstrated a twofold improvement in reproducibility over the manual method. The study also validated the software-delineated joint margins through a comparison with gold standard hand-delineated contours performed by an expert reader using a mouse tool on the digital images. Conrozier and colleagues[42] described an "edge-based algorithm" to perform joint-delineation to examine the effect of tibial plateau alignment and different patient positioning protocols on the sensitivity to change for JSW.

More recently, a class of technologies known as "statistical shape models"[43] has been used to segment the anatomy of the knee joint in radiographs. This approach uses multivariate statistics to derive the allowable shape of an object from a set of examples. Seise and colleagues[44] describes an adaptation of the original "active shape model"[45] approach to the automated segmentation of the tibia and the rims of the tibial plateaus in digitized radiographs. Although segmentation of the femoral condyles is also described, the extension of the method to a measurement of JSW is not. A different, but related, statistical modeling approach was described by Lacey and colleagues[46] for the determination of JSW and other measurements. This approach requires the operator to initialize the statistical model using a set of six approximate landmarks. The result is an annotation of the femoral condyles and the tibial plateaus from the tibial spines to the outer margin of the joint in each compartment. A software application based on this approach was tested as a workflow tool in which no manual correction of the resulting annotation was performed on 640 knee radiographs from the Osteoarthritis Initiative[47] database. In this study, 10% of the radiographs were not analyzed because they were either of poor quality or else significant manual correction to the annotation was required.

An interactive analysis system termed "knee images digital analysis" described by Marijnissen and colleagues[48] uses weight-bearing semiflexed MTP radiographs[24] and an aluminum step-wedge for calibration. The software determines a range of parameters including medial and lateral JSW, subchondral bone density, knee align-ment, and size of osteophytes. The analysis begins with a suggestion by the software of a framework of four lines that define the position of the joint, which may be reposi-tioned by the user. This framework is then used to support the interactive placement of circles marking positions at which to measure JSW and the other parameters. The entire interactive process takes approximately 10 minutes. The system was tested by two operators using radiographs of 20 healthy knees and 55 showing signs of OA and demonstrated a small interoperator variation in the measurement.

MinJSW Versus Mean JSW and JSW at Specific Locations

Because the current software-based methods delineate the full extent of the joint, a logical next step was to make a systematic study of JSW. The determination of a mean JSW or a joint space area has been studied in either a constant area or a region of interest and its performance compared with that of minJSW. MinJSW was found more reproducible and more sensitive to change than mean JSW or a joint space area.[49,50] Although in some reports mean JSW has been suggested to perform better, minJSW remains the most generally used and accepted outcome measurement for OA progression.[33,51,52]

Another approach that was more recently described is the determination of JSW at more general positions along the joint interface (**Figs. 6** and **7**). This generally requires the use of robust anatomic landmarks so that consistent locations can be established both cross-sectional and longitudinally. In (see **Fig. 5**) the inner landmarks are the tips of the tibial spines. For each compartment, the outer landmark is defined as being midway between a landmark at the outer extent of the tibial fossa and the edge of the tibial plateau, which is usually found as point of maximum curvature at the edge of the compartment. Duryea and colleagues[52] found improved reproducibility of loca-tion-specific JSW compared with software measurements of minJSW. More recent publications have also shown an improved responsiveness over minJSW for more severely diseased knees imaged using a fixed-flexion protocol.[53-55] There has also been a study undertaken to compare fixed-position JSW as measured in radiographs with a similar measure derived from MRI data from the same subject, again using images from the Osteoarthritis Initiative database.[56] In this comparative study, measurements from both modalities showed statistically significant progression of OA but in different populations. This may be because the radiographs, unlike MRI,

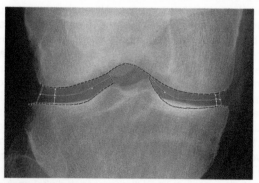

Fig. 6. Delineation of femoral and tibial margins allows the calculation of medial JSW along a normalized distance across the medial and lateral compartments from the tibial spine to the medial and lateral margins of the tibia (*in pink*); the minJSW is also shown (*in yellow*).

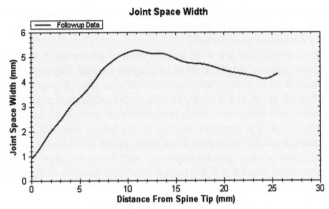

Fig. 7. The corresponding JSW plot for (see **Fig. 6**) from which can be derived fixed-position JSW at any position in the compartment.

are weight-bearing and measure changes caused by structures other than the carti-lage, but it is unclear whether the two approaches quantify the same progression in pathology but with poor agreement, or are sensitive to different manifestations of the disease. A recent study has also examined location-specific JSW in the lateral compartment and found improved responsiveness in a subset of OA knees exhibiting valgus malalignment.[57]

IMPLICATIONS FOR RESEARCH AND PRACTICE

A fair appraisal of alternative protocols for standardized knee radiography must take into account several practical limitations of fluoroscopically assisted techniques when they are exported for use in medical centers active in clinical research. Many established clinical research centers do not support the fluoroscopic equipment required for a weight-bearing knee examination. In the United States, even where such equipment is available, a manpower shortage among radiology technologists makes maintenance of quality control of radiographs with respect to positioning criteria difficult. Ethical and practical considerations (eg, cumulative radiation expo-sure, willingness of subjects) may limit the capacity of investigators to attain uniformly high technical quality by precluding repetition of substandard examinations. Finally, fluoroscopic positioning increases the cost of a radiographic knee examination three-fold to fourfold. These reservations notwithstanding, the benefits associated with fluo-roscopically assisted knee radiography, with respect to quality and reproducibility of radioanatomic positioning of the tibiofemoral joint space and resulting sensitivity to JSN, are commensurate with the costs. Where fluoroscopy is unavailable, however, a fixed-flexion protocol modified to include iterative acquisitions with small adjust-ments of beam angle to achieve parallel radioanatomic alignment of the medial tibial plateau[22,29] is recommended.

The advances in standardized knee radiography that have made clinical trials of purported disease-modifying OA drugs feasible can also benefit clinical practice. The conventional extended view knee radiograph is still used by clinicians to docu-ment evidence of marginal tibiofemoral osteophytes, on which the diagnosis of knee OA is based. Continued use of this view for diagnostic purposes is not contrain-dicated by the information presented in this analysis. The clinician should know, however, that the extended knee radiograph cannot be relied on to afford an accurate or reliable representation of the tibiofemoral joint space. The radiographic severity of knee OA (ie, the extent of JSN in the presence of marginal osteophytes) may not be apparent in the extended knee view.[58]

Most clinical radiology departments are capable of producing a PA radiograph of the knee in Lyon schuss position with 10-degree caudal angulation of the x-ray beam (ie, a fixed-flexion radiograph, with or without use of a positioning frame). A radiograph satisfying these standards offers two distinct advantages over the conventional extended knee view. First, knee flexion is more likely to reveal cartilage loss that is common to the posterior aspect of the femur. Second, the fixed-flexion view is more likely than the extended knee view, albeit not certain, to represent the joint space in parallel or near-parallel alignment with the x-ray beam. These strengths should result in greater accuracy in the evaluation of the severity of structural changes of tibiofemoral OA. They should also provide an image of the knee that is more reliably reproduced in future assessments of disease progression.

As in other fields, software techniques to evaluate knee radiography have become increasingly more advanced as time has passed. Earlier approaches were simple digital calipers or used modifications to commercial image processing software. Later attempts used a targeted approach based on low-level programming algorithms specially designed for the task of delineating the joint margins. This process had been aided by the advent of more powerful processors and research into more sophisticated algorithms. Computer-aided diagnosis in such areas as mammography, chest, and neurologic imaging continues to be a very active field. It is likely that the future development of image processing software to assess knee radiography for OA will draw from work in these other areas. Some of the systems described here already include software to assess additional structural features, such as osteophytes, bone alignment, and subchondral sclerosis, and will likely begin to include more abstract analysis of the shape and appearance or bone texture of the joint.

Before the advent of fully digital modalities, such as computed radiography and digital radiography, digitized radiographic images were created by capturing the illuminated image with a digital camera or using a specialized radiographic film digitizer. The new fully digital modalities have the potential to integrate seamlessly with these software approaches through hospital PACS infrastructure for research studies and for patient care once these methods reach the clinic. This may be particularly true for digital radiography, which produces an image file directly on the hard disk of a computer without the need for any intermediate steps. Many clinical digital radiography systems designed for chest or abdominal imaging use detectors with inferior spatial resolution, however, compared with the traditional digitized film-screen system. Given the similarity in size of the breast and knee, and the need for high spatial resolution for both imaging tasks, it may be advisable to design future digital imaging systems for skeletal radiography using mammography detectors.

SUMMARY

OA is the most common form of arthritis and one of the leading causes of disability in elders. With little currently available in the treatment of this disease, better understanding of responsive and valid end points is essential to identifying potential new interventions for treatment of this disease. Over the past two decades, numerous knee radiography protocols have been developed with various levels of complexity and performance as it relates to detecting change. Sensitivity to JSN is improved when radioanatomic alignment of the medial tibial plateau is achieved. The development of a fully automated algorithm where no reader interaction is used to make the assessment could be considered the ultimate goal of these efforts. It is unlikely, however, that a 100% accurate software approach will ever be achieved particularly for more advanced in severity or poorly positioned knees. The use of reader as a quality assurance and correction step using a graphical user interface permits a method to evaluate all images in a study. There are currently a large number of epidemiologic and clinical trials underway in OA collecting both plain radiographic and MRI data. Investigations that try to identify the most valid and responsive set of end points are ongoing for these studies. Before recommending the widespread use of one particular imaging construct in structure-modifying clinical trials it is essential that clinicians have this information and an established relationship with clinical end points, such as pain, function, and need for joint replacement.

REFERENCES

1. Altman R, Asch E, Bloch D, et al. Development of criteria for the classification and reporting of osteoarthritis. Arthritis Rheum 1986;29:1039-49.
2. Altman R, Alarcon D, Appelrouth D, et al. The American College of Rheumatology Subcommittee on Criteria for Osteoarthritis. The American College of Rheumatology criteria for the classification and reporting of osteoarthritis of the hip. Arthritis Rheum 1991;34:505-11.
3. Spector TD, Hart DJ, Byrne J, et al. Definition of osteoarthritis of the knee for epidemiological studies. Ann Rheum Dis. 1993;52:790-4.
4. Altman R, Hochberg M, Murphy W, et al. Atlas of individual radiographic features in osteoarthritis. Osteoarthritis Cartilage 1995;3(Suppl A):3-70.
5. Scott WW Jr, Lethbridge-Cejku M, Reichle R, et al. Reliability of grading scales for individual radiographic features of osteoarthritis of the knee. The Baltimore Longitudinal Study of Aging Atlas of Knee Osteoarthritis. Invest Radiol 1993;28: 497-501.
6. Kellgren JH, Lawrence JS. Radiographic assessment of osteoarthritis. Ann Rheum Dis 1957;16:494-502.
7. Mazzuca SA, Brandt KD. Is knee radiography useful for studying the efficacy of a disease-modifying osteoarthritis drug in humans? Rheum Dis Clin North Am 2003;29:819-30.
8. Mazzuca SA, Brandt KD, Buckwalter KA, et al. Pitfalls in the accurate measurement of joint space narrowing in semiflexed, anteroposterior radiographic imaging of the knee. Arthritis Rheum 2004;50:2508-15.
9. Hunter DJ, Zhang YQ, Tu X, et al. Change in joint space width: hyaline articular cartilage loss or alteration in meniscus? Arthritis Rheum 2006;54(8):2488-95.
10. Brandt KD, Mazzuca SA, Conrozier T, et al. Which is the best radiologic/radiographic protocol for a clinical trial of a structure-modifying drug in patients with knee osteoarthritis? Proceedings of January 17-18, 2002 workshop in Toussus-le-Noble, France. J Rheumatol 2002;29:1308-20.
11. Mazzuca SA, Brandt KD, Dieppe PA, et al. Effect of alignment of the medial tibial plateau and x-ray beam on apparent progression of osteoarthritis in the standing anteroposterior knee radiograph. Arthritis Rheum 2001;44:1786-94.
12. Buckland-Wright JC, Macfarlane DG, Williams SA, et al. Accuracy and precision of joint space width measurements in standard and macroradiographs of osteoarthritic knees. Ann Rheum Dis 1995;54:872-80.
13. Ahlback S. Osteoarthritis of the knee: a radiographic investigation. Acta Radiol 1968;277(Suppl):7-72.

14. Leach RE, Gregg T, Siber FJ. Weight bearing radiography in osteoarthritis of the knee. Radiology 1970;97:265–8.
15. Burnett S, Hart DJ, Cooper C, et al. A radiographic atlas of osteoarthritis. London: Springer-Verlag; 1994.
16. Mazzuca SA, Brandt KD, Katz BP. Is conventional radiography suitable for evaluation of a disease-modifying drug in patients with knee osteoarthritis? Osteoarthritis Cartilage 1997;5:217–26.
17. Mazzuca SA, Brandt KD, Buckwalter KA, et al. Knee pain reduces joint space width in conventional standing anteroposterior radiographs of osteoarthritic knees. Arthritis Rheum 2002;46:1223–7.
18. Messieh SS, Fowler PJ, Munro T. Anteroposterior radiographs of the osteoarthritic knee. J Bone Joint Surg Br 1990;72:639–40.
19. Hellio Le Graverand M-P, Brandt KD, Mazzuca SA, et al. Head-to-head comparison of the Lyon schuss and fixed flexion radiographic techniques: long-term reproducibility in normal knees and sensitivity to change in osteoarthritic knees. Ann Rheum Dis 2008;67:1562–6.
20. Mazzuca SA, Brandt KD, Buckland-Wright JC, et al. Field test of the reproducibility of automated measurements of medial tibiofemoral joint space width derived from standardized knee radiographs. J Rheumatol 1999;26:1359–65.
21. Piperno M, Hellio Le Graverand M-P, Conrozier T, et al. Quantitative evaluation of joint space width in femorotibial osteoarthritis: comparison of three radiographic views. Osteoarthritis Cartilage 1998;6:252–9.
22. Mazzuca SA, Hellio LeGraverand M-P, Vignon E, et al. Performance of a non-fluoroscopically assisted substitute for the Lyon schuss knee radiograph: quality and reproducibility of positioning and sensitivity to joint space narrowing in osteoarthritic knees. Osteoarthritis Cartilage 2008;16:1555–9.
23. Hellio Le Graverand M-P, Buck RJ, Wyman BT, et al. Change in regional cartilage morphology and joint space width in osteoarthritis participants versus healthy controls: a multicenter study using 3.0 Tesla MRI and Lyon schuss radiography. Ann Rheum Dis 2008 Dec 22 [Epub ahead of print].
24. Buckland-Wright JC, Wolfe F, Ward RJ, et al. Substantial superiority of semiflexed (MTP) views in knee osteoarthritis: a comparative radiographic study, without fluoroscopy, of standing extended, semiflexed (MTP), and schuss views. J Rheumatol 1999;26:2664–74.
25. Mazzuca SA, Brandt KD, Buckwalter KA, et al. Field test of the reproducibility of the semiflexed metatarsophalangeal (MTP) view in repeated radiographic examinations of subjects with osteoarthritis of the knee. Arthritis Rheum 2002;46:109–13.
26. Mazzuca SA, Brandt KD, Buckwalter KA. Longitudinal comparison of the metatarsophalangeal and semiflexed anteroposterior views: detection of radiographic joint space narrowing in osteoarthritic knees. Arthritis Rheum 2002;46(Suppl 9):S150.
27. Hellio Le Graverand MP, Mazzuca S, Lassere M, et al. Radiography Working Group of the OARSI-Omeract Imaging Workshop. Assessment of the radioanatomic positioning of the osteoarthritic knee in serial radiographs: comparison of three acquisition techniques. Osteoarthritis Cartilage 2006;14(Suppl):A37–43.
28. Peterfy C, Li J, Zaim S, et al. Comparison of fixed-flexion positioning with fluoroscopic semi-flexed positioning for quantifying radiographic joint-space width in the knee: test-retest reproducibility. Skeletal Radiol 2003;32:128–32.
29. Charles HC, Kraus VB, Ainslie M, et al. Optimization of the fixed-flexion radiograph. Osteoarthritis Cartilage 2007;15:1221–4.

30. Nevitt MC, Peterfy C, Guermazi A, et al. Longitudinal performance evaluation and validation of fixed-flexion radiography of the knee for detection of joint space loss. Arthritis Rheum. 2007;56(5):1512–20.
31. Sawitzke AD, Shi H, Finco MF, et al. The effect of glucosamine and/or chondroitin sulfate on the progression of knee osteoarthritis: a report from the glucosamine/chondroitin arthritis intervention trial. Arthritis Rheum. 2008; 58(10):3183–91.
32. Chondrometry LM. Quantitative evaluation of joint space width and rate of joint space loss in osteoarthritis of the hip. Rev Rhum Engl Ed 1995;62(3):155–8.
33. Ravaud P, Chastang C, Auleley GR, et al. Assessment of joint space width in patients with osteoarthritis of the knee: a comparison of 4 measuring instruments. J Rheumatol 1996;23(10):1749–55.
34. Laoussadi S, Menkes CJ. Mesure visuelle de l'interligne articulaire du genou et de la hanche a l'aide d'une loupe graduee. Rev Rhum Mal Osteoartic 1991;58: 678 [in French].
35. Vyborny CJ, Giger ML, Nishikawa RM. Computer-aided detection and diagnosis of breast cancer. Radiol Clin North Am 2000;38(4):725–40.
36. Dacre JE, Coppock JS, Herbert KE, et al. Development of a new radiographic scoring system using digital image analysis. Ann Rheum Dis 1989;48(3): 194–200.
37. Dacre JE, Huskisson EC. The automatic assessment of knee radiographs in osteoarthritis using digital image analysis. Br J Rheumatol 1989;28(6):506–10.
38. Conrozier T, Vignon E. Quantitative radiography in osteoarthritis: computerized measurement of radiographic knee and hip joint space. Baillieres Clin Rheumatol 1996;10(3):429–33.
39. Lynch JA, Buckland-Wright JC, Macfarlane DG. Precision of joint space width measurement in knee osteoarthritis from digital image analysis of high definition macroradiographs. Osteoarthritis Cartilage 1993;1(4):209–18.
40. Lynch JA. Textural and geometric measurement of changes in joint structure from high definition macroradiographs of osteoarthritic knees. London: University of London (UMDS); 1993.
41. Duryea J, Li J, Peterfy CG, et al. Trainable rule-based algorithm for the measurement of joint space width in digital radiographic images of the knee. Med Phys 2000;27(3):580–91.
42. Conrozier T, Favret H, Mathieu P, et al. Influence of the quality of tibial plateau alignment on the reproducibility of computer joint space measurement from Lyon schuss radiographic views of the knee in patients with knee osteoarthritis. Osteoarthritis Cartilage 2004;12(10):765–70.
43. Cootes TF, Taylor CJ. Anatomical statistical models and their role in feature extraction. Br J Radiol 2004;77(Spec No 2):S133–9.
44. Seise M, McKenna SJ, Ricketts IW, et al. Learning active shape models for bifurcating contours. IEEE Trans Med Imaging 2007;26(5):666–77.
45. Cootes TF, Taylor CJ, Cooper DH, et al. Active shape models: their training and application. Comput Vis Image Underst 1995;61(1):38–59.
46. Lacey T, Haslam J, et al. Automated radiographic measurements in the medial tibiofemoral compartment of the knee: intra-operator reproducibility. Proc ACR/ARHP Scientific Meeting, Boston, 6-11 November 2007. 1695, S665.
47. Osteoarthitis Initiative (OAI). Available at: http://www.oai.ucsf.edu/.
48. Marijnissen AC, Vincken KL, Vos PA, et al. Knee Images Digital Analysis (KIDA): a novel method to quantify individual radiographic features of knee osteoarthritis in detail. Osteoarthritis Cartilage 2008;16(2):234–43.

49. Conrozier T, Lequesne M, Favret H, et al. Measurement of the radiological hip joint space width: an evaluation of various methods of measurement. Osteoarthritis Cartilage 2001;9:281–6.

50. Vignon E. Radiographic issues in imaging the progression of hip and knee osteoarthritis. J Rheumatol Suppl 2004;70:36–44.

51. Bruyere O, Henrotin YE, Honore A, et al. Impact of the joint space width measurement method on the design of knee osteoarthritis studies. Aging Clin Exp Res 2003;15:136–41.

52. Duryea J, Zaim S, Genant HK. New radiographic-based surrogate outcome measures for osteoarthritis of the knee. Osteoarthritis Cart 2003;11:102–10.

53. Chu E, DiCarlo JC, Peterfy C, et al. Fixed-location joint space width measurement increases sensitivity to change in osteoarthritis. Osteoarthritis Cartilage 2007;15:S192.

54. Neuman G, Hunter D, Nevitt M, et al. Location specific radiographic joint space width for osteoarthritis progression. Osteoarthritis Cartilage 2009;17(6):761–5.

55. Wyman B, Buck R, Vignon E, et al. Comparison of one year change in minimum joint space width to fixed location joint space measurements in Lyon schuss X-rays from the A9001140 study. Osteoarthritis Cartilage 2008;16(Suppl 4):S164.

56. Lacey T, Brett A, Williams TG, et al. Comparison of x-ray and MRI in the determination of OA progression in the knee measured at a fixed-load-bearing position in the medical compartment. Osteoarthritis Cart 2008;16(Suppl 4):S176.

57. Duryea J, Hunter DJ, Nevitt MC, et al. Study of location specific lateral compartment radiographic joint space width for knee osteoarthritis progression: analysis of longitudinal data from the Osteoarthritis Initiative (OAI). Osteoarthritis Cartilage 2008;16:S168.

58. Merle-Vincent F, Vignon E, Brandt K, et al. Superiority of the Lyon-schuss view over the standing anteroposterior view for detecting joint space narrowing, especially in the lateral tibiofemoral compartment, in early knee osteoarthritis. Ann Rheum Dis 2007;66(6):747–55.

Usefulness of Ultrasound in Osteoarthritis

Helen I. Keen, MBBS, FRACP[a],
Philip G. Conaghan, MBBS, PhD, FRACP, FRCP[b],*

KEYWORDS

- Ultrasonography • Osteoarthritis • Synovitis
- Osteophytes • Cartilage

Osteoarthritis (OA) refers to a group of joint disorders with a variety of causes but common clinical and pathologic features. The disease is difficult to define succinctly due to its complex pathologic nature and heterogeneous clinical presentation. For OA epidemiologic studies, OA is usually defined according to radiographic changes. These changes can be graded according to existing criteria, which generally focus on the presence of joint space narrowing, osteophytes, subchondral bone sclerosis, subchondral bone cysts, and bone end deformity.[1] Radiographic features of OA do not correlate, however, with symptoms of OA at the individual patient level[2–6]; thus, the value of conventional radiography (CR) has limitations in the clinical setting. Additionally, the use of radiographs in the clinical trials setting has limitations.[7] For these reasons, novel imaging techniques are being tested and used as an adjuvant to CR in the investigation and management of OA in the clinical setting and in investigational studies. Ultrasonography is one of these techniques and is the focus of this review.

ULTRASONOGRAPHY IN PRACTICE

Ultrasonography of joints is well developed and has become part of mainstream practice thanks largely to the development of modern ultrasonographic technologies. For superficial joints, higher frequency probes are appropriate (>7.5 MHz) whereas deeper placed joints, such as the hip, may require the use of lower frequency probes. Modern

---

A version of this article originally appeared in the 47:4 issue of Radiologic Clinics of North America.
[a] School of Medicine and Pharmacology, University of Western Australia, Medical Research Foundation Building, Level 3, Rear 50 Murray Street, Perth, Western Australia 6000, Australia
[b] NIHR Leeds Musculoskeletal Biomedical Research Unit and Section of Musculoskeletal Diseases, Leeds Institute of Molecular Medicine, University of Leeds, Leeds, UK.
* Corresponding author. Section of Musculoskeletal Diseases, Chapel Allerton Hospital, Chapeltown Road, Leeds LS7 4SA, UK
E-mail address: p.conaghan@leeds.ac.uk (P.G. Conaghan).

Rheum Dis Clin N Am 35 (2009) 503–519
doi:10.1016/j.rdc.2009.09.002
0889-857X/09/$ – see front matter © 2009 Elsevier Inc. All rights reserved.

machines can use beam steering and compound imaging technologies to allow wider fields of view. Many machines also permit extended field-of-view scanning. Although a larger field of view offers no additional diagnostic information, it can make anatomic demonstration of the larger joints easier and offers advantages when trying to demonstrate findings on hard copy images to colleagues. Ultrasonography has limitations for assessing joint disease, particularly for the assessment of OA. Fundamental to this is the inability of ultrasonography to visualize the majority of the articular surface in most joints due to a limited sonographic window; in many joints it is not possible to usefully visualize the majority of articular cartilage lesions seen in OA. The second limitation is the inability of ultrasonography to demonstrate intrinsic bone abnormalities, such as marrow lesions, cysts, and sclerosis.

ULTRASONOGRAPHY OF SYNOVIAL JOINT PATHOLOGY

Synovial joints affected by OA display common pathologic features on imaging. Although anatomic differences exist with respect to the site of pathology or what can be visualized by ultrasonography due to the physical limitations of the modality, it is first worth considering the generic structures and pathology of the synovial joint that can be imaged in OA.

Definitions of synovial pathologies demonstrable by ultrasonography in OA of synovial joints are reviewed as is evidence regarding the validity of ultrasonography in assessing each of these pathologies. Although the definitions of ultrasonography-detectable pathology that are discussed occasionally require a lesion to be imaged in two planes, imaging in two planes should be considered in all examinations to minimize potential effects of artifact and confirm pathology (**Fig. 1**).

Synovium

Normal synovium is between only 1 and 3 cells thick; however, it becomes hypertrophied as a result of inflammation, allowing detection by current-generation ultrasonography technology.[8,9] An ultrasonography definition of synovial hypertrophy was developed by the Outcome Measures in Rheumatoid Arthritis Clinical Trials (OMERACT) ultrasonography task force (**Figs. 2** and **3** demostrate acqusition issues):

> "Abnormal hypoechoic (relative to subdermal fat, but sometimes may be isoechoic or hyperechoic) intraarticular tissue that is non displaceable and poorly compressible and which may exhibit Doppler signal."[10]

Although this definition was developed for application to rheumatoid arthritis (RA), it may be generalizable to other forms of arthritis, particularly given that OA and RA synovial inflammation largely differ quantitatively rather than qualitatively.[11,12]

Ultrasonography has been demonstrated to have criterion and construct validity in detecting synovial hypertrophy. The criterion validity of ultrasonography-detected grayscale synovial morphology has been demonstrated compared with direct visualization by arthroscopy.[8,9,13] Construct validity has been demonstrated against MRI at the knee, acromioclavicular joint, and small joints of the hands and feet.[14–21]

It has also been convincingly demonstrated that ultrasonography is better able to detect synovitis than clinical examination. This has been demonstrated in the knee and the small joints of the hands and feet using MRI as the comparator.[8,21–24] Of clinical relevance, ultrasonography is able to detect grayscale synovitis in joints thought to be clinically quiescent.[25–27] In addition to morphologic changes, synovial vascularity as detected by Doppler signal also has validity.[28–30] Intra-articular Doppler signal

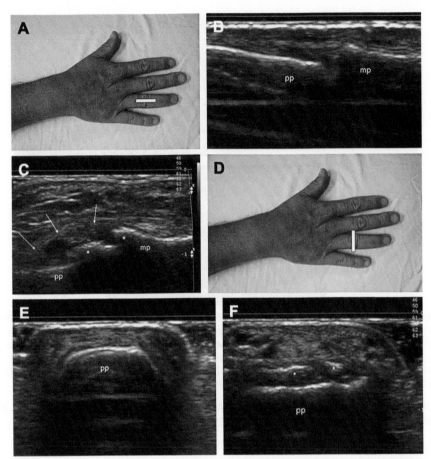

Fig. 1. Images of normal and osteoarthritic small joints of the hand with appearance of osteophytes in two planes. (*A*) Position of probe footprint, longitudinal. (*B*) Longitudinal ultrasonography image shows the cortical bone of the proximal (pp) and middle (mp) phalanx. (*C*) Longitudinal ultrasonography image demonstrates the cortical bone of the proximal (pp) and middle (mp) phalanx, with osteophyte (*) proximal and distal to the joint and synovial hypertrophy (arrows). (*D*) Position of probe footprint, transverse. (*E*) Transverse ultrasonography image shows the cortical bone of the proximal (pp) phalanx. (*F*) Transverse ultrasonography image demonstrates the cortical bone of the proximal (pp) phalanx, with osteophytes marked (*).

demonstrated in knee and hip joints has been shown to correlate with histologic vascularity and inflammatory infiltrates.[28–30]

Most of the validity data (discussed previously) are derived from the literature on inflammatory arthritis, with a paucity of information specific to the validity of ultrasonography in detecting synovitis in OA. It has been demonstrated, however, to correlate moderately with MRI and direct visualization by arthroscopy at the knee joint,[18,31] and again detect more synovial hypertrophy than clinical examination in OA knees and hands.[24,32] Additionally, Doppler signal in OA correlates with histologic evidence of vascularity in OA knees and hips.[29,30] When using Doppler imaging to assess synovial vascularity in any joint, it is important to realize that the vessels detected in synovium are compressible and the lightest transducer pressure possible must be used to avoid

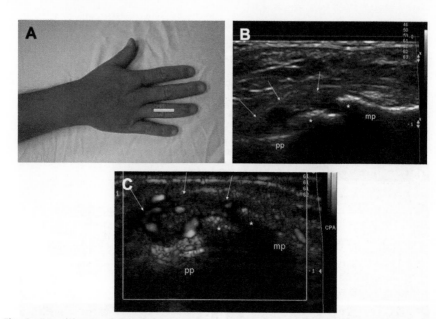

Fig. 2. Dorsal longitudinal ultrasonography images of the proximal interphalangeal (PIP) joint. (*A*) Position of probe footprint. (*B*) Grayscale ultrasonography image of an osteoarthritic PIP joint demonstrates the proximal phalanx (pp) and middle phalanx (mp) with associated synovial hypertrophy (*arrows*) and osteophytes (*). (*C*) Power Doppler image of the same osteoarthritic PIP joint demonstrates the vascularity within the region of synovial hypertrophy (*arrows*) as indicated by the flash of color.

obliterating any evidence of vascular flow. A gel standoff or water bath can be used but generally liberal use of acoustic jelly is sufficient to avoid excess transducer pressure.

Synovial Fluid

Fluid collections within the joint are readily detected by ultrasonography. The OMER-ACT ultrasonography task force defines synovial fluid (see **Fig. 3**) as

Abnormal hypoechoic or anechoic (relative to subdermal fat, but sometimes may be isoechoic or hyperechoic) intra-articular material that is displaceable and compressible, but does not exhibit Doppler signal.[10]

Few studies have focused on the validity of ultrasonography in detecting synovial fluid in isolation from synovial hypertrophy; they are often considered together in published studies. Studies have demonstrated, however, that ultrasonography-detected hypoechoic collections can be demonstrated to be synovial fluid on aspiration.[33,34] Additionally, ultrasonography-detected synovial fluid has been validated against MRI in the small joints of the hands and wrists[35] and ankles, although more fluid was required to detect effusions by ultrasonography than MRI.[36] This may in part account be due to the ability of fluid to pool in sonographically inaccessible recesses within the joint. One way to improve visualization of subtle effusions is to ensure the joint is moved into different positions as it is examined, which may move any fluid to areas where it can be visualized.

A further problem can be distinguishing joint fluid from synovium, which is of low reflectivity itself. Clues are that Doppler signal may be detected in synovium but not effusion and that the fluid appears compressible because it can be displaced into other areas of the joint in contrast to synovium. This is why the compressibility and absence

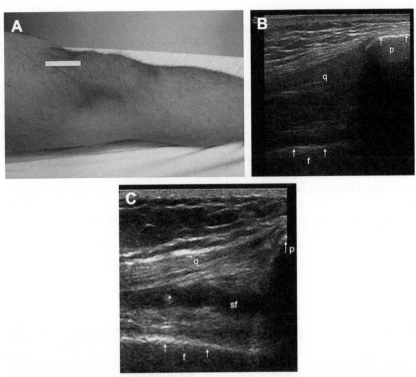

Fig. 3. Sagittal ultrasonography image of the suprapatellar pouch. (*A*) Position of probe footprint. (*B*) Longitudinal ultrasonography appearance of a normal knee demonstrates the cortical (*arrows*) bone of the patella (p) and distal femur (f) and quadriceps tendon. (*C*) Longitudinal ultrasonography image of an osteoarthritic knee shows hypoechoic collection of synovial fluid in the supra patellar sac (sf) and villous synovial hypertrophy extending into the fluid collection (*).

of Doppler signal are important elements of the definition of an effusion (discussed previously). In deep joints, such as the hip, where Doppler signal may be difficult to detect and compression is not possible, it can be difficult to make the distinction. In cases where this is critical, such as the need to exclude infection, attempted joint aspiration may be required. Ultrasonography is better able to detect effusions than clinical examination, although most of this evidence arises from studies of the knee joint.[8,24,37–42]

Bone Cortex

The highly echogenic cortical bone surface is readily demonstrated with ultrasonography even though the internal structure of the bone is not seen. Normally it appears as a continuous smooth bright line allowing easy visualization of any abnormalities,[43] such as erosions,[44,45] irregularities,[45,46] osteophytes,[43,45,47–49] and enthesophytes.[50] Little is known, however, about the validity of ultrasonography-detected cortical changes in OA, and most of the evidence relates to pathologic and structures changes seen in inflammatory arthritis.

Osteophytes are one of the cardinal features of OA and are commonly described in the ultrasonography OA literature.[43,45,47–49] There are no published consensus statements regarding ultrasound definitions, however. This is perhaps because osteophytes are so frequently recognized on ultrasonography and their appearances are not considered as controversial as other features of arthropathy. Recently used definitions include "A single or multiple characteristic irregularities of the bone profile, located at the edges of the joint surfaces"[43] and "cortical protrusions seen in 2 planes" (see **Figs. 1** and **2; Fig. 4**).[51]

There is also little evidence of the validity of ultrasonography in detecting osteophytes. Given the sensitivity and specificity of ultrasonography in detecting cortical erosions in RA, it is likely to have a similar ability to detect osteophytes. In a recently published study looking at small joint OA in the hand, ultrasonography detected more osteophytes than CR.[52] This is most likely a reflection of the multiplanar imaging capability of ultrasonography and, in particular, its ability to image joints in the dorsal longitudinal plane, which is not routinely done with CR.

Erosions are the most commonly studied ultrasonography-detected cortical abnormality in the rheumatologic ultrasonography literature. Although they are a feature of a subtype of hand OA and MRI studies suggest that they may be seen more frequently in OA than CR suggests,[53] they are much less commonly appreciated than in RA. The OMERACT ultrasonography task force published a definition of rheumatoid erosions: "An intra-articular discontinuity of the bone surface that is visible in 2 perpendicular planes."[10]

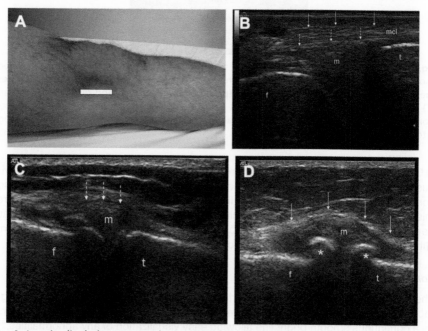

Fig. 4. Longitudinal ultrasonography images of the medial joint line. (*A*) Position of probe footprint. (*B*) Ultrasonography image of a normal knee shows distal femur (f), proximal tibia (t), triangular outline of the medial meniscus (m) (*dashed arrows*) and the linear echoes produced by the medial collateral ligament (mcl) (*solid arrows*). (*C*) Ultrasonography image shows medial meniscal extrusion (m) (*dashed arrows*). (*D*) Ultrasonography image in knee OA demonstrates medial meniscal extrusion (m) with resulting displacement of the medial collateral ligament (*arrows*) and obvious osteophytes (*) proximal and distal to the joint line.

The ability of ultrasonography to detect RA erosions has been validated against CR, CT, and MRI, largely focusing on the small joints of the hands and feet but also in the wrists, knees, and shoulder joints.[17,21,22,54–56] In RA, ultrasonography can detect small erosions earlier in the disease process than CR.[21,54,56] This may have implications for studying cortical changes in OA before development of radiographic evidence of disease. The only study to examine the validity of ultrasonography in detecting erosions in OA of the small joints of the hand found ultrasonography to be inferior to CR.[44] This is in contrast to the findings in RA and is likely related to the different pathologic processes involved in the two diseases. The presence of osteophyte formation at the joint margins may shield erosions from view[42] as they can hide other periarticular features normally well visualized. Additionally, although RA erosions are characteristically juxta-articular, the location of erosions in OA is classically recognized as central, and the central area of the joint is poorly visualized using ultrasonography.

Other cortical abnormalities in OA that have been described as detectable by ultrasonography, such as cortical irregularity and enthesophytes, are not well reported in the literature.[45,46,50] Two studies have addressed the sensitivity of ultrasonography in diagnosing OA based on features including cortical irregularity compared with CT and MRI. In these studies, although ultrasonography was sensitive to the detection of OA, the use of bone remodeling as a diagnostic tool had poor specificity.[19,57]

Cartilage

Hyaline cartilage is readily identified on ultrasonography provided that an acoustic window is available. In some joints, particular maneuvers can be made to improve the area of articular cartilage visualized. For instance, a larger proportion of the femoral trochlear cartilage can be identified with the knee maximally flexed, and plantar flexion of the ankle exposes more of the cartilage over the talus for examination. Flexion of the small joints of fingers, including the metacarpophalangeal joints, allows a more extensive assessment of the cartilage over proximal joint surface.

Normal hyaline cartilage appears as a homogenous low reflective layer closely paralleling the subchondral bone (**Fig. 5**). Abnormalities described in OA seen on ultrasonography include[43,47,58]

- Loss of the sharpness of the cartilage margins
- Heterogeneity
- Irregularities in thickness

In vitro models have demonstrated reliability of ultrasonography in detecting cartilage thickness[59,60] compared with histologic examination. Additionally, ultrasonography compares reasonably to MRI in detecting femoral condylar cartilage thickness in in vivo studies.[18,31,61] The clinical relevance of noninvasive ultrasonography-detected cartilage changes is uncertain. Generally, only peripheral, non–load-bearing regions of cartilage can be visualized using noninvasive B-mode ultrasonography.

Tendons and Ligaments

The ultrasound appearances of tendons and ligaments are well described.[62] Ultrasonography-detected ligamentous abnormalities have been described in arthritis[63] and tendon tears resulting from attrition of the tendon on osteophyte or bony irregularity may be associated with OA and identified by ultrasonography.[64] Perhaps of most relevance to OA is inflammation of the tendon or ligament enthesis (enthesitis). Although

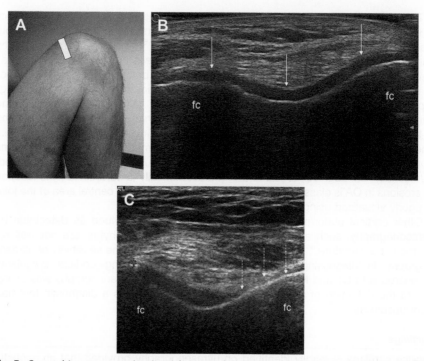

Fig. 5. Coronal images over the distal femur in full flexion. (*A*) Position of probe footprint. (*B*) Ultrasonography image demonstrates a smooth regular homogenous band of cartilage (*arrows*) overlying the distal femoral condyles (fc). (*C*) Ultrasonography image shows pathologic cartilage band, irregular thickness, increased echogenicity, and loss of clarity of the cartilage margins (*dashed arrows*).

not specifically for OA, enthesitis has been defined by the OMERACT ultrasonography task force as:

> Abnormally hypoechoic (loss of normal fibrillar architecture) and/or thickened tendon or ligament at it's bony attachment (may occasionally contain hyperechoic foci consistent with calcification), seen in 2 perpendicular planes that may exhibit Doppler signal and/or bony changes including enthesophytes, erosions, or irregularity.[10]

There is a paucity of published information about the validity of ultrasonography in detecting enthesitis, with little investigation in OA specifically, although ultrasonography has been demonstrated to detect more sites of entheseal disease in OA than CR in the foot[65] and more than CR or clinical examination at the shoulder.[46]

IMAGING SPECIFIC JOINTS

Guidelines for the acquisition of ultrasonography images of synovial joints for rheumatology have been published by the European League Against Rheumatism ultrasonography task force[66] and are reviewed according to joint, along with changes commonly detected in OA by ultrasonography and, where available, the relative frequency of the changes.

Shoulder

The capabilities of ultrasonography in the diagnosis of shoulder pathology and, specifically, rotator cuff disease are well recognized, and the various positions for examining the shoulder, along with appropriate dynamic maneuvers, are well described.[67] A comprehensive examination includes examination of the glenohumeral joint from its posterior aspect and from the axilla.[66] As the shoulder joint is considered to include the acromioclavicular joint and the sternoclavicular joint, these can also be imaged.

OA of the glenohumeral joint is often a result of longstanding rotator cuff pathology, in particular tears that allow superior migration of the humeral head and subsequent contact with the inferior surface of the acromion. The ultrasonography appearance of these changes includes thinning and tears of the rotator cuff, irregularity of the bony cortex of the humeral head, particularly superiorly, and inferior osteophytes.[64] There may also be fluid within the subacromial bursa or glenohumeral joint.[64] The glenoid labrum can be appreciated as a homogenous, but slightly hyperechoic, appearance, akin to the menisci of the knee. Due to the normal anatomic structure of the labrum, identifying different portions of the labrum requires specific positioning maneuvers and the use of probes of varying frequencies. The posterior labrum is most superficial and most easily visualized, and identification is further aided by the presence of a glenohumeral joint effusion. Pathology, such as tears, can be visualized by ultrasonography, although superior lesions are difficult to appreciate with ultrasonography due to acoustic shadowing by the acromion.[64]

OA of the acromioclavicular joint appears as narrowing of the joint space between the acromion and the clavicle, irregularity and bony prominence of the juxta-articular cortical bones, including osteophyte formation, and synovial hypertrophy with low levels of Doppler signal within the joint capsule (**Fig. 6**). Inferior osteophytes on the

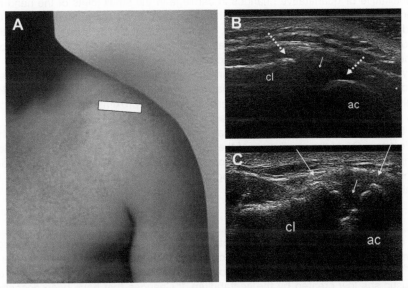

Fig. 6. Longitudinal image of the acromioclavicular joint. (*A*) Position of probe footprint. (*B*) Ultrasonography image shows normal acromioclavicular joint. There is a smooth uniform appearance of the cortical bone (*dashed arrows*) at the joint line (*small arrow*). (*C*) Ultrasonography image shows osteoarthritic acromioclavicular joint. There are raised cortical bone (*arrows*) and irregularities surrounding the joint line (*small arrow*). Clavicle (cl), acromion (ac).

acromioclavicular joint can cause trauma to the supraspinatus tendon and, although these are not seen at ultrasonography, the tendon damage may be visible.[64]

Imaging of the sternoclavicular joint is a common request for investigating the cause of a localized mass over this joint. OA is common at this joint, particularly in middle-aged women, characterized by joint space narrowing, cortical osteophytosis, and cysts.[64]

Hand

The palmar and dorsal surfaces of the hand and wrist joints should be imaged in longitudinal and transverse planes, and medial and lateral longitudinal views of the small joints should also be obtained. In OA, most of the pathology is seen over the small joints of the hand and base of thumb rather than the thenar and hypothenar eminences.

The most commonly affected regions (as detected by ultrasonography) in OA of the small joints of the hand are the base of thumb and distal and proximal interphalangeal joints (as would be expected from epidemiologic studies of the distribution of hand OA).[52] Involvement of metacarpophalangeal joints may be more common than appreciated, however, by assessing CR images of OA.[52]

Ultrasonography-detected osteophytes are commonly seen on the dorsal aspect of the hand, in the midline protruding along the longitudinal plane of the phalanx (see **Fig. 2**).[52] This is not well appreciated on CR as the standard dorsiplanar and dorsiplanar oblique planes do not allow imaging of this region. Erosive changes in OA of the small joints of the hand have been described with ultrasonography; however, as discussed previously, the only study assessing the validity of ultrasonography-detected erosions in OA of the small joints of the hand found ultrasonography inferior to CR.[44]

Qualitative or quantitative changes in cartilage in the small joints of the hand are often appreciated with ultrasonography. The prevalence of osteophytes in OA producing acoustic shadows, however, can hamper this and accurate quantification is not possible. A surrogate of joint space loss was examined with ultrasonography in the small joints of the hand and found problematic.[52]

Synovial hypertrophy and fluid is commonly seen in association with osteophytes in hand OA (see **Fig. 2**), with Doppler signal less often appreciated and generally in low levels.[32] Occasionally, florid Doppler signal in a distal or proximal interphalangeal joint may mimic a more inflammatory process, such as psoriatic arthritis.

It has recently been hypothesized that ligamentous pathology may have a pathogenic role in OA of the small joints of the hand,[68] and although the collateral ligament complexes can be visualized on ultrasonography, the reliability and the clinical and pathologic significance of ultrasonography detected changes is yet to be established.

Hip

The deep anatomic location and physical structure of the hip joint means that clinical examination is not reliably able to detect synovial pathology or the bone changes of OA.[66] Similarly, visualization by ultrasonography is limited, particularly due to the acoustic shadow created by the acetabulum.[64] Changes that have been described in OA of the hip include synovial hypertrophy or effusion causing distension of the hip joint capsule, osteophytes (most commonly arising from the anterior inferior margin of the femoral head), and flattening of the profile of the normal curved, visible portion of the femoral head.[48,64] Just deep to the joint capsule, where the capsule inserts into the acetabulum, the labrum can be visualized as a homogenous hyperechoic structure. Pathology, such as labral tears, can be detected with ultrasonography, and cystic, mucoid degeneration of labral fissures can be appreciated as circumscribed, hypoechoic lesions with a lobulated appearance that are not easily compressible.[64]

Knee

At the knee joint, the typical features of synovial hypertrophy, effusion, osteophytes, and cartilage thinning have been described. In addition, meniscal extrusion and tears may be visualized, with associated displacement of the collateral ligaments.

Recommendations for acquisition of images of the knee joint have been described by the European League Against Rheumatism.[66] It is recommended that the knee initially be imaged with patients supine in the neutral or slightly flexed position (30°) for lateral and anterior images, then in the prone position for posterior images. Slight flexion with quadriceps contraction aids visualization of the suprapatella pouch (SPP), and maximal flexion aids visualization of the trochlear cartilage. The standard scans should include imaging in the transverse and longitudinal planes of the suprapatella region, infrapatella region, and posterior knee (medial and lateral). Additionally, the knee should be imaged longitudinally over the medial and lateral aspects of the joint.[66]

In OA, synovial hypertrophy in the SPP can be readily visualized as flattened thickened synovium or with frond-like protrusions into the pouch.[8] Ultrasonography-detected synovial hypertrophy is common in knee OA but the prevalence ranges depending on the definition used and study population examined (see **Fig. 3**). Synovial fluid is easily detected in the SPP, especially with the aid of dynamic maneuvers and can aid visualization of synovial hypertrophy through transmitting sound to the underlying sac wall (see **Fig. 3**). In addition to imaging the SPP in the midline, it is important to image the lateral and medial recesses as these may be the only sites of synovial hypertrophy or effusion.[69,70] Synovial hypertrophy and small amounts of fluid can also be found in the lateral and medial longitudinal planes surrounding the medial and lateral joint lines. Enthesophytes extending into the quadriceps and patella tendons can also be identified by ultrasonography.

Imaging of the popliteal fossa can allow identification of popliteal cysts associated with OA. These appear as a hypoechoic or anechoic mass arising between the semimembranosus and medial head of gastrocnemius tendons.[64] They may have a heterogeneous echoic appearance as they can be filled with debris from the communication knee joint.[64] Leakage of fluid from the cyst is characterized by fluid within the surrounding tissue and a beaked appearance of the cyst distally. Complete rupture and emptying of the cyst may be indicated only by the detection of residual fluid between the heads of the semimembranosus tendon and medial gastrocnemius.[64]

Cartilage pathology can be appreciated in the trochlea of the distal femur, with the knee in full flexion (see **Fig. 5**).[64] Changes, such as thinning, heterogeneity, and loss of clarity (described previously), can be seen. The changes, in particular thinning, are generally more pronounced in OA than in inflammatory arthritis.[64] As discussed previously, however, the clinical significance of these ultrasonography-detected changes in the hyaline cartilage of the knee are uncertain. The peripheral superficial aspects of menisci can also be visualized with ultrasonography, allowing some meniscal pathology, such as cysts, extrusion, or horizontal tears, to be visualized.[63,64] Meniscal extrusion is a significant component of the joint space narrowing as seen radiographically in knee OA and has been demonstrated to be associated with ultrasonography-detectable displacement of the medial collateral ligament and some pain parameters in knee OA (see **Fig. 4**).[63]

Ultrasonography-detected osteophytes are a common feature of knee OA, commonly seen around the medial and lateral joint line, originating from the distal femur or proximal tibia (see **Fig. 4**). The other relatively common place to detect osteophytes by ultrasonography is over the distal femoral condyles with the knee fully flexed to distally displace the patella. Enthesophytes can be seen protruding from the patella into the quadriceps or patella tendons.

Ankle

Due to the anatomy of the ankle joint, imaging of the joint cavity is limited by ultrasonography.[64] Dynamic imaging of the ankle joint while a patient dorsi- and plantarflexes the foot aids detection of pathology.[64] Synovial hypertrophy and fluid in OA can be detected anteriorly assuming the pathology is of sufficient severity.[36] Large effusions displace the anterior capsular fat pad inferiorly, aiding diagnosis.[36] Large effusions can also be visualized posteriorly and may be seen to surround the flexor hallucis tendon as the tendon sheath communicates with the ankle joint in the majority of cases.

The chondral surface of the talus can be visualized by plantar flexing the ankle joint,[64] allowing cartilage pathology to be identified. Osteophytes are most commonly seen extending from the distal tibia or talus and can result in anterior impingement of the ankle.[64] Osteophytes may also result in tendon impingement about the ankle.

Forefoot

OA in the forefoot is most commonly found in the first metatarsophalangeal joint (**Fig. 7**).[64] Again, typical ultrasound findings include cortical irregularity (including

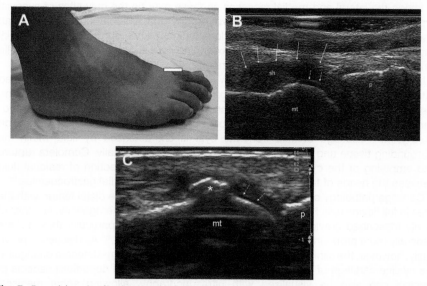

Fig. 7. Dorsal longitudinal images of the first metatarsophalangeal joint. (*A*) Position of probe footprint. (*B*) Ultrasonography image shows metatarsal (mt) and proximal phalanx (p) joint with associated synovial hypertrophy (sh) considered to be within normal range (*solid arrows*). The metatarsal articular cartilage is indicated by the small dashed arrows. (*C*) Ultrasonography image shows osteoarthritic metatarsophalangeal joint with osteophyte (*) and cartilage thinning (*dashed arrows*).

osteophytes), synovial hypertrophy, and effusion (although a small amount of fluid or synovial hypertrophy is considered within the normal range in this load-bearing joint).[64] Cartilage changes can also be appreciated in the first metatarsophalangeal joint, although as with other joints, the reliability and significance of changes are not yet established.

FUTURE RESEARCH ENDEAVORS

Ultrasonography offers several advantages in the assessment of OA in clinical practice. As an adjuvant to conventional methods of assessing joints, it allows sensitive and specific identification of soft tissue and bone changes (including vascularity). In contrast to radiographs, it does not require ionizing radiation, can image the joint in multiple planes, and allows dynamic assessment of moving structures.[71] In the hands of a clinician skilled in image acquisition and interpretation, ultrasonography can be performed in the clinical setting, becoming part of the clinical assessment.[71] This, in addition to its relative patient friendliness and low cost compared with CT and MRI, makes it a useful clinical tool.[71] Acquisition of ultrasonography skills takes time, practice, and ongoing maintenance of competency, however.[71] Additionally, it can be time consuming to perform in the clinical setting. The quality of the images obtained and the interpretation of the images depends on the skills and experience of a technician.[71] Visualization of certain structures is limited by the intrinsic properties of the technique and current technology (discussed later). Another consideration is that ultrasonography should be used as an adjuvant to routine clinical assessment and investigations to aid the diagnosis and management of disease rather than as a stand-alone diagnostic test.[71] Although there is a great deal of published data regarding the validity of ultrasonography in inflammatory arthritis,[72,73] the validity of ultrasonography OA requires further work, with particular focus on the pathology that can be detected.[74] In particular, areas needing refinement and confirmation include definitions of pathology in OA, assessment of the criterion and construct validity of these definitions, and development of standardized, universally applicable scoring systems with good reliability and demonstrable sensitivity to change. The benefits of ultrasonography over other CR include the ability to image soft tissue structures and the potential to detect small or early structural lesions. Hence, these types of pathology should be the focus of investigation by ultrasonography; perhaps there will be a role for studying preradiographic OA.

The significance of ultrasonography-detected pathology in OA needs further investigation. Given the discordance between radiographic structural changes and symptoms in OA,[2–6] the clinical importance of ultrasonography-detected structural changes, with regards to symptoms, prognosis, outcome, and response, to therapy needs investigation. If ultrasonography-detected structural changes bear no relationship to any of these domains, then the utility of ultrasonography in OA is likely to be limited. In reality, such endeavors will likely increase utility of ultrasonography in the clinical setting and in the clinical trial setting of OA.

REFERENCES

1. Zhang Y, Jordan JM. Epidemiology of osteoarthritis. Rheum Dis Clin North Am 2008;34(3):515–29.
2. Hart D, Spector T, Egger P, et al. Defining osteoarthritis of the hand for epidemiological studies: the Chingford study. Ann Rheum Dis 1994;53(4):220–3.
3. Spector TD, Hart DJ, Byrne J, et al. Definition of osteoarthritis of the knee for epidemiological studies. Ann Rheum Dis 1993;52(11):790–4.

4. Felson DT, Naimark A, Anderson J, et al. The prevalence of knee osteoarthritis in the elderly. The Framingham Osteoarthritis Study. Arthritis Rheum 1987;30(8): 914–8.

5. Felson DT. An update on the pathogenesis and epidemiology of osteoarthritis. Radiol Clin North Am 2004;42(1):1–9.

6. Sonne-Holm S, Jacobsen S. Osteoarthritis of the first carpometacarpal joint: a study of radiology and clinical epidemiology. Results from the Copenhagen Osteoarthritis Study. Osteoarthritis Cartilage 2006;14(5):496–500.

7. Guermazi A, Eckstein F, Hellio Le Graverand-Gastineau MP, et al. Osteoarthritis: current role of imaging. Med Clin North Am 2009;93(1):101–26.

8. Karim Z, Wakefield R, Quinn M, et al. Validation and reproducibility of ultrasonography in the detection of synovitis in the knee: a comparison with arthroscopy and clinical examination. Arthritis Rheum 2004;50(2):387–94.

9. Fiocco U, Cozzi L, Rubaltelli L, et al. Long-term sonographic follow-up of rheumatoid and psoriatic proliferative knee joint synovitis. Br J Rheumatol 1996;35(2):155–63.

10. Wakefield RJ, Balint PV, Szkudlarek M, et al. Musculoskeletal ultrasound including definitions for ultrasonographic pathology [erratum appears in J Rheumatol 2006 Feb;33(2):440 Note: Bruyn, George [corrected to Bruyn, George AW]]. J Rheumatol 2005;32(12):2485–7.

11. Haraoui B, Pelletier JP, Cloutier JM, et al. Synovial membrane histology and immunopathology in rheumatoid arthritis and osteoarthritis. In vivo effects of anti-rheumatic drugs. Arthritis Rheum 1991;34(2):153–63.

12. Peter JB, Pearson CM, Marmor L. Erosive osteoarthritis of the hands. Arthritis Rheum 1966;9(3):365–88.

13. Rubaltelli L, Fiocco U, Cozzi L, et al. Prospective sonographic and arthroscopic evaluation of proliferative knee joint synovitis. J Ultrasound Med 1994;13(11):855–62.

14. Scheel A. A novel ultrasonographic synovitis scoring system suitable for analyzing finger joint inflammation in rheumatoid arthritis. Arthritis Rheum 2005; 52(3):733–43.

15. Backhaus M, Kamradt T, Sandrock D, et al. Arthritis of the finger joints: a comprehensive approach comparing conventional radiography, scintigraphy, ultrasound, and contrast-enhanced magnetic resonance imaging. Arthritis Rheum 1999;42(6):1232–45.

16. Beckers C, Jeukens X, Ribbens C, et al. (18)F-FDG PET imaging of rheumatoid knee synovitis correlates with dynamic magnetic resonance and sonographic assessments as well as with the serum level of metalloproteinase-3. Eur J Nucl Med Mol Imaging 2006;33(3):275–80, Epub 2005 Oct 25.

17. Scheel AK, Schmidt WA, Hermann KG, et al. Interobserver reliability of rheumatologists performing musculoskeletal ultrasonography: results from a EULAR "Train the trainers" course. Ann Rheum Dis 2005;64(7):1043–9.

18. Tarhan S, Unlu Z. Magnetic resonance imaging and ultrasonographic evaluation of the patients with knee osteoarthritis: a comparative study. Clin Rheumatol 2003;22(3):181–8.

19. Alasaarela E, Tervonen O, Takalo R, et al. Ultrasound evaluation of the acromioclavicular joint. J Rheumatol 1997;24(10):1959–63.

20. Eich G, Halle F, Hodler J, et al. Juvenile chronic arthritis: imaging of the knees and hips before and after intraarticular steroid injection. Pediatr Radiol 1994;24(8):558–63.

21. Szkudlarek M, Narvestad E, Klarlund M, et al. Ultrasonography of the metatarsophalangeal joints in rheumatoid arthritis: comparison with magnetic resonance imaging, conventional radiography, and clinical examination. Arthritis Rheum 2004;50(7):2103–12.

22. Szkudlarek M. Ultrasonography of the metacarpophalangeal and proximal inter-phalangeal joints in rheumatoid arthritis: a comparison with magnetic resonance imaging, conventional radiography and clinical examination. Arthritis Res Ther 2006;8(2):R52, Epub 2006 Mar 6.
23. Cellerini M, Salti S, Trapani S, et al. Correlation between clinical and ultrasound assessment of the knee in children with mono-articular or pauci-articular juvenile rheumatoid arthritis. Pediatr Radiol 1999;29(2):117–23.
24. D'Agostino MA, Conaghan P, Le Bars M, et al. EULAR report on the use of ultra-sonography in painful knee osteoarthritis. Part 1: prevalence of inflammation in osteoarthritis. Ann Rheum Dis 2005;64(12):1703–9, Epub 2005 May 5.
25. Hau M, Schultz H, Tony HP, et al. Evaluation of pannus and vascularization of the metacarpophalangeal and proximal interphalangeal joints in rheumatoid arthritis by high-resolution ultrasound (multidimensional linear array). Arthritis Rheum 1999;42(11):2303–8.
26. Bajaj S, Lopez-Ben R, Oster R, et al. Ultrasound detects rapid progression of erosive disease in early rheumatoid arthritis: a prospective longitudinal study. Skeletal Radiol 2007;36(2):123–8, Epub 2006 Oct 11.
27. Wakefield RJ, Green MJ, Marzo-Ortega H, et al. Should oligoarthritis be reclassi-fied? Ultrasound reveals a high prevalence of subclinical disease [see comment]. Ann Rheum Dis 2004;63(4):382–5.
28. Schmidt WA, Volker L, Zacher J, et al. Colour Doppler ultrasonography to detect pannus in knee joint synovitis. Clin Exp Rheumatol 2000;18(4):439–44.
29. Walther M, Harms H, Krenn V, et al. Synovial tissue of the hip at power Doppler US: correlation between vascularity and power Doppler US signal. Radiology 2002;225(1):225–31.
30. Walther M, Harms H, Krenn V, et al. Correlation of power Doppler sonography with vascularity of the synovial tissue of the knee joint in patients with osteoarthritis and rheumatoid arthritis. Arthritis Rheum 2001;44(2):331–8.
31. Ostergaard M, Court-Payen M, Gideon P, et al. Ultrasonography in arthritis of the knee. A comparison with MR imaging. Acta Radiol 1995;36(1):19–26.
32. Keen HI, Wakefield RJ, Grainger AJ, et al. An ultrasonographic study of osteoar-thritis of the hand: synovitis and its relationship to structural pathology and symp-toms. Arthritis Rheum 2008; 59(12):1756–63.
33. Iagnocco A, Coari G. Usefulness of high resolution US in the evaluation of effu-sion in osteoarthritic first carpometacarpal joint. Scand J Rheumatol 2000; 29(3):170–3.
34. Balint PV, Kane D, Hunter J, et al. Ultrasound guided versus conventional joint and soft tissue fluid aspiration in rheumatology practice: a pilot study. J Rheuma-tol 2002;29(10):2209–13.
35. Hoving J, Buchbinder R, Hall S, et al. A comparison of magnetic resonance imaging, sonography, and radiography of the hand in patients with early rheuma-toid arthritis. J Rheumatol 2004;31(4):663–75.
36. Jacobson JA, Andresen R, Jaovisidha S, et al. Detection of ankle effusions: comparison study in cadavers using radiography, sonography, and MR imaging. AJR Am J Roentgenol 1998;170(5):1231–8.
37. van Holsbeeck M, van Holsbeeck K, Gevers G, et al. Staging and follow-up of rheumatoid arthritis of the knee. Comparison of sonography, thermography, and clinical assessment. J Ultrasound Med 1988;7(10):561–6.
38. Kane D. Ultrasonography is superior to clinical examination in the detection and localization of knee joint effusion in rheumatoid arthritis. J Rheumatol 2003;30(5): 966–71.

39. Toolanen G, Lorentzon R, Friberg S, et al. Sonography of popliteal masses. Acta Orthop Scand 1988;59(3):294–6.
40. Fam AG, Wilson SR, Holmberg S. Ultrasound evaluation of popliteal cysts on osteoarthritis of the knee. J Rheumatol 1982;9(3):428–34.
41. Andonopoulos A, Yarmenitis S, Sfountouris H, et al. Baker's cyst in rheumatoid arthritis: an ultrasonographic study with a high resolution technique. Clin Exp Rheumatol 1995;13(5):633–6.
42. Gompels B, Darlington L. Evaluation of popliteal cysts and painful calves with ultrasonography: comparison with arthrography. Ann Rheum Dis 1982;41(4): 355–9.
43. Delle Sedie A, Riente L, Bombardieri S. Limits and perspectives of ultrasound in the diagnosis and management of rheumatic diseases. Mod Rheumatol 2008;18: 125–31.
44. Iagnocco A, Filippucci E, Ossandon A, et al. High resolution ultrasonography in detection of bone erosions in patients with hand osteoarthritis. J Rheumatol 2005; 32(12):2381–3.
45. Grassi W. Sonographic imaging of the distal phalanx. Semin Arthritis Rheum 2000;29(6):379–84.
46. Falsetti P, Frediani B, Filippou G, et al. Enthesitis of proximal insertion of the deltoid in the course of seronegative spondyloarthritis. An atypical enthesitis that can mime impingement syndrome. Scand J Rheumatol 2002;31(3):158–62.
47. Grassi W, Filippucci E, Farina A. Ultrasonography in osteoarthritis. Semin Arthritis Rheum 2005;34(6 Suppl 2):19–23.
48. Qvistgaard E, Torp-Pedersen S, Christensen R, et al. Reproducibility and inter-reader agreement of a scoring system for ultrasound evaluation of hip osteoarthritis. Ann Rheum Dis 2006;65(12):1613–9.
49. Robinson P, Keenan AM, Conaghan PG. Clinical effectiveness and dose response of image-guided intra-articular corticosteroid injection for hip osteoarthritis. Rheumatology (Oxford) 2007;46(2):285–91.
50. Frediani B, Falsetti P, Storri L, et al. Ultrasound and clinical evaluation of quadricipital tendon enthesitis in patients with psoriatic arthritis and rheumatoid arthritis. Clin Rheumatol 2002;21(4):294–8.
51. Keen HI, Lavie F, Wakefield RJ, et al. The development of a preliminary ultrasonographic scoring system for features of hand osteoarthritis. Ann Rheum Dis 2008;67(5):651–5.
52. Keen HI, Wakefield RJ, Grainger A, et al. Can ultrasonography improve on radiographic assessment in osteoarthritis of the hands? A comparison between radiographic and ultrasonographic detected pathology. Ann Rheum Dis 2008;67(8): 1116–20.
53. Grainger AJ, Farrant JM, O'connor PJ, et al. MR imaging of erosions in interphalangeal joint osteoarthritis: is all osteoarthritis erosive? Skeletal Radiol 2007;36(8): 737–45.
54. Wakefield R, Gibbon W, Conaghan P, et al. The value of sonography in the detection of bone erosions in patients with rheumatoid arthritis: a comparison with conventional radiography. Arthritis Rheum 2000;43(12):2762–70.
55. Magnani M, Salizzoni E, Mule R, et al. Ultrasonography detection of early bone erosions in the metacarpophalangeal joints of patients with rheumatoid arthritis. Clin Exp Rheumatol 2004;22(6):743–8.
56. Lopez-Ben R, Bernreuter WK, Moreland LW, et al. Ultrasound detection of bone erosions in rheumatoid arthritis: a comparison to routine radiographs of the hands and feet. Skeletal Radiol 2004;33(2):80–4.

57. Brandlmaier I, Bertram S, Rudisch A, et al. Temporomandibular joint osteoarthrosis diagnosed with high resolution ultrasonography versus magnetic resonance imaging: how reliable is high resolution ultrasonography? J Oral Rehabil 2003; 30(8):812–7.

58. Grassi W. Sonographic imaging of normal and osteoarthritic cartilage. Semin Arthritis Rheum 1999;28(6):398–403.

59. Myers SL, Dines K, Brandt DA, et al. Experimental assessment by high frequency ultrasound of articular cartilage thickness and osteoarthritic changes. J Rheumatol 1995;22(1):109–16.

60. Jurvelin JS, Rasanen T, Kolmonen P, et al. Comparison of optical, needle probe and ultrasonic techniques for the measurement of articular cartilage thickness. J Biomech 1995;28(2):231–5.

61. Jonsson K, Buckwalter K, Helvie M, et al. Precision of hyaline cartilage thickness measurements. Acta Radiol 1992;33(3):234–9.

62. Grobbelaar N, Bouffard JA. Sonography of the knee, a pictorial review. Semin Ultrasound CT MR 2000;21(3):231–74.

63. Naredo E, Cabero F, Palop MJ, et al. Ultrasonographic findings in knee osteoarthritis: a comparative study with clinical and radiographic assessment. Osteoarthritis Cartilage 2005;13:568–74.

64. Bianchi S, Martinoli C. Ultrasound of the musculoskeletal system. Berlin: Springer; 2007.

65. Falsetti P, Frediani B, Fioravanti A, et al. Sonographic study of calcaneal entheses in erosive osteoarthritis, nodal osteoarthritis, rheumatoid arthritis and psoriatic arthritis. Scand J Rheumatol 2003;32(4):229–34.

66. Backhaus M, Burmester GR, Gerber T, et al. Guidelines for musculoskeletal ultrasound in rheumatology. Ann Rheum Dis 2001;60(7):641–9.

67. Allen GM, Wilson DJ. Ultrasound of the shoulder. Eur J Ultrasound 2001;14(1): 3–9.

68. Tan AL, Toumi H, Benjamin M, et al. Combined high-resolution magnetic resonance imaging and histological examination to explore the role of ligaments and tendons in the phenotypic expression of early hand osteoarthritis. Ann Rheum Dis 2006;65(10):1267–72 [see comment].

69. Song IH, Hermann KG, Scheel AK, et al. Comparison of the efficacy of contrast-enhanced ultrasonography and magnetic resonance imaging in detecting synovial process in patients with knee osteoarthritis compared to healthy subjects. Arthritis Rheum 2006;54(Suppl):s262.

70. Song IH, Althoff CE, Hermann KG, et al. Knee osteoarthritis efficacy of a new method of contrast-enhanced musculoskeletal ultrasonography in detection of synovitis in patients with knee osteoarthritis in comparison with magnetic resonance imaging. Ann Rheum Dis 2008;67(1):19–25.

71. Wakefield RJ, Gibbon WW, Emery P. The current status of ultrasonography in rheumatology. Rheumatology 1999;38(3):195–8.

72. Joshua F, Edmonds J, Lassere M. Power Doppler ultrasound in musculoskeletal disease: a systematic review. Semin Arthritis Rheum 2006;36(2):99–108.

73. Joshua F, Lassere M, Bruyn G, et al. Summary findings of a systematic review of the ultrasound assessment of synovitis. J Rheumatol 2007;34(4):839–47.

74. Keen HI, Wakefield RJ, Conaghan PG. A systematic review of ultrasonography in osteoarthritis. Ann Rheum Dis 2009;68(5):611–9.

Magnetic Resonance Imaging-Based Semiquantitative and Quantitative Assessment in Osteoarthritis

Frank W. Roemer, MD[a,b,c,*], Felix Eckstein, MD[d,e],
Ali Guermazi, MD[a,c]

KEYWORDS

- Magnetic resonance imaging • Osteoarthritis • Knee
- Quantitative and semi-quantitative assessment

Over the last 2 decades magnetic resonance imaging (MRI) has established itself as the most important imaging modality in assessing joint pathology in the clinical and research environment. The tomographic viewing perspective of MRI obviates morphologic distortion, magnification, and superimposition. MRI is uniquely able to directly depict all tissues of the joint. This allows the joint to be evaluated as a whole organ, and provides a much more detailed picture of the changes associated with osteoarthritis (OA) than is possible with other techniques.

In relation to knee OA, MRI studies initially focused on the assessment of articular cartilage as the main outcome measure in clinical and epidemiologic studies.[1–7]

A version of this article originally appeared in the 47:4 issue of Radiologic Clinics of North America.

Disclosure: A.G. is president of Boston Imaging Core Lab, LLC (BICL), Boston, MA, a company providing radiological image assessment services. He is shareholder of Synarc, Inc. F.W.R. is shareholder of BICL. F.E. is co-owner and CEO of Chondrometrics GmbH; he provides consulting services to Pfizer Inc, Merck Serono Inc, Wyeth Inc, Novo Nordisk Inc, and Novartis Inc.

[a] Quantitative Imaging Center, Department of Radiology, Boston University School of Medicine, FGH Building, 3rd floor, 820 Harrison Avenue, Boston, MA 02118, USA

[b] Department of MRI, Stenglinstr 2, 86156 Augsburg, Germany

[c] Boston Imaging Core Lab, LLC 580 Harrison Avenue, 4th Floor, Boston, MA 02118, USA

[d] Institute of Anatomy & Musculoskeletal Research, Paracelsus Medical University, Strubergasse 21, A 5020 Salzburg Austria

[e] Chondrometrics GmbH, Ulrichshöglerstre 23, D 83404 Ainring, Germany

* Corresponding author.

E-mail address: froemer@bu.edu (F. W. Roemer).

Rheum Dis Clin N Am 35 (2009) 521–555
doi:10.1016/j.rdc.2009.08.006
0889-857X/09/$ – see front matter © 2009 Elsevier Inc. All rights reserved.

rheumatic.theclinics.com

Several methodologies have been introduced and validated to assess many properties of articular cartilage using MRI, including compositional and biochemical analysis,[8–11] cartilage thickness and volume measurements (see discussion later in this article), as well as semiquantitative analysis of surface damage, which allows cross-sectional and longitudinal evaluation[12–15] (**Fig. 1**). In addition, the great potential of MRI for the assessment of other joint structures that are involved in the OA process was soon recognized.[16–20] Validated tools for whole organ (or synonymously whole joint) assessment of the OA joint were subsequently introduced, which help in discriminating different patterns of intra-articular involvement in OA.[13,21–23] Furthermore, MRI detects pathology of preradiographic OA at a much earlier stage of the disease than conventional radiography is able to detect.[24]

While MRI has enormous potential, methods of standardized whole organ analysis of joints are still in their infancy. Semiquantitative (SQ) whole organ scoring was originally introduced by Peterfy and colleagues in 1999[23] and has since been applied to a multitude of OA studies. The analyses based on SQ scoring have deeply added to the understanding of the pathophysiology and natural history of OA as well as the clinical implications of structural changes assessed.[15,25–33] Semiquantitative scoring of MRI is a valuable method for performing multifeature assessment of the knee, using conventional MRI acquisition techniques that are applied in a clinical environment. Such approaches score, in a semiquantitative manner, a variety of features that are currently believed to be relevant to the functional integrity of the knee or that are potentially involved in the pathophysiology of OA, or both. These articular features include articular cartilage integrity, subarticular bone marrow abnormalities, subchondral cysts, subarticular bone attrition, marginal and central osteophytes (**Fig. 2**), medial and lateral meniscal integrity, anterior and posterior cruciate ligament integrity, medial and lateral collateral ligament integrity, synovitis and effusion, and intra-articular loose bodies, as well as periarticular cysts (**Fig. 3**) and bursitis.

In this article, the authors review the different semiquantitative approaches for MRI-based whole organ assessment of knee OA and also discuss practical aspects of whole joint assessment. Alternative SQ scoring approaches are presented. The second part of the article focuses on quantitative approaches in OA, particularly

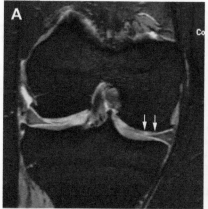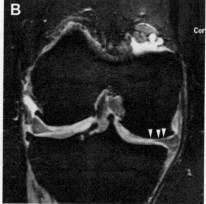

Fig. 1. Progressive cartilage loss in a 6-month interval. (*A*) Baseline coronal Double-Echo Steady-State (DESS) imaging sequence shows diffuse thinning of cartilage in the central medial femur (*arrows*). (*B*) Follow-up image depicts subtle, but definite progression of cartilage damage (*arrowheads*).

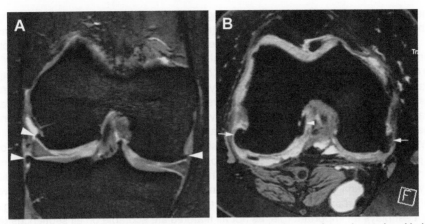

Fig. 2. Osteophytes. (*A*) Coronal DESS image shows marginal osteophytes (*arrowheads*). (*B*) Axial image shows additional posterior osteophytes (*arrows*) and notch osteophyte (*small arrowhead*).

measurement of (subregional) cartilage loss. Risk factors identified by quantitative measurement technology are also discussed.

SEMIQUANTITATIVE ASSESSMENT OF JOINT IN OSTEOARTHRITIS
Whole Joint Assessment on Magnetic Resonance Imaging of the Knee

Whole organ assessment of scoring different joint structures on MRI has shown adequate reliability, specificity, and sensitivity, as well as an ability to detect lesion progression.[13,21,27,34,35] To date, 3 SQ scoring systems for whole organ assessment of knee OA have been published and have been applied in epidemiologic studies or clinical trials: the Whole Organ Magnetic Resonance Imaging Score (WORMS),[13] the Knee Osteoarthritis Scoring System (KOSS),[21] and the Boston-Leeds Osteoarthritis

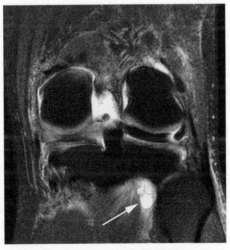

Fig. 3. Periarticular cysts. Tibiofibular joint cyst is depicted on coronal proton density (PD) fat-suppressed (fs) image (*arrow*).

Knee Score (BLOKS).[22] Additional scoring tools have been introduced, covering joint pathology that may not be adequately assessed by the aforementioned systems or offer alternative approaches. Examples are the assessment of synovitis on contrast-enhanced MRI or detailed evaluation of the intercondylar tibial region.[36,37] To date, no study has been performed that compares directly the established scoring systems concerning longitudinal sensitivity to change and correlating the different systems to clinical outcomes. As a reference standard such as histology is not available, true superiority of one system over the other will probably not be proven. The 3 different scoring systems are summarized in **Table 1**.

When deciding which scoring system should be applied for the assessment of a given study, many aspects have to be considered. The most important factors are certainly the outcome measures that are relevant to the study. Second, resources have to be taken into account, as assessment using a complete whole organ score will differ from scoring only certain selected features. Lastly, the available image data set plays an important role, as not all features are scorable on all sequences or with any given sequence protocol. For example, none of the scoring systems incorporates contrast-enhanced MRI.

When estimating the time involved to apply any of these SQ systems and consequently the resources needed for assessment of a given study, the imaging protocol (especially number of sequences and individual images), the quality of images, and the degree of joint abnormalities due to OA has to be taken into account. Time needed for scoring cross-sectionally will differ from longitudinal scoring, and number of time points to be assessed needs to be considered. The method of documenting the scores (manually or electronically) is a crucial factor when estimating effort and resources required for the specific research endeavor.

To date no data are available concerning whether several consecutive MRI examinations from the same subject should be evaluated semiquantitatively in known chronologic order, or if the images should be presented with the reader blinded to the sequence in which they were acquired (ie, the order of films is not revealed).[38] Studies evaluating blinded versus nonblinded reading to date have been performed only for radiographic SQ assessment of spinal fractures and in rheumatoid arthritis (RA) subjects.[39–42] The primary rationale behind blinding to sequence is to reduce reader bias toward finding change in the expected direction. However, as long as readers are blinded to treatment assignment in a clinical trial it is not necessary to blind them to the chronologic sequence of the image data, as possible bias cannot influence the trial results. If the research aim is not treatment but rather the natural history, and the question is how often progression or other change occurs, blinding might be of advantage. If films are read with known chronology in these studies, a reader could have the inclination to overread progression, although the experience from RA has shown otherwise.[38]

Whole Organ Magnetic Resonance Imaging Score

Peterfy and colleagues[13] published WORMS in 2004. Many epidemiologic studies and clinical trials have used WORMS to semiquantitatively assess several OA features of the knee.[15,43–45] WORMS uses a complex subregional division of the different knee compartments: the patella is divided into the medial and lateral facet. The medial and lateral femur and tibial plateau, respectively, are subdivided into an anterior, central, and posterior subregion (**Fig. 4**). Finally, the subspinous tibial region that is not covered by cartilage is defined as an additional distinct subregion. The following features are covered by the WORMS system: cartilage, subchondral bone marrow lesions, subchondral cysts, osteophytes, bone attrition, meniscal status, a combined effusion/synovitis score, and collateral and cruciate ligaments. In addition, several periarticular features are evaluated such as meniscal and popliteal cysts, periarticular bursitis, and loose bodies (**Fig. 5**).

Compared with the other systems, WORMS uses a strict subregional rather than a lesion-oriented approach to the scoring especially of cartilage, bone marrow lesions (BMLs), and subchondral cysts. This approach has the possible advantage of summing several lesions per subregion, and may facilitate reading and subsequent analyses. Using a lesional approach,[19,21,22] definition of the exact number of individual lesions is sometimes difficult, as lesions may be directly adjacent to each other, or will be merging or splitting in longitudinal assessments. WORMS is the only SQ scoring system that assesses subchondral bone attrition, which is defined as flattening or depression of the articular surface not related to trauma (**Fig. 6**).

Knee Osteoarthritis Scoring System

The KOSS system, introduced by Kornaat and colleagues,[21] covers similar MRI-detected OA features as WORMS, but the following differences have to be mentioned. Cartilage status, subchondral BMLs, and cysts are scored individually for each subregion, and each score is differentiated by size of the lesion. Osteophytes are differentiated into marginal, intercondylar, and central. Although KOSS uses a more complex meniscal score concerning tear morphology than WORMS, it does not describe regional subdivision, or partial or total meniscal maceration/resection. Meniscal subluxation is scored in addition to meniscal morphology (**Fig. 7**). Effusion is scored in a similar fashion to WORMS (**Fig. 8**). KOSS uses a different subregional division than WORMS and differentiates the patellar crest (crista patellae), the medial and lateral patellar facet, the medial and lateral trochlear articular facet, the medial and lateral femoral condyle (excluding the trochlear groove), and the medial and lateral tibial plateau.

Boston-Leeds Osteoarthritis Knee Score

The BLOKS system was published by Hunter and colleagues in 2008.[22] Concerning the subregional division of the articular surfaces, BLOKS uses a similar approach to that of KOSS, focusing on the weight-bearing components versus the patellofemoral joint (**Fig. 9**). As in WORMS, the patella is subdivided into the medial and lateral facets (**Fig. 10**). BMLs and cysts are scored in a complex manner, taking into account size of BML, percentage of involved subchondral surface area of BML, and percentage of BML that is cystic. Thus, subchondral cysts are defined as cystic portions of BML and are not assessed separately as in the other 2 scoring systems (**Fig. 11**). The lesional approach for BMLs allows for superior longitudinal analysis of individual lesions, especially concerning percentage of lesion that is cystic or noncystic. On the other hand, the definition of each individual lesion is time consuming, and the ill-delineated nature of these lesions makes differentiation between individual lesions in certain instances difficult.

Cartilage scoring is conducted by reporting 2 scores. Score 1 describes percentage of any cartilage loss in the subregion and percentage of cartilage damage that represents full-thickness loss. The second cartilage score describes cartilage status at defined locations on specific landmark-defined image sections in the coronal plane, and differentiates partial and full-thickness cartilage loss. Signal changes in the Hoffa fat pad are scored as a surrogate for synovitis.[46] BLOKS uses a complex scoring system to assess the meniscal status including tears (**Fig. 12**), signal changes (**Fig. 13**), and meniscal extrusion.

Table 1
Comparison of 3 different semiquantitative scoring systems of knee osteoarthritis

	BLOKS	KOSS	WORMS
Number of knees scored in original publication	10 knees (71 knees for validity exercise of BML scoring)	25 knees	19 knees
MRI protocol of original publication (all publications used 1.5 T systems)	For reliability exercise (10 knees): sag/cor T2w FS, sag T1 SE, axial/cor 3D FLASH For validity of BML assessment: sag PD/T2w Cor/axial PD/T2w FS	Cor/sag T2w and PDw, sag 3D SPGR, axial PD and axial T2w FS	Axial T1w SE, cor T1w SE, sag T1w SE, sag T2w FS, sag 3D SPGR
Subregional division of knee	9 subregions: Medial/lateral patella, medial/lateral trochlea, medial, lateral weight-bearing femur, medial/lateral weight-bearing tibia, subspinous tibia	9 subregions: medial patella, patellar crest, lateral patella, medial/lateral trochlea, medial/lateral femoral condyle, medial/lateral tibial plateau	15 subregions: medial/lateral patella, medial/lateral femur (anterior/central/posterior), medial/lateral tibia (anterior/central/posterior), subspinous tibia
Interreader reliability	Performed on 10 knees w-kappa between 0.51 (meniscal extrusion) and 0.79 (meniscal tear)	Performed on 25 knees w-kappa between 0.57 (osteochondral defects) and 0.88 (bone marrow edema)	Performed on 19 knees ICC between 0.74 (bone marrow abnormalities and synovitis/effusion) and 0.99 (cartilage)
Intrareader reliability	Not presented	Performed on 25 knees w-kappa between 0.56 (intrasubstance meniscal degeneration) and 0.91 (bone marrow edema and Baker cyst)	Not presented
Scored MR features			
Cartilage	Two different scores Score 1: Subregional approach. A. percentage of any cartilage loss in subregion. B. percentage of full-thickness cartilage loss in subregion Score 2: Site-specific approach. scoring of cartilage thickness at 11 specific locations (not subregions) from 0 (none) to 2 (full-thickness loss)	Subregional approach: focal and diffuse defects are differentiated. Depth of lesions is scored from 0 to 3. Diameter of lesion is scored from 0 to 3. Osteochondral defects are scored separately	Subregional approach: Scores from 0 to 6 depending on depth and extent of cartilage loss. Intrachondral cartilage signal additionally scored as present/absent

Bone marrow lesions	Scoring of individual lesions 3 different aspects of BMLs are scored: a. Size of BML scored from 0 to 3 concerning percentage of subregional bone volume b. Percentage of surface area adjacent to subchondral plate c. Percentage of BML that is noncystic	Scoring of individual lesions from 0 to 3 concerning maximum diameter of lesion	Summed BML size/volume for subregion from 0 to 3 in regard to percentage of subregional bone volume
Subchondral cysts	Scored together with BMLs	Scoring of individual lesions from 0 to 3 concerning maximum diameter of lesion	Summed cyst size/volume for subregion from 0 to 3 in regard to percentage of subregional bone volume
Osteophytes	Scored at 12 sites from 0 to 3	Scored from 0 to 3. Marginal, intercondylar and central osteophytes are differentiated. Locations/sites of osteophyte scoring not forwarded	Scored at 16 sites from 0 to 7
Bone attrition		Not scored	Scored in 14 subregions from 0 to 3
Effusion	Scored from 0 to 3	Scored from 0 to 3	Scored from 0 to 3
Synovitis	a. Scoring of size of signal changes in Hoffa fat pad b. Five additional sites scored as present/absent (details of scoring not described)	Synovial thickening scored as present/absent on sagittal T1w SPGR sequence (location not described)	Combined effusion/synovitis score
Meniscal status	Anterior horn, body, posterior horn scored separately in medial/lateral meniscus Presence/absence scored: – intrameniscal signal – vertical tear – horizontal tear – complex tear – root tear – macerated – meniscal cyst	No subregional division of meniscus described. Presence/absence of following tears: – horizontal tear – vertical tear – radial tear – complex tear – bucket-handle tear – meniscal intrasubstance degeneration scored from 0 to 3	Anterior horn, body, posterior horn scored separately in medial/lateral meniscus tears from 0 to 4: 1. Minor radial or parrot beak tear 2. Nondisplaced tear or prior surgical repair 3. Displaced tear or partial resection 4. Complete maceration/destruction or complete resection

(continued on next page)

Table 1
(continued)

	BLOKS	KOSS	WORMS
Meniscal extrusion	Scored as medial and lateral extrusion on coronal image and anterior extrusion for medial/lateral meniscus on sagittal image from 0 to 3	Scored on coronal image from 0 to 3	Not scored
Ligaments	Cruciate ligaments scored as normal or complete tear. Associated insertional BMLs are scored in tibia and in femur	Not scored	Cruciate ligaments and collateral ligaments scored as intact or torn
Periarticular features	Patella tendon: no signal change and signal abnormality. The following features are scored as present or absent: − pes anserine bursitis − iliotibial band signal − Popliteal cyst − infrapatellar bursa − prepatellar bursa Ganglion cysts of the TFJ, meniscus, ACL, PCL, semimembranosus, semitendinosus, other	Only popliteal cysts scored from 0 to 3	Popliteal cysts, anserine bursitis, semimebranosus bursa meniscal cyst, infrapatellar bursitis, prepatellar bursitis, tibiofibular cyst scored from 0 to 3
Loose bodies	Scored as absent/present	Not scored	Scored from 0 to 3

Abbreviations: 3D FLASH, 3-dimensional fast low-angle shot sequence; 3D SPGR, 3-dimensional spoiled gradient echo sequence; 1.5 T, 1.5 Tesla; ACL, anterior cruciate ligament; BLOKS, Boston–Leeds Osteoarthritis Knee Score; BML, bone marrow lesion; cor, coronal; ICC, intraclass correlation coefficient; KOSS, Knee Osteoarthritis Scoring System; PCL, posterior cruciate ligament; PDw, proton density weighted; sag, sagittal; T1w SE, T1-weighted spin echo sequence; T2w FS, T2-weighted fat-suppressed sequence; TFJ, tibiofibular joint; w-kappa, weighted kappa; WORMS, Whole Organ Magnetic Imaging Score.

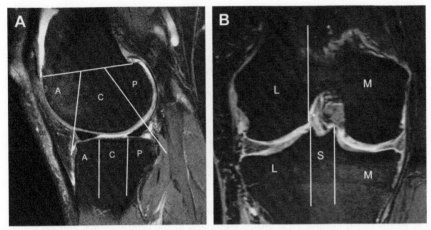

Fig. 4. Subregional division of the knee joint in Whole Organ Magnetic Resonance Imaging Score (WORMS). (*A*) Sagittal intermediate-weighted (IW) fs image. The tibial plateau is subdivided into an anterior (A), central (C), and posterior (P) subregion defined by meniscal coverage. The femur is subdivided in to an anterior (A), central (C), and posterior (P) portion defined by the anterior and posterior margins of the meniscus. (*B*) Coronal DESS image. In the coronal plane the tibia is divided into the medial (M) and lateral (L) tibial plateau, and the subspinous region (S) that is not covered by articular cartilage. The femur is divided into lateral (L) and medial (M), the femoral notch being considered part of the medial femur.

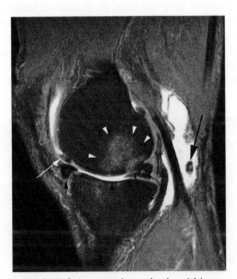

Fig. 5. Loose body. On sagittal PD fs image a loose body within a popliteal (Baker) cysts is visualized (*large black arrow*). Other typical MRI features of advanced knee OA are depicted in addition: a large subchondral bone marrow lesion in the weight-bearing region of the medial femur (*white arrowheads*), an anterior osteophyte of the medial femur (*white arrow*), diffuse full-thickness cartilage loss of the central medial tibia (*black arrowhead*), anterior extrusion of the anterior horn of the medial meniscus (*short black arrow*), and a horizontal tear of the posterior horn of the medial meniscus (*thin black arrow*).

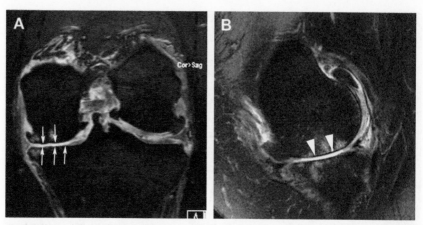

Fig. 6. Attrition. (*A*) Coronal DESS image. Flattening of the central medial femoral condyle and tibial plateau is depicted (*arrows*). (*B*) Sagittal IW fs image. Flattening of the central medial condyle is shown (*arrowheads*).

Reliability

Excellent reliability data have been published for all 3 whole organ SQ scoring systems. A comparative overview of the reliability exercises is presented in **Table 2**. The usual range of these exercises represents good to excellent agreement between 2 independent radiologists after an intensive training and validation exercise. However, it has to be kept in mind that these numbers are highly dependent on the MRI protocol and on the experience of the individual expert readers. The numbers presented in **Table 2** reflect only the data on published features; for example, the cruciate ligaments are scored with BLOKS or Baker cysts are assessed with WORMS, but these features were not included in the reliability exercises. Intraobserver data have been published only for the KOSS system and showed comparable results to the interobserver reliability. Additional reliability exercises were performed for aspects of the WORMS system in the Multicenter Osteoarthritis (MOST) study, and have been published.[27,29,31,32]

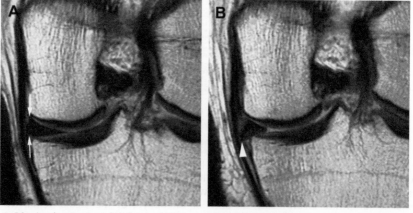

Fig. 7. Meniscal extrusion. (*A*) Coronal IW image. Regular position of meniscus is observed at baseline (*arrows*). (*B*) Incident meniscal extrusion is observed at 12-month follow-up (*arrowheads*).

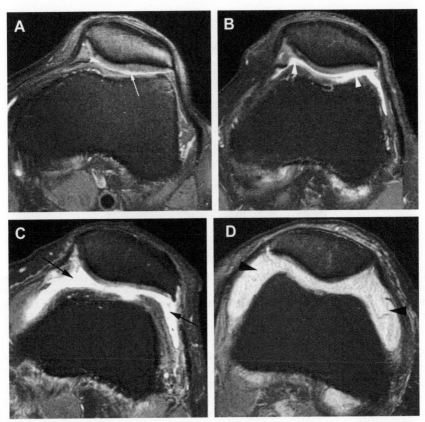

Fig. 8. Joint effusion. The 3 whole joint scoring systems assess amount of joint effusion in a similar fashion according to the degree of joint capsule distention. (*A*) Axial PD fs image shows physiologic amount of effusion (*white arrow*). (*B*) Axial PD fs image depicts grade 1 joint effusion (*white arrowheads*). (*C*) Grade 2 effusion is visualized (*black arrows*). (*D*) Axial PD fs image shows an extensive grade 3 joint effusion with marked distension of the joint capsule (*black arrowheads*).

Additional Semiquantitative Scoring Systems

Additional methods to score tissue pathology on MRI in knee OA have been suggested. Examples are presented in this section to illustrate these alternative approaches.

Several semiquantitative grading schemes for the evaluation of articular cartilage have been proposed, with most of them being derived from the surgery-based scoring method suggested by Outerbridge in 1961.[47] Arthroscopic scoring systems usually assess cartilage macroscopically on a scale from 0 to 4, based on visual evaluation and direct probing.[48] MRI-adapted modifications of these systems grade the depth of articular cartilage damage and differentiate between surface defects of less or more than 50% of cartilage thickness, but rarely incorporate involved area of superficial or full-thickness defects [49–52] Biswal and colleagues[14] suggested a similar scoring system to that of WORMS, grading cartilage on a 6-point scale and also incorporating lesion size.

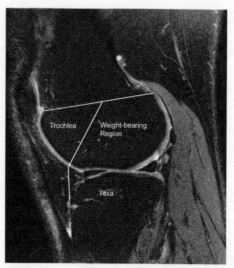

Fig. 9. Subregional division in Boston-Leeds Osteoarthritis Knee Score (BLOKS) and Knee Osteoarthritis Scoring System (KOSS). Sagittal IW fs image. The femur is subdivided into the femoral trochlea and the weight-bearing region. The medial and lateral tibial plateaus are each defined as one subregion.

Synovitis is frequently present in OA; it may predict other structural changes in OA, and correlate with pain and other clinical outcomes.[20,53] Quantitative MRI markers of synovitis include the volume of synovial tissue and fluid, and synovial enhancement following intravenous injection of contrast material. As the published whole organ scoring systems are based on nonenhanced MRI, only indirect surrogate imaging features may be used to estimate the degree of synovitis. One of these is joint effusion, as a reflection of inflammatory synovial activation of the joint.[32] However, synovitis has

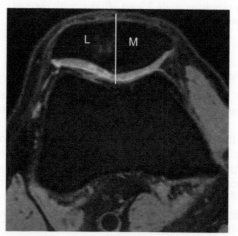

Fig. 10. Subregional division of the patella. In WORMS and BLOKS the patella is divided into the medial (M) and lateral (L) facet, the patellar crest being defined as medial. In KOSS the patella crest is a separate entity, and thus the patella has 3 subregions.

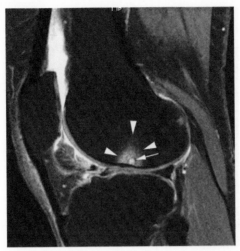

Fig. 11. Bone marrow lesion (BML). Sagittal IW fs image shows BML with cystic (*arrow*) and noncystic (*arrowheads*) portion in the central part of the lateral femoral condyle.

been scored semiquantitatively in the absence of gadolinium–diethylenetriamine penta-acetic acid,[20,53] as signal alterations in the infrapatellar fat pad on noncontrast MRI correlated with mild chronic synovitis on histologic analysis.[46] This surrogate assessment seems to be nonspecific, albeit sensitive.[54] Other differential diagnoses such as nonspecific edema or chronic fibrotic changes might present with a similar aspect on MRI.[55] Another scoring system assessing synovitis on nonenhanced images has been introduced recently.[56] Validation data comparing the system with an established reference standard such as histology or contrast-enhanced MRI was not forwarded.[57] A detailed whole joint synovitis scoring system measuring synovial thickness on T1-weighted fat-suppressed, contrast-enhanced images was presented recently.

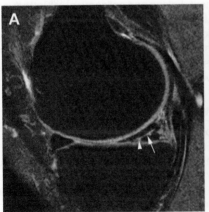
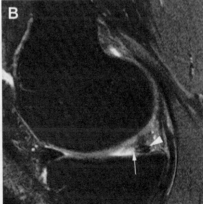

Fig. 12. Meniscal damage. (*A*) Sagittal IW fs image. Horizontal tear (*small arrow*) extending to the inferior meniscal surface (*small arrowhead*) is shown. (*B*) Meniscal maceration. Missing central portion of meniscus (*large arrow*). In addition, horizontal tear is depicted (*large arrowhead*).

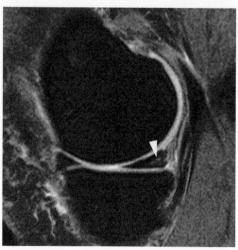

Fig. 13. Mucoid intrameniscal degeneration. Sagittal IW fs image shows intrameniscal signal change in the posterior horn of the medial meniscus (*arrowhead*).

Synovitis is assessed at 11 defined joint locations and scored semiquantitatively from 0 to 3 (**Fig. 14**). Good reliability and a correlation with pain could be proven.[37] In a recent publication considering microscopic analysis as gold standard, only the MRI total synovitis score performed on injected images correlated with synovial membrane inflammation, with histology as the reference standard.[58]

There are few MRI scoring systems published that evaluate ligaments of the knee joint in OA. One report scored the medial collateral ligament for no, weak, and high signal intensity on coronal and axial sections.[17] Another study used a classification system based on ligamentous injury grading of 0 to 3, ranging from edema on one side of the ligament fibers to edema on both sides, and edema with ligamentous disruption.[59] However, it has to be kept in mind that this classification assesses traumatic injury and is not necessarily applicable to OA joints.

Concerning bone marrow lesion assessment, Felson and colleagues[19,26] introduced a lesional approach to be graded from 0 to 3. Expanding this scoring method and incorporating the number of slices that depict a specific lesion was suggested by other research groups.[52,60] One publication recently assessed BMLs using software cursors applied to the greatest diameter of each lesion.[61] A drawback seems to be that large diameters do not necessarily reflect BML volume.

Sequence Protocols for Semiquantitative Whole Organ Assessment

When designing any imaging protocol for whole organ assessment, one has to consider which articular tissues will be included in the assessment and which measurement methods will be applied to assess the individual tissue or feature. Full anatomic coverage has to be supported by the MR system. Other quality parameters such as signal homogeneity, correct image orientation, sufficient signal to noise ratio, and spatial resolution, as well as the minimization of technical artifacts have to be taken into account. Length of the protocol based on the number of sequences applied, the number of acquisitions per sequence, spatial resolution, and type of sequence needs to be determined to find a compromise between patient comfort and tolerance, costs, and image quality.

Table 2
Published inter- and intraobserver reliability results for reading of MRI features using different whole joint scoring systems

Joint Feature	WORMS Interreader Agreement (ICC)	KOSS Interreader (ICC [95% CI]/w-kappa)	KOSS Intrareader (ICC [95% CI]/w-kappa)	BLOKS Interreader (w-kappa [95% CI])
BML size	0.74	0.91 [0.88–0.93]/0.88	0.93 [0.91–0.94]/0.91	0.72 [0.58–0.87]
BML % area (BLOKS only)	N/A	N/A	N/A	0.69 [0.55–0.82]
% of lesion BML (BLOKS only)	N/A	N/A	N/A	0.72 [0.58–0.87]
Osteophytes	0.97	0.71 [0.67–0.76]/0.67	0.76 [0.72–0.80]/0.79	0.65 [0.52–0.77]
Cartilage morphology	0.99	0.64 [0.58–0.69]/0.57	0.78 [0.74–0.81]/0.67	0.72 [0.59–0.85]
Cartilage 2 (BLOKS only)	N/A	N/A	N/A	0.73 [0.60–0.85]
Osteochondral defects (KOSS only)	N/A	0.63 [0.55–0.70]/0.66	0.87 [0.83–0.90]/0.87	N/A
Synovitis	0.74	0.74 [0.58–0.85]	0.81 [0.69–0.89]/0.77	0.62 [0.05–1.00]
Effusion	See synovitis; scores combined	See synovitis; scores combined	See synovitis; scores combined	0.61 [0.05–0.85]
Meniscal extrusion/subluxation	N/A	0.67 [0.57–0.75]/0.65	0.82 [0.75–0.86]/0.82	0.51 [0.24–0.78]
Meniscal signal/Intrasubstance degeneration	N/A	0.78 [0.68–0.85]/0.66	0.76 [0.66–0.83]/0.56	0.68 [0.44–0.93]
Meniscal tear	0.87	0.70 [0.61–0.77]/0.70	0.78 [0.70–0.83]/0.78	0.79 [0.40–1.00]
Ligaments	1.0	N/A	N/A	N/A
Subchondral cysts	0.94	0.87 [0.83–0.89]/0.83	0.90 [0.87–0.92]/0.87	Part of % BML score
Baker cysts	N/A	0.89 [0.76–0.95]/0.80	0.96 [0.90–0.98]/0.91	N/A

Abbreviations: 95% CI, 95% confidence interval; BLOKS, Boston-Leeds Osteoarthritis Knee Score; ICC, intraclass correlation coefficient; KOSS, Knee Osteoarthritis Scoring System; N/A, not applicable; w-kappa, weighted kappa; WORMS, Whole Organ Magnetic Resonance Imaging Score.

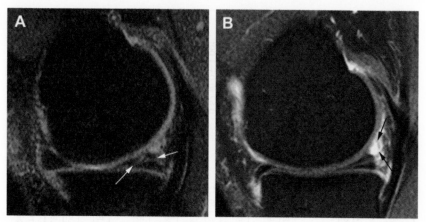

Fig. 14. Localized synovitis. (*A*) Sagittal PD fs image shows horizontal meniscal tear extending to the inferior surface and posterior aspect of the posterior horn of the medial meniscus (*arrows*). (*B*) T1-weighted fs image after intravenous contrast administration shows marked perimeniscal enhancement, reflecting synovitic thickening (*black arrows*) not depicted on the nonenhanced sequence.

Suggestions for MRI protocols focusing on whole organ assessment have been described in detail in an Osteoarthritis Research Society International (OARSI)/ Outcome Measures in Rheumatology Clinical Trials (OMERACT) consensus review by Peterfy and colleagues.[62] A minimalist protocol still allowing for assessment of most articular features that are included in whole organ scoring would consist of proton density–weighted or T2-weighted fat-suppressed sequences in 3 orthogonal planes, which has provided reliable image quality with data that has markedly improved the understanding of disease progression.[63,64] A detailed description of the rationales for choosing the protocol for the Osteoarthritis Initiative (OAI) has been reported recently[65] (**Fig. 15**).

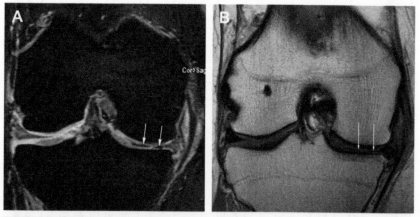

Fig. 15. Susceptibility. (*A*) Coronal DESS sequence. Discrete calcification of chondral surface in the weight-bearing region of the medial tibiofemoral compartment is depicted (*arrows*). (*B*) On coronal IW sequence calcification may not be appreciated, and is only delineable in the knowledge of the findings on the DESS image (*long white arrows*).

Image Quality

Sufficient image quality is crucial for SQ whole organ assessment. MRIs need to be acquired in a standardized fashion, adhering to protocol requirements.[62] An example of how to acquire optimal image data, what kind of problems are to be encountered, and how to deal with them is presented in the publicly available OAI MRI operations manual.[66] Despite sufficient anatomic coverage, field homogeneity, absence of motion artifacts, and sufficient fat suppression in fat-saturated sequences are paramount for reliable SQ scoring of OA joints. Knowledge of additional possible artifacts such as susceptibility (including metallic artifacts), vascular pulsation, and aliasing is crucial.[62] Examples of possible artifacts and of commonly encountered image quality impairment are presented in **Fig. 16**.

Semiquantitative Scoring of Other Joints

At present, most research teams using MRI-based SQ assessment of OA focus on the knee joint. Reasons for this are size of the joint, with relatively thick articular cartilage in comparison to other diarthrodial joints, high prevalence of knee OA, and joint anatomy that allows convenient assessment of most structures in 2 orthogonal planes. SQ assessment of facet joint OA on multidetector computed tomography scans has been introduced.[67] An SQ system to assess early hip OA was recently presented.[68] To the authors' knowledge, additional MRI- or CT-based SQ assessment of OA of other joints has not been performed to date (**Fig. 17**).

QUANTITATIVE MEASUREMENT OF CARTILAGE IN OSTEOARTHRITIS

Quantitative measurement of the cartilage exploits the 3D nature of MRI data sets to assess tissue dimensions (ie, volume, thickness, or others) or signal as continuous variables (**Fig. 18**). The strength of this approach is that it is less observer dependent and more objective than scoring methods, and that relatively small changes in cartilage morphology over time, which occur over larger areas, may be detected, although they are not apparent to the naked eye. Recently it was reported that quantitative measures[69] were more powerful in revealing significant relationships between OA risk factors (meniscal damage and malalignment) and knee cartilage loss than SQ measures (ie, WORMS).[23] In turn, the disadvantages of quantitative measurement are that they require specialized software and are relatively time intensive, because tissue boundaries need to be segmented through series of slices by trained personnel. Also, quantitative measurements are less sensitive to small focal changes within larger structures (ie, focal lesions), which are more readily picked by expert readers. It was shown, for instance, that MRI-based SQ assessment of cartilage status differed significantly between participants with and without radiographic OA, whereas quantitative measures of cartilage thickness displayed only small differences.[33] Therefore, both approaches have their particular strengths and should ideally be used in complementary fashion. The second part of this article therefore focuses on quantitative measurement technology as applied to cartilage morphology in the knee (volume and thickness). Quantitative methods for assessing cartilage composition (ie, delayed gadolinium-enhanced MRI of cartilage, T2, T1rho, and others),[70] bone (ie, subchondral trabecular structure),[70] the meniscus,[15] or cartilage volume and thickness in other joints have also been published, but are not considered here for reasons of brevity.

For quantitatively measuring the cartilage, the bone-cartilage interface and the cartilage surface need to be segmented by a trained user, with or without assistance from (semi)automatic segmentation software[71–79] and input devices.[80] Expert quality control, however, is very important to warrant consistent and accurate analysis, and

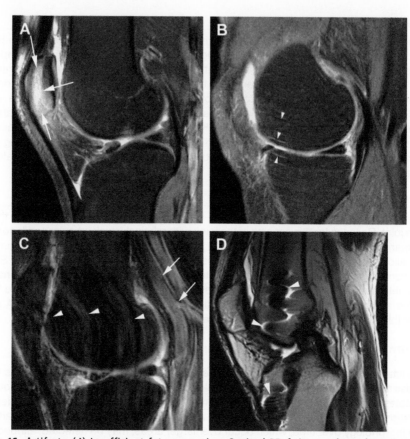

Fig. 16. Artifacts. (*A*) Insufficient fat suppression. Sagittal PD fs image shows hyperintense bone marrow within the patella that is consistent with bone marrow edema. However, the association of high signal extending across adjacent tissue compartments (prepatellar soft tissues and Hoffa fat pad) suggests failed fat suppression as an alternative cause. This artifact reduces the diagnostic accuracy of this scan for assessment of patellar BMLs. (*B*) Motion artifact. Sagittal PD fs image of the medial tibiofemoral compartment. Repetitive bandlike high- and low-intensity signal changes are observed in the anterior femur and tibia (*small arrowheads*). These changes are a result of motion during the sequence acquisition and will impair assessment of the subchondral bone marrow in these subregions. (*C*) Pulsation artifact. Mid-sagittal PD fs image shows marked pulsation artifacts from the popliteal artery (*arrows*) in the phase-encoding direction (anterior-posterior), obscuring the articular anatomy of the knee. Bandlike repetition artifacts of the vessel will impair bone marrow assessment in the adjacent femur and tibia (*arrowheads*). (*D*) Susceptibility artifacts after reconstructive surgery. Sagittal T2-weighted fast spin echo image shows severe metallic artifacts in femur and tibia associated with surgical anterior cruciate ligament repair and intraosseous marrow implant after diaphyseal femoral fracture (*arrowheads*).

the time required for segmentation (or the correction of computer-generated segmentation) generally takes several hours per joint. In a next step, a variety of morphologic cartilage parameters can be computed, such as the size of the total area of subchondral bone (tAB), the area of the cartilage surface (AC), the denuded (dAB) and cartilage-covered (cAB) subchondral bone area, the cartilage thickness over the tAB

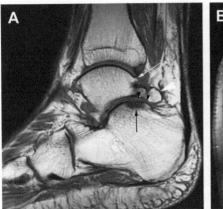
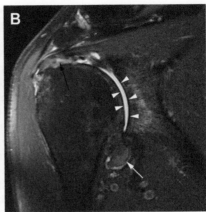

Fig. 17. Osteoarthritis of other joints. (*A*) Sagittal T1-weighted image shows severe OA of the subtalar joint. Note cartilage loss (*black arrowheads*) and subchondral calcaneal BML (*black arrow*). In addition, osteophytes at the posterior tibiotalar (*white arrow*) and subtalar joints (*white arrowhead*) are depicted. (*B*) Coronal PD fs image of shoulder OA. Diffuse humeral and glenoidal cartilage loss is depicted (*arrowheads*). In addition, an articular-sided partial tear of the supraspinatus tendon is shown (*black arrow*). Note huge osteophyte at the caudal humeral head (*white arrow*).

(ThCtAB), the cAB (ThCcAB) or anatomically defined subregions,[81–83] the cartilage volume (VC), the cartilage volume normalized to the tAB (VCtAB), cartilage signal intensity,[84–86] and others. A consensus-based nomenclature and definition for these and other outcome measures was proposed by a group of experts[87] and is used throughout this review.

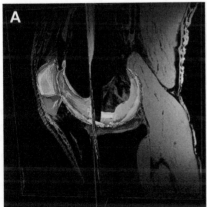
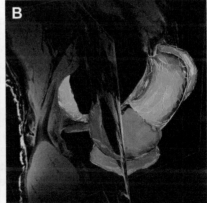

Fig. 18. Three-dimensional reconstruction of human knee cartilage obtained from a sagittal SPGR/FLASH (spoiled gradient recalled echo acquisition in the steady state/fast low-angle shot) data set; medial view (*A*) and view from posterior and lateral (*B*): The segmented cartilage of the trochlea femoris is displayed in *turquoise*, that of the weight-bearing and posterior part of the medial femoral condyle in *yellow* and *orange*, respectively, that of the weight-bearing and posterior part of the lateral femoral condyle in *red* and *violet*, respectively, and that of the medial and lateral tibia in *blue* and *green*, respectively.

Most of the quantitative studies in OA have focused on the volume of the cartilage (VC), but this outcome measure has several limitations: The ability to discriminate between OA and healthy subjects is limited, because people with larger bones display larger VC,[88,89] creating wide overlap between the groups. Men have larger joint surfaces than women (and hence also larger VC), even after adjustment for body height and weight,[90] and VC is thus difficult to compare between men and women. In longitudinal studies, the subchondral bone area has been shown to increase with aging in healthy reference subjects, and even more so in OA patients.[91–93] Such effects may mask a reduction in cartilage thickness in OA, because of the expansion of the bone and cartilage layer that partially compensates for losses in cartilage thickness, if the VC is measured. Therefore, alternative outcomes have been suggested, such as the VCtAB or the ThCtAB.[88,94] Buck and colleagues[95] reported that almost all of the variability observed in cross-sectional and longitudinal studies of healthy and OA participants can be described by tAB, ThC (either ThCtAB or ThCcAB), and dAB, which provide independent and complete information on cartilage morphology status and its changes with time.

Several studies reported reference values of cartilage morphology in healthy volunteers[88,96–98] or templates for comparison of cartilage thickness distribution patterns between healthy reference subjects and OA patients.[94,99] Some reports found that the sensitivity to change or ThCtAB or VCtAB was higher than for VC,[100,101] whereas others found comparable standardized response means (SRMs) for VC, VCtAB, or ThCtAB.[102,103] Quantitative measures of surface curvature and joint incongruity[104–106] have been explored and reported to be associated with cartilage loss (at 0.2 T).[107] Cartilage homogeneity was also reported to be significantly different between subjects without and with radiographic OA at 0.2 T,[84,108] although other validated MRI techniques of composition cartilage imaging have often been less successful in discriminating healthy volunteers and subjects with OA.[70]

Imaging Protocols for Quantitative Measurement of Cartilage in Osteoarthritis

Imaging protocols for quantitative analysis of cartilage morphology and their validation has been summarized previously.[70,109–115] Water-excitation (or fat-suppressed) T1-weighted spoiled gradient recalled echo acquisition in the steady state (SPGR) or fast low-angle shot (FLASH) at 1.5 or 3 T represent the current gold standard,[62,111,113] but double-echo steady-state imaging (DESS) with water excitation has recently been cross-calibrated with FLASH, because of the faster acquisition time and lower slice thickness, and because of its use in the OA Initiative (http://www.niams.nih.gov/ne/oi/).[65,116–119]

The technical accuracy (validity) and test-retest precision (reproducibility) of quantitative cartilage measurements at 1.5 T have been summarized previously.[70,111] Imaging at 1.0 T was found to be consistent with 1.5 T, albeit less precise (reproducible).[120] Quantitative cartilage measurement at 0.2 T has been proposed[71,72,84,105–107] but has not been validated versus external standards or measurement at higher field strength. Cartilage imaging at 3 T has been cross-calibrated with 1.5 T, and lower precision errors than for 1.5 T imaging were reported when acquiring thinner (coronal) slices[121] Precision errors at 3 T were observed to be similar for different vendors in a multicenter trial, and measurements were relatively stable over a 3-month observation period.[92] The stability of geometric (phantom) measurements was also satisfactory over a 3-year period in the OAI.[122] Results from DESS (at 3 T, as used in the OAI) were found to be consistent with FLASH and displayed similar test-retest precision errors.[117–119] Comparative studies[100,102,119] also found similar rates of and sensitivity to change, but no larger face-to-face comparison has yet been published.

Rate of Change and Sensitivity to Change in Osteoarthritis

Reports on longitudinal changes of cartilage morphology in subjects with OA[70,82,100,102,111,123–133] have revealed somewhat variable results (between 0%[123,130] and 7%[125] annual change) for annual cartilage loss.[70,111,134] Recent analyses of a first release of 160 participants of the OAI progression cohort found relatively small rates of progression; the rates were higher in the weight-bearing medial femur than in the medial tibia,[100,102,132,133] but this was not a consistent finding across other cohorts, particularly not when focusing on the SRM. It has therefore been suggested that the aggregate thickness in the tibia and weight-bearing femur be reported.[100,101,118,131,135] Estimates of tibial cartilage loss over 2 years were found to correlate with those over 4.5 years. This result suggests that changes in cartilage volume measured over 2 years predict long-term cartilage loss.[129] The ratio of medial compartment versus lateral compartment cartilage loss was reported to be 1.4:1 in knees with neutral biomechanical alignment, 3.7:1 in varus knees, and 1:6.0 in valgus knees,[101] confirming that knee alignment is an important determinant of medial versus lateral cartilage loss. After anterior cruciate ligament injury,[136] a reduction of cartilage thickness was observed in the trochlea, but there was an increase in the weight-bearing medial femur. This finding may be attributed to cartilage swelling or hypertrophy observed as a sign of early OA.[137–141]

Only weak correlations between MRI-detected cartilage loss and OA progression in radiography have been reported,[126,130,142] but a recent publication found a higher correlation when the longitudinal reduction in radiographic joint space width was compared with cartilage loss in the central aspect of the femorotibial joint.[82] Whereas some studies found a higher rate and sensitivity to change of cartilage morphology compared with radiography,[126,128,143] a recent 2-year study reported a somewhat higher SRM (−0.62) for Lyon Schuss (but not for fixed flexion [−0.20]) radiography versus cartilage thickness of the medial tibia as measured with MRI (−0.59).[131] It was hypothesized that during weight-bearing radiography, slightly swollen cartilage may be compressed mechanically and meniscal extrusion may be increased.[18,30,144]

Spatial Patterns of Cartilage Loss as Derived from Subregional Cartilage Analysis

Two studies[82,132] reported that the rate of change in cartilage morphology in the central aspects of the femorotibial joint exceeded that in total cartilage plates, but found that the SRM was not substantially improved because of the higher variability (standard deviation) of the (central) regional changes.[103] Three studies in different cohorts[101,131,132] recently examined the spatial pattern of femorotibial cartilage loss based on the technology proposed by Wirth and colleagues (**Fig. 19**).[81] In a small meta-analysis,[145] the medial femorotibial compartment, the central part of the weight-bearing femoral condyle, was found to be the "most progressive" region (the one with the greatest average cartilage loss; see **Fig. 19**), followed by the external medial tibia, the external medial femur, and the central medial tibia (see **Fig. 19**). Laterally, the central, internal, and posterior lateral tibial regions were most strongly affected by cartilage loss, where only very small changes (if any) were observed in the lateral femur (see **Fig. 19**). Of note, the central subregion of the lateral weight-bearing femoral condyle was the one with the least average thinning in the lateral femorotibial compartment, whereas the central subregion of the medial weight-bearing femoral condyle was the one with the greatest average thinning in the medial femorotibial compartment (see **Fig. 19**). However, in line with other observations,[103] the sensitivity to change in the subregions was not consistently higher than in the total plates across studies.[145] Yet, the analysis of the "central" medial compartment

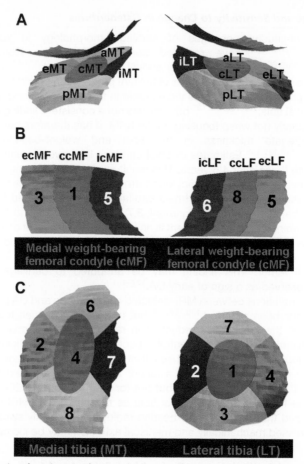

Fig. 19. Anatomic subregions in the weight-bearing femorotibial joint as described by Wirth and colleagues,[81] and results of a meta-analysis[145] of subregional progression rates in 3 cohorts[101,131,132] in the medial and in the lateral femorotibial compartment, respectively: 1, subregion with the greatest rate of thinning in OA participants within each compartment; 2, subregions with the second greatest rate of thinning, and so forth; 8, region with the least amount of thinning (or the greatest amount of thickening) across OA participants and studies. (*A*) Posterior view onto the weight-bearing femorotibial joint showing the medial and lateral weight-bearing part of the femoral condyle (*top*) and the medial (MT) and lateral tibia (LT) (*bottom*): c, central subregion; p, posterior subregion; e, external subregion; a, anterior subregion; I, internal subregion. (*B*) Inferior view onto the central medial (cMF) and lateral (cLF) (weight-bearing) part of the femoral condyle: central subregions (*red*); internal subregions (*blue*), external subregions (*green*). (*C*) Superior view onto the medial (MT) and lateral (LT) tibia: c, central subregions (*red*); I, internal subregions (*blue*); e, external subregions (*green*); p, posterior subregion (*yellow*); a, anterior subregion (*turquoise*).

(central tibia and central weight-bearing femur taken together; cMFTC) consistently produced greater SRMs than analysis of the entire compartment (medial tibia and weight-bearing medial femur; MFTC).

One important reason why certain subregions do not display a higher sensitivity to change than others is the spatial heterogeneity of the cartilage loss between OA participants. Alignment, for instance, determines the relationship of cartilage loss in the medial versus lateral compartment,[69,101] and the local biomechanical environment (ie, individual joint shape, meniscus lesions, individual neuromuscular control patterns, and others) may be responsible for certain subregions to progress faster than others in certain subjects. Buck and colleagues[146] therefore proposed a novel strategy for more efficiently measuring changes in cartilage thickness in OA, by uncoupling the magnitude of thickness change from the specific anatomic location in which it is measured. The strategy provides ordered values of subregional cartilage thickness change in the medial femorotibial compartment (8 subregions), ranked according to the direction and magnitude of change. In each participant, the subregion with the greatest cartilage loss was assigned to a rank 1, the one with the second greatest cartilage loss to rank 2, and so on, and the subregion with the smallest cartilage loss or with the greatest cartilage thickness increase to rank 8. This grading was performed independently for each subject, and the results for various subcohorts were not only averaged across the subregions but also across the ordered values (ranks). Comparing the rate of change in participants with different radiographic (Kellgren Lawrence; KL) grades,[147] the investigators reported the minimal P value for the differences in 2-year change in medial cartilage thickness of OA participants with medial joint space narrowing (KL grade 3) and healthy reference subjects (KL grade 0) to be 0.001 using the new ordered values approach; 4 ordered medial subregions (ranks) differed significantly between both groups. With the conventional approach, in contrast, only one medial subregion differed significantly between OA participants with medial joint space narrowing and the healthy reference cohort ($P = .037$). The investigators concluded that the novel ordered values approach was more sensitive in detecting cartilage thinning in KL grade 3 versus KL grade 0 participants, and speculated that the new method may be particularly useful in the context of other comparisons, for example, a group treated with a disease-modifying OA drug versus one treated with a placebo.[146]

Correlation of Cartilage Loss with Pain, Clinical Outcome, and Treatment Response

Wluka and colleagues[148] found no significant relationship between baseline pain and tibial cartilage loss over 2 years, but a significant correlation between the increase in symptoms and a reduction in cartilage volume over the observations period. Raynauld and colleagues,[126] in contrast, report a borderline significant relationship between baseline pain and femorotibial cartilage loss over 2 years, but no correlation between the increase in symptoms and a reduction in cartilage volume. A recent study using the OAI cohort did not identify a relationship between pain at baseline and femorotibial cartilage loss the following year.[100]

The rate of change in cartilage volume over 2 years was found to be significantly associated with total knee arthroplasty (TKA) at year 4[149]: For every 1% increase in the rate of cartilage loss there was a 20% increased risk of undergoing TKA. Participants in the highest tertile of tibial cartilage loss had 7.1 higher odds of TKA than those in the lowest tertile. In contrast, radiographic scores of OA did not predict TKA in this study. This finding is important, because it links cartilage loss, as a potential surrogate measure of disease progression, to a clinical outcome, that is, how a patient feels or functions, or how long the knee "survives". Raynauld and colleagues[143] recently reported that licofelone significantly reduced cartilage loss over time, and that MRI was superior to radiographs in demonstrating a structure-modifying effect in this multicenter trial. However, no structure- or disease-modifying OA drug (SMOAD or DMOAD) has yet been approved by regulatory agencies.

Risk Factors of Cartilage Loss

This section focuses exclusively on studies that have reported correlations between risk factors of progression and *quantitative* measures of cartilage morphology, but not those that have relied on SQ or quantitative assessment of joint space width, or increases in SQ MRI scores.

- **High body mass index**[82,100,126,128,132,150–152]
- **Meniscal extrusion and tears/damage**[82,127,128]: Sharma and colleagues[69] found a significant relationship of cartilage loss with meniscal tears, but not with meniscal extrusion. Raynauld and colleagues[61] reported that selecting a subcohort of participants with meniscal tears/extrusion did not improve the ability to identify treatment effects of a potentially structure-modifying drug, because of the larger standard deviation of the change in the participants with meniscal pathology. Meniscal tears were frequently observed in asymptomatic subjects[28,153] and were found to be associated with greater tibial plateau bone area, but not with reduced tibial cartilage volume, in a 2-year longitudinal study.[153]
- **Knee malalignment**[69,89,101,154]: Teichtahl and colleagues[155] showed increasing varus malalignment between baseline and follow-up to be associated with an increase in the rate of medial tibial cartilage loss, whereas it did not significantly affect the rate of loss of the lateral tibia. The investigators concluded that these findings suggest that methods to reduce progression of varus alignment may also delay the progression of medial tibiofemoral OA. Frontal plane knee valgus malalignment also appeared to be correlated with patellar cartilage loss.[156] In a largely nonarthritic cohort, in contrast, no correlation between cartilage loss and malalignment was identified.[157]
- **Advanced radiographic OA**, as evidenced by higher grades of KLG,[147] decreased joint space width, or increased joint space narrowing (JSN)[133]: In contrast, one study found increased cartilage loss with higher baseline cartilage volume[124] stating cartilage loss was greater in the early phase of OA. However, a recent study[158] performed a direct side comparison in participants from the OAI, whereby one symptomatic knee had JSN (OARSI grades 1 to 3) and the contralateral (also symptomatic) knee did not. The investigators found the rate of change and SRM over 1 year to be higher in the JSN knees, the effect becoming even stronger with increasing OARSI JSN grades.
- **Bone marrow alterations**[82,128]: Raynauld and colleagues[61] reported that although BMLs and cysts did not increase significantly in size over 24 months in an OA cohort, there was a significant correlation between size change of bone marrow lesions and cysts with the loss of cartilage volume in the medial femorotibial compartment. A relationship between very large BMLs and lateral tibial cartilage loss was also reported in asymptomatic persons.[159,160]
- **Focal cartilage lesions or defects**, as graded by visual scoring[161,162]: Cartilage defects at baseline appeared to be associated with longitudinal measurement of quantitative cartilage loss in the same compartment in OA subjects, although the second of these 2 studies[162] only found a significant relationship in the femoro-patellar, but not in the femorotibial joint. Other studies reported that the presence of cartilage defects predicted knee cartilage loss also in asymptomatic individuals without radiographic knee OA.[163,164]
- **Denuded areas of bone**: A recent study[133] reported that radiographic markers of advanced OA (JSN and subchondral bone sclerosis), low cartilage thickness at baseline, and particularly denuded areas of bone (dAB) at baseline were

significant predictors of cartilage loss in the affected (medial) compartment. Moreover, denuded areas have been shown to be associated with pain at baseline, and to predict incident pain (in subjects without pain at baseline) over a 2-year follow-up interval, with and without correcting for BMLs.[165,166]

Other factors such as age, sex, pain, function, physical activity levels, synovitis (effusion), sex hormone levels, serum or urine biomarkers, and joint laxity were not consistently found to be associated with cartilage loss as measured quantitatively with MRI, and studies have produced partially contradictory results. Hunter and colleagues[167] studied whether thin cartilage (in the contralateral knee) was a predisposing factor for radiographic OA, but observed no difference in cartilage thickness between premorbid knees (no radiographic change, but radiographic OA in the contralateral knee) and knees of a non-OA subsample. The investigators suggested that the initial pathology in OA may be focal cartilage loss and adjacent swelling, this being consistent with observations by Reichenbach and colleagues,[33] who found that focal cartilage lesions (WORMS scores) discriminate better between normal subjects and those with early radiographic OA than quantitative measures of cartilage thickness.

FUTURE DIRECTIONS

The OAI is a recent large research study jointly sponsored by public institutions such as the National Institutes of Health and the National Institute of Arthritis and Musculoskeletal and Skin Diseases, and the pharmaceutical industry, with almost 5000 participants being studied for a period of 4 years using 3 T MRI (approximately 1500 with symptomatic and radiographic OA and approximately 3500 with risk factors of OA). Year-4 acquisitions have begun and baseline, year-1, and year-2 follow-up MRI data have been made publicly available for substantial parts of the cohort. These results and others of large epidemiologic studies will allow the research community to make rapid progress in understanding the risk factors involved in quantitative cartilage loss and bone changes in OA. Most importantly, it will make it possible to determine which imaging biomarkers best predict clinical outcomes, such as real or virtual TKA, so that these can be used as surrogate measures of disease progression in therapeutic intervention trials.

SUMMARY

With several large, currently ongoing epidemiologic studies, huge amounts of image data are being acquired and, in the case of the OAI, made publicly available. These data will allow the research community ample opportunity to use SQ, quantitative, and compositional MRI assessment to deepen knowledge on risk factors for disease development and progression. In addition, novel analytical approaches will have to be developed to define those subcohorts that will be of relevance for answering specific research questions to increase knowledge on disease progression. As resources are limited, it seems unlikely that in the near future complete assessment of the MRI data sets will become feasible (especially in the OAI). Interdisciplinary collaboration will be crucial in determining which imaging biomarkers will superiorly predict clinical outcomes. Several reliable SQ scoring approaches have been introduced that offer the possibility of whole joint assessment, or assessment of only certain features pertinent to the research focus of a given study. MRI-based SQ and quantitative assessment of knee OA have proved to be a powerful and applicable methodology that has profoundly contributed to the understanding of disease characterization and its natural history.

REFERENCES

1. Eckstein F, Schnier M, Haubner M, et al. Accuracy of cartilage volume and thickness measurements with magnetic resonance imaging. Clin Orthop Relat Res 1998;(352):137–48.
2. Burgkart R, Glaser C, Hyhlik-Durr A, et al. Magnetic resonance imaging-based assessment of cartilage loss in severe osteoarthritis: accuracy, precision, and diagnostic value. Arthritis Rheum 2001;44:2072–7.
3. Cicuttini F, Forbes A, Asbeutah A, et al. Comparison and reproducibility of fast and conventional spoiled gradient-echo magnetic resonance sequences in the determination of knee cartilage volume. J Orthop Res 2000;18:580–4.
4. Gahunia HK, Babyn P, Lemaire C, et al. Osteoarthritis staging: comparison between magnetic resonance imaging, gross pathology and histopathology in the rhesus macaque. Osteoarthritis Cartilage 1995;3:169–80.
5. Broderick LS, Turner DA, Renfrew DL, et al. Severity of articular cartilage abnormality in patients with osteoarthritis: evaluation with fast spin-echo MR vs arthroscopy. AJR Am J Roentgenol 1994;162:99–103.
6. Chan WP, Lang P, Stevens MP, et al. Osteoarthritis of the knee: comparison of radiography, CT, and MR imaging to assess extent and severity. AJR Am J Roentgenol 1991;157:799–806.
7. Blackburn WD Jr, Bernreuter WK, Rominger M, et al. Arthroscopic evaluation of knee articular cartilage: a comparison with plain radiographs and magnetic resonance imaging. J Rheumatol 1994;21:675–9.
8. Burstein D, Bashir A, Gray ML. MRI techniques in early stages of cartilage disease. Invest Radiol 2000;35:622–38.
9. Burstein D, Velyvis J, Scott KT, et al. Protocol issues for delayed Gd(DTPA) (2-)-enhanced MRI (dGEMRIC) for clinical evaluation of articular cartilage. Magn Reson Med 2001;45:36–41.
10. Gray ML, Burstein D, Lesperance LM, et al. Magnetization transfer in cartilage and its constituent macromolecules. Magn Reson Med 1995;34:319–25.
11. Kimelman T, Vu A, Storey P, et al. Three-dimensional T1 mapping for dGEMRIC at 3.0 T using the Look Locker method. Invest Radiol 2006;41:198–203.
12. Sowers MF, Hayes C, Jamadar D, et al. Magnetic resonance-detected subchondral bone marrow and cartilage defect characteristics associated with pain and X-ray-defined knee osteoarthritis. Osteoarthritis Cartilage 2003;11:387–93.
13. Peterfy CG, Guermazi A, Zaim S, et al. Whole-Organ Magnetic Resonance Imaging Score (WORMS) of the knee in osteoarthritis. Osteoarthritis Cartilage 2004;12:177–90.
14. Biswal S, Hastie T, Andriacchi TP, et al. Risk factors for progressive cartilage loss in the knee: a longitudinal magnetic resonance imaging study in forty-three patients. Arthritis Rheum 2002;46:2884–92.
15. Hunter DJ, Zhang YQ, Niu JB, et al. The association of meniscal pathologic changes with cartilage loss in symptomatic knee osteoarthritis. Arthritis Rheum 2006;54:795–801.
16. Zanetti M, Bruder E, Romero J, et al. Bone marrow edema pattern in osteoarthritic knees: correlation between MR imaging and histologic findings. Radiology 2000;215:835–40.

17. Pham XV, Monteiro I, Judet O, et al. Magnetic resonance imaging changes in periarticular soft tissues during flares of medial compartment knee osteoarthritis. Preliminary study in 10 patients. Rev Rhum Engl Ed 1999;66:398–403.
18. Gale DR, Chaisson CE, Totterman SM, et al. Meniscal subluxation: association with osteoarthritis and joint space narrowing. Osteoarthritis Cartilage 1999;7:526–32.
19. Felson DT, Chaisson CE, Hill CL, et al. The association of bone marrow lesions with pain in knee osteoarthritis. Ann Intern Med 2001;134:541–9.
20. Hill CL, Gale DG, Chaisson CE, et al. Knee effusions, popliteal cysts, and synovial thickening: association with knee pain in osteoarthritis. J Rheumatol 2001; 28:1330–7.
21. Kornaat PR, Ceulemans RY, Kroon HM, et al. MRI assessment of knee osteoarthritis: Knee Osteoarthritis Scoring System (KOSS)–inter-observer and intra-observer reproducibility of a compartment-based scoring system. Skeletal Radiol 2005;34:95–102.
22. Hunter DJ, Lo GH, Gale D, et al. The reliability of a new scoring system for knee osteoarthritis MRI and the validity of bone marrow lesion assessment: BLOKS (Boston Leeds Osteoarthritis Knee Score). Ann Rheum Dis 2008;67:206–11.
23. Peterfy CG, White D, Tirman P, et al. Whole-organ evaluation of the knee in osteoarthritis using MRI (abstract). Ann Rheum Dis 1999;38:342.
24. Guermazi A, Hunter DJ, Roemer FW, et al. Magnetic resonance imaging prevalence of different features of knee osteoarthritis in persons with normal knee x-rays. Arhritis Rheum 2007;56(Suppl):S128.
25. Hernandez-Molina G, Neogi T, Hunter DJ, et al. The association of bone attrition with knee pain and other MRI features of osteoarthritis. Ann Rheum Dis 2008;67: 43–7.
26. Felson DT, McLaughlin S, Goggins J, et al. Bone marrow edema and its relation to progression of knee osteoarthritis. Ann Intern Med 2003;139:330–6.
27. Felson DT, Niu J, Guermazi A, et al. Correlation of the development of knee pain with enlarging bone marrow lesions on magnetic resonance imaging. Arthritis Rheum 2007;56:2986–92.
28. Englund M, Guermazi A, Gale D, et al. Incidental meniscal findings on knee MRI in middle-aged and elderly persons. N Engl J Med 2008;359:1108–15.
29. Englund M, Guermazi A, Roemer FW, et al. Meniscal tear in knees without surgery and the development of radiographic osteoarthritis among middle-aged and elderly persons: the Multicenter Osteoarthritis Study. Arthritis Rheum 2009;60:831–9.
30. Hunter DJ, Zhang YQ, Tu X, et al. Change in joint space width: hyaline articular cartilage loss or alteration in meniscus? Arthritis Rheum 2006;54:2488–95.
31. Roemer FW, Guermazi A, Javaid MK, et al. Change in MRI-detected subchondral bone marrow lesions is associated with cartilage loss: the MOST Study. A longitudinal multicentre study of knee osteoarthritis. Ann Rheum Dis 2009; 68:1461–5.
32. Roemer FW, Guermazi A, Hunter DJ, et al. The association of meniscal damage with joint effusion in persons without radiographic osteoarthritis: the Framingham and MOST osteoarthritis studies. Osteoarthritis Cartilage 2009;17:748–53.
33. Reichenbach S, Yang M, Eckstein F, et al. Do cartilage volume or thickness distinguish knees with and without mild radiographic osteoarthritis? The Framingham Study. Ann Rheum Dis 2009; Feb 4th [Epub ahead of print].
34. Hunter DJ, Gerstenfeld L, Bishop G, et al. Bone marrow lesions from osteoarthritis knees are characterized by sclerotic bone that is less well mineralized. Arthritis Res Ther 2009;11:R11.

35. Englund M, Niu J, Guermazi A, et al. Effect of meniscal damage on the development of frequent knee pain, aching, or stiffness. Arthritis Rheum 2007;56: 4048–54.

36. Hernandez-Molina G, Guermazi A, Niu J, et al. Central bone marrow lesions in symptomatic knee osteoarthritis and their relationship to anterior cruciate ligament tears and cartilage loss. Arthritis Rheum 2008;58:130–6.

37. Guermazi A, Roemer FW, Crema MD, et al. Assessment of synovitis in knee osteoarthritis on contrast-enhanced MRI using a novel comprehensive semi-quantitative scoring system. Arthritis Rheum 2008;58:S696–7.

38. Felson DT, Nevitt MC. Blinding images to sequence in osteoarthritis: evidence from other diseases. Osteoarthritis Cartilage 2009;17:281–3.

39. van Der Heijde D, Boonen A, Boers M, et al. Reading radiographs in chronological order, in pairs or as single films has important implications for the discriminative power of rheumatoid arthritis clinical trials. Rheumatology (Oxford) 1999; 38:1213–20.

40. Salaffi F, Carotti M. Interobserver variation in quantitative analysis of hand radiographs in rheumatoid arthritis: comparison of 3 different reading procedures. J Rheumatol 1997;24:2055–6.

41. Ross PD, Huang C, Karpf D, et al. Blinded reading of radiographs increases the frequency of errors in vertebral fracture detection. J Bone Miner Res 1996;11: 1793–800.

42. Bruynesteyn K, Van Der Heijde D, Boers M, et al. Detecting radiological changes in rheumatoid arthritis that are considered important by clinical experts: influence of reading with or without known sequence. J Rheumatol 2002;29:2306–12.

43. Amin S, Guermazi A, Lavalley MP, et al. Complete anterior cruciate ligament tear and the risk for cartilage loss and progression of symptoms in men and women with knee osteoarthritis. Osteoarthritis Cartilage 2008;16:897–902.

44. Reichenbach S, Guermazi A, Niu J, et al. Prevalence of bone attrition on knee radiographs and MRI in a community-based cohort. Osteoarthritis Cartilage 2008;16:1005–10.

45. Hunter DJ, Zhang Y, Niu J, et al. Increase in bone marrow lesions associated with cartilage loss: a longitudinal magnetic resonance imaging study of knee osteoarthritis. Arthritis Rheum 2006;54:1529–35.

46. Fernandez-Madrid F, Karvonen RL, Teitge RA, et al. Synovial thickening detected by MR imaging in osteoarthritis of the knee confirmed by biopsy as synovitis. Magn Reson Imaging 1995;13:177–83.

47. Outerbridge RE. The etiology of chondromalacia patellae. J Bone Joint Surg Br 1961;43:752–7.

48. Noyes FR, Stabler CL. A system for grading articular cartilage lesions at arthroscopy. Am J Sports Med 1989;17:505–13.

49. Sonin AH, Pensy RA, Mulligan ME, et al. Grading articular cartilage of the knee using fast spin-echo proton density-weighted MR imaging without fat suppression. AJR Am J Roentgenol 2002;179:1159–66.

50. Disler DG, McCauley TR, Wirth CR, et al. Detection of knee hyaline cartilage defects using fat-suppressed three-dimensional spoiled gradient-echo MR imaging: comparison with standard MR imaging and correlation with arthroscopy. AJR Am J Roentgenol 1995;165:377–82.

51. Duc SR, Pfirrmann CW, Schmid MR, et al. Articular cartilage defects detected with 3D water-excitation true FISP: prospective comparison with sequences commonly used for knee imaging. Radiology 2007;245:216–23.

52. Ding C, Garnero P, Cicuttini F, et al. Knee cartilage defects: association with early radiographic osteoarthritis, decreased cartilage volume, increased joint surface area and type II collagen breakdown. Osteoarthritis Cartilage 2005;13:198–205.

53. Hill CL, Hunter DJ, Niu J, et al. Synovitis detected on magnetic resonance imaging and its relation to pain and cartilage loss in knee osteoarthritis. Ann Rheum Dis 2007;66:1599–603.

54. Roemer FW, Guermazi A, Zhang Y, et al. Hoffa's fat pad: evaluation on unenhanced MR images as a measure of patellofemoral synovitis in osteoarthritis. AJR Am J Roentgenol 2009;192:1696–700.

55. Saddik D, McNally EG, Richardson M. MRI of Hoffa's fat pad. Skeletal Radiol 2004;33:433–44.

56. Pelletier JP, Raynauld JP, Abram F, et al. A new non-invasive method to assess synovitis severity in relation to symptoms and cartilage volume loss in knee osteoarthritis patients using MRI. Osteoarthritis Cartilage 2008;16(Suppl 3):S8–13.

57. Roemer FW, Hunter DJ, Guermazi A. Semiquantitative assessment of synovitis in osteoarthritis on non contrast-enhanced MRI. Osteoarthritis Cartilage 2009;17: 820–1 [author reply 822–4].

58. Loeuille D, Rat AC, Goebel JC, et al. Magnetic resonance imaging in osteoarthritis: which method best reflects synovial membrane inflammation? Correlations with clinical, macroscopic and microscopic features. Osteoarthritis Cartilage 2009;17:186–92.

59. Bergin D, Keogh C, O'Connell M, et al. Atraumatic medial collateral ligament oedema in medial compartment knee osteoarthritis. Skeletal Radiol 2002;31:14–8.

60. Davies-Tuck ML, Wluka AE, Wang Y, et al. The natural history of cartilage defects in people with knee osteoarthritis. Osteoarthritis Cartilage 2008;16:337–42.

61. Raynauld JP, Martel-Pelletier J, Berthiaume MJ, et al. Correlation between bone lesion changes and cartilage volume loss in patients with osteoarthritis of the knee as assessed by quantitative magnetic resonance imaging over a 24-month period. Ann Rheum Dis 2008;67:683–8.

62. Peterfy CG, Gold G, Eckstein F, et al. MRI protocols for whole-organ assessment of the knee in osteoarthritis. Osteoarthritis Cartilage 2006;14(Suppl A):A95–111.

63. Roemer FW, Guermazi A, Lynch JA, et al. Short tau inversion recovery and proton density-weighted fat suppressed sequences for the evaluation of osteoarthritis of the knee with a 1.0 T dedicated extremity MRI: development of a time-efficient sequence protocol. Eur Radiol 2005;15:978–87.

64. Roemer FW, Zhang Y, Niu J, et al. Tibiofemoral joint osteoarthritis: risk factors for mr-depicted fast cartilage loss over a 30-month period in the multicenter osteoarthritis studies. Radiology 2009;252:772–80.

65. Peterfy CG, Schneider E, Nevitt M. The osteoarthritis initiative: report on the design rationale for the magnetic resonance imaging protocol for the knee. Osteoarthritis Cartilage 2008;16:1433–41.

66. Available at: http://www.oai.ucsf.edu/datarelease/OperationsManuals.asp. Accessed June 13, 2009.

67. Kalichman L, Li L, Kim DH, et al. Facet joint osteoarthritis and low back pain in the community-based population. Spine (Phila Pa 1976) 2008;33:2560–5.

68. Kress I, Mamisch TC, Werlen S, et al. MRI-based morphologic grading system for early hip osteoarthritis. Boston: OARSI Workshop on Imaging-based Measures in Osteoarthritis; 2008 [abstract book, page 40].

69. Sharma L, Eckstein F, Song J, et al. Relationship of meniscal damage, meniscal extrusion, malalignment, and joint laxity to subsequent cartilage loss in osteoarthritic knees. Arthritis Rheum 2008;58:1716–26.

70. Eckstein F, Burstein D, Link TM. Quantitative MRI of cartilage and bone: degenerative changes in osteoarthritis. NMR Biomed 2006;19:822–54.
71. Folkesson J, Dam EB, Olsen OF, et al. Segmenting articular cartilage automatically using a voxel classification approach. IEEE Trans Med Imaging 2007;26:106–15.
72. Folkesson J, Dam E, Olsen OF, et al. Automatic segmentation of the articular cartilage in knee MRI using a hierarchical multi-class classification scheme. Med Image Comput Comput Assist Interv Int Conf Med Image Comput Comput Assist Interv 2005;8:327–34.
73. Pathak SD, Ng L, Wyman B, et al. Quantitative image analysis: software systems in drug development trials. Drug Discov Today 2003;8:451–8.
74. Kauffmann C, Gravel P, Godbout B, et al. Computer-aided method for quantification of cartilage thickness and volume changes using MRI: validation study using a synthetic model. IEEE Trans Biomed Eng 2003;50:978–88.
75. Cashman PM, Kitney RI, Gariba MA, et al. Automated techniques for visualization and mapping of articular cartilage in MR images of the osteoarthritic knee: a base technique for the assessment of microdamage and submicro damage. IEEE Trans Nanobioscience 2002;1:42–51.
76. Lynch JA, Zaim S, Zhao J, et al. Cartilage segmentation of 3D MRI scans of the osteoarthritic knee combining user knowledge and active contours. Proc SPIE 2000;3979:925–35.
77. Cohen ZA, McCarthy DM, Kwak SD, et al. Knee cartilage topography, thickness, and contact areas from MRI: in-vitro calibration and in-vivo measurements. Osteoarthritis Cartilage 1999;7:95–109.
78. Stammberger T, Eckstein F, Michaelis M, et al. Interobserver reproducibility of quantitative cartilage measurements: comparison of B-spline snakes and manual segmentation. Magn Reson Imaging 1999;17:1033–42.
79. Solloway S, Hutchinson CE, Waterton JC, et al. The use of active shape models for making thickness measurements of articular cartilage from MR images. Magn Reson Med 1997;37:943–52.
80. McWalter EJ, Wirth W, Siebert M, et al. Use of novel interactive input devices for segmentation of articular cartilage from magnetic resonance images. Osteoarthritis Cartilage 2005;13:48–53.
81. Wirth W, Eckstein F. A technique for regional analysis of femorotibial cartilage thickness based on quantitative magnetic resonance imaging. IEEE Trans Med Imaging 2008;27:737–44.
82. Pelletier JP, Raynauld JP, Berthiaume MJ, et al. Risk factors associated with the loss of cartilage volume on weight-bearing areas in knee osteoarthritis patients assessed by quantitative magnetic resonance imaging: a longitudinal study. Arthritis Res Ther 2007;9:R74.
83. Koo S, Gold GE, Andriacchi TP. Considerations in measuring cartilage thickness using MRI: factors influencing reproducibility and accuracy. Osteoarthritis Cartilage 2005;13:782–9.
84. Qazi AA, Folkesson J, Pettersen PC, et al. Separation of healthy and early osteoarthritis by automatic quantification of cartilage homogeneity. Osteoarthritis Cartilage 2007;15:1199–206.
85. Hohe J, Faber S, Stammberger T, et al. A technique for 3D in vivo quantification of proton density and magnetization transfer coefficients of knee joint cartilage. Osteoarthritis Cartilage 2000;8:426–33.
86. Hohe J, Faber S, Muehlbauer R, et al. Three-dimensional analysis and visualization of regional MR signal intensity distribution of articular cartilage. Med Eng Phys 2002;24:219–27.

87. Eckstein F, Ateshian G, Burgkart R, et al. Proposal for a nomenclature for magnetic resonance imaging based measures of articular cartilage in osteoarthritis. Osteoarthritis Cartilage 2006;14:974–83.
88. Burgkart R, Glaser C, Hinterwimmer S, et al. Feasibility of T and Z scores from magnetic resonance imaging data for quantification of cartilage loss in osteoarthritis. Arthritis Rheum 2003;48:2829–35.
89. Eisenhart-Rothe RV, Graichen H, Hudelmaier M, et al. Femorotibial and patellar cartilage loss in patients prior to total knee arthroplasty, heterogeneity, and correlation with alignment of the knee. Ann Rheum Dis 2006;65(1):69–73.
90. Otterness IG, Eckstein F. Women have thinner cartilage and smaller joint surfaces than men after adjustment for body height and weight. Osteoarthritis Cartilage 2007;15:666–72.
91. Wang Y, Ding C, Wluka AE, et al. Factors affecting progression of knee cartilage defects in normal subjects over 2 years. Rheumatology (Oxford) 2006;45:79–84.
92. Eckstein F, Buck RJ, Burstein D, et al. Precision of 3.0 Tesla quantitative magnetic resonance imaging of cartilage morphology in a multicentre clinical trial. Ann Rheum Dis 2008;67:1683–8.
93. Eckstein F, Hudelmaier M, Cahue S, et al. Medial-to-lateral ratio of tibiofemoral subchondral bone area is adapted to alignment and mechanical load. Calcif Tissue Int 2009;84:186–94.
94. Cohen ZA, Mow VC, Henry JH, et al. Templates of the cartilage layers of the patellofemoral joint and their use in the assessment of osteoarthritic cartilage damage. Osteoarthritis Cartilage 2003;11:569–79.
95. Buck R, Wyman B, Hellio Le Graverand-Gastineau MP, et al. An efficient subset of morphological measures for articular cartilage in the healthy and diseased human knee. Magn Reson Med 2009; conditionally accepted for publication.
96. Hudelmaier M, Glaser C, Hohe J, et al. Age-related changes in the morphology and deformational behavior of knee joint cartilage. Arthritis Rheum 2001;44: 2556–61.
97. Eckstein F, Reiser M, Englmeier KH, et al. In vivo morphometry and functional analysis of human articular cartilage with quantitative magnetic resonance imaging—from image to data, from data to theory. Anat Embryol (Berl) 2001; 203:147–73.
98. Beattie KA, Duryea J, Pui M, et al. Minimum joint space width and tibial cartilage morphology in the knees of healthy individuals: a cross-sectional study. BMC Musculoskelet Disord 2008;9:119.
99. Tameem HZ, Selva LE, Sinha US. Morphological atlases of knee cartilage: shape indices to analyze cartilage degradation in osteoarthritic and non-osteoarthritic population. Conf Proc IEEE Eng Med Biol Soc 2007;2007:1310–3.
100. Eckstein F, Maschek S, Wirth W, et al. One year change of knee cartilage morphology in the first release of participants from the Osteoarthritis Initiative progression subcohort: association with sex, body mass index, symptoms and radiographic osteoarthritis status. Ann Rheum Dis 2009;68:674–9.
101. Eckstein F, Wirth W, Hudelmaier M, et al. Patterns of femorotibial cartilage loss in knees with neutral, varus, and valgus alignment. Arthritis Rheum 2008;59: 1563–70.
102. Hunter DJ, Niu J, Zhang Y, et al. Change in cartilage morphometry: a sample of the progression cohort of the Osteoarthritis Initiative. Ann Rheum Dis 2009;68: 349–56.
103. Raynauld JP, Martel-Pelletier J, Abram F, et al. Analysis of the precision and sensitivity to change of different approaches to assess cartilage loss by

quantitative MRI in a longitudinal multicentre clinical trial in patients with knee osteoarthritis. Arthritis Res Ther 2008;10:R129.

104. Hohe J, Ateshian G, Reiser M, et al. Surface size, curvature analysis, and assessment of knee joint incongruity with MRI in vivo. Magn Reson Med 2002;47:554–61.

105. Dam EB, Folkesson J, Pettersen PC, et al. Automatic morphometric cartilage quantification in the medial tibial plateau from MRI for osteoarthritis grading. Osteoarthritis Cartilage 2007;15:808–18.

106. Folkesson J, Dam EB, Olsen OF, et al. Accuracy evaluation of automatic quantification of the articular cartilage surface curvature from MRI. Acad Radiol 2007; 14:1221–8.

107. Folkesson J, Dam EB, Olsen OF, et al. Automatic quantification of local and global articular cartilage surface curvature: biomarkers for osteoarthritis? Magn Reson Med 2008;59:1340–6.

108. Qazi AA, Dam EB, Nielsen M, et al. Osteoarthritic cartilage is more homogeneous than healthy cartilage: identification of a superior region of interest colocalized with a major risk factor for osteoarthritis. Acad Radiol 2007;14:1209–20.

109. Gray ML, Eckstein F, Peterfy C, et al. Toward imaging biomarkers for osteoarthritis. Clin Orthop Relat Res 2004;(427 Suppl):S175–81.

110. Mosher TJ, Dardzinski BJ. Cartilage MRI T2 relaxation time mapping: overview and applications. Semin Musculoskelet Radiol 2004;8:355–68.

111. Eckstein F, Cicuttini F, Raynauld JP, et al. Magnetic resonance imaging (MRI) of articular cartilage in knee osteoarthritis (OA): morphological assessment. Osteoarthritis Cartilage 2006;14(Suppl A):A46–75.

112. Eckstein F, Hudelmaier M, Putz R. The effects of exercise on human articular cartilage. J Anat 2006;208:491–512.

113. Gold GE, Burstein D, Dardzinski B, et al. MRI of articular cartilage in OA: novel pulse sequences and compositional/functional markers. Osteoarthritis Cartilage 2006;14(Suppl A):A76–86.

114. Mosher TJ. Musculoskeletal imaging at 3T: current techniques and future applications. Magn Reson Imaging Clin N Am 2006;14:63–76.

115. Burstein D. MRI for development of disease-modifying osteoarthritis drugs. NMR Biomed 2006;19:669–80.

116. Hardy PA, Recht MP, Piraino D, et al. Optimization of a dual echo in the steady state (DESS) free-precession sequence for imaging cartilage. J Magn Reson Imaging 1996;6:329–35.

117. Eckstein F, Hudelmaier M, Wirth W, et al. Double echo steady state magnetic resonance imaging of knee articular cartilage at 3 Tesla: a pilot study for the Osteoarthritis Initiative. Ann Rheum Dis 2006;65:433–41.

118. Eckstein F, Kunz M, Hudelmaier M, et al. Impact of coil design on the contrast-to-noise ratio, precision, and consistency of quantitative cartilage morphometry at 3 Tesla: a pilot study for the osteoarthritis initiative. Magn Reson Med 2007;57: 448–54.

119. Eckstein F, Kunz M, Schutzer M, et al. Two year longitudinal change and test-retest-precision of knee cartilage morphology in a pilot study for the osteoarthritis initiative. Osteoarthritis Cartilage 2007;15:1326–32.

120. Inglis D, Pui M, Ioannidis G, et al. Accuracy and test-retest precision of quantitative cartilage morphology on a 1.0 T peripheral magnetic resonance imaging system. Osteoarthritis Cartilage 2007;15:110–5.

121. Eckstein F, Charles HC, Buck RJ, et al. Accuracy and precision of quantitative assessment of cartilage morphology by magnetic resonance imaging at 3.0T. Arthritis Rheum 2005;52:3132–6.

122. Schneider E, NessAiver M, White D, et al. The osteoarthritis initiative (OAI) magnetic resonance imaging quality assurance methods and results. Osteoarthritis Cartilage 2008;16:994–1004.
123. Gandy SJ, Dieppe PA, Keen MC, et al. No loss of cartilage volume over three years in patients with knee osteoarthritis as assessed by magnetic resonance imaging. Osteoarthritis Cartilage 2002;10:929–37.
124. Wluka AE, Stuckey S, Snaddon J, et al. The determinants of change in tibial cartilage volume in osteoarthritic knees. Arthritis Rheum 2002;46: 2065–72.
125. Cicuttini FM, Wluka AE, Wang Y, et al. Longitudinal study of changes in tibial and femoral cartilage in knee osteoarthritis. Arthritis Rheum 2004;50:94–7.
126. Raynauld JP, Martel-Pelletier J, Berthiaume MJ, et al. Quantitative magnetic resonance imaging evaluation of knee osteoarthritis progression over two years and correlation with clinical symptoms and radiologic changes. Arthritis Rheum 2004;50:476–87.
127. Berthiaume MJ, Raynauld JP, Martel-Pelletier J, et al. Meniscal tear and extrusion are strongly associated with progression of symptomatic knee osteoarthritis as assessed by quantitative magnetic resonance imaging. Ann Rheum Dis 2005;64:556–63.
128. Raynauld JP, Martel-Pelletier J, Berthiaume MJ, et al. Long term evaluation of disease progression through the quantitative magnetic resonance imaging of symptomatic knee osteoarthritis patients: correlation with clinical symptoms and radiographic changes. Arthritis Res Ther 2006;8:R21.
129. Wluka AE, Forbes A, Wang Y, et al. Knee cartilage loss in symptomatic knee osteoarthritis over 4.5 years. Arthritis Res Ther 2006;8:R90.
130. Bruyere O, Genant H, Kothari M, et al. Longitudinal study of magnetic resonance imaging and standard X-rays to assess disease progression in osteoarthritis. Osteoarthritis Cartilage 2007;15:98–103.
131. Graverand MPHL, Buck RJ, Wyman BT, et al. Change in regional cartilage morphology and joint space width in osteoarthritis participants versus healthy controls—a multicenter study using 3.0 Tesla MRI and Lyon Schuss radiography. Ann Rheum Dis 2008 Dec 22nd [Epub ahead of print].
132. Wirth W, Hellio Le Graverand MP, Wyman BT, et al. Regional analysis of femorotibial cartilage loss in a subsample from the Osteoarthritis Initiative progression subcohort. Osteoarthritis Cartilage 2009;17:291–7.
133. Eckstein F, Wirth W, Hudelmaier MI, et al. Relationship of compartment-specific structural knee status at baseline with change in cartilage morphology: a prospective observational study using data from the osteoarthritis initiative. Arthritis Res Ther 2009;11:R90.
134. Guermazi A, Burstein D, Conaghan P, et al. Imaging in osteoarthritis. Rheum Dis Clin North Am 2008;34:645–87.
135. Raynauld JP, Kauffmann C, Beaudoin G, et al. Reliability of a quantification imaging system using magnetic resonance images to measure cartilage thickness and volume in human normal and osteoarthritic knees. Osteoarthritis Cartilage 2003;11:351–60.
136. Frobell RB, Le Graverand MP, Buck R, et al. The acutely ACL injured knee assessed by MRI: changes in joint fluid, bone marrow lesions, and cartilage during the first year. Osteoarthritis Cartilage 2009;17:161–7.
137. Watson PJ, Carpenter TA, Hall LD, et al. Cartilage swelling and loss in a spontaneous model of osteoarthritis visualized by magnetic resonance imaging. Osteoarthritis Cartilage 1996;4:197–207.

138. Calvo E, Palacios I, Delgado E, et al. High-resolution MRI detects cartilage swelling at the early stages of experimental osteoarthritis. Osteoarthritis Cartilage 2001;9:463–72.

139. Calvo E, Palacios I, Delgado E, et al. Histopathological correlation of cartilage swelling detected by magnetic resonance imaging in early experimental osteoarthritis. Osteoarthritis Cartilage 2004;12:878–86.

140. Vignon E, Arlot M, Hartmann D, et al. Hypertrophic repair of articular cartilage in experimental osteoarthrosis. Ann Rheum Dis 1983;42:82–8.

141. Adams ME, Brandt KD. Hypertrophic repair of canine articular cartilage in osteoarthritis after anterior cruciate ligament transection. J Rheumatol 1991; 18:428–35.

142. Cicuttini F, Hankin J, Jones G, et al. Comparison of conventional standing knee radiographs and magnetic resonance imaging in assessing progression of tibiofemoral joint osteoarthritis. Osteoarthritis Cartilage 2005;13:722–7.

143. Raynauld JP, Martel-Pelletier J, Bias P, et al. Protective effects of licofelone, a 5-lipoxygenase and cyclo-oxygenase inhibitor, versus naproxen on cartilage loss in knee osteoarthritis: a first multicentre clinical trial using quantitative MRI. Ann Rheum Dis 2009;68:938–47.

144. Adams JG, McAlindon T, Dimasi M, et al. Contribution of meniscal extrusion and cartilage loss to joint space narrowing in osteoarthritis. Clin Radiol 1999;54: 502–6.

145. Eckstein F, Guermazi A, Roemer FW. Quantitative MR imaging of cartilage and trabecular bone in osteoarthritis. Radiol Clin North Am 2009;47:655–73.

146. Buck RJ, Wyman BT, Le Graverand MP, et al. Does the use of ordered values of subregional change in cartilage thickness improve the detection of disease progression in longitudinal studies of osteoarthritis? Arthritis Rheum 2009;61:917–24.

147. Kellgren JH, Lawrence JS. Radiological assessment of osteo-arthrosis. Ann Rheum Dis 1957;16:494–502.

148. Wluka AE, Wolfe R, Stuckey S, et al. How does tibial cartilage volume relate to symptoms in subjects with knee osteoarthritis? Ann Rheum Dis 2004;63:264–8.

149. Cicuttini FM, Jones G, Forbes A, et al. Rate of cartilage loss at two years predicts subsequent total knee arthroplasty: a prospective study. Ann Rheum Dis 2004;63:1124–7.

150. Cicuttini F, Wluka A, Wang Y, et al. The determinants of change in patella cartilage volume in osteoarthritic knees. J Rheumatol 2002;29:2615–9.

151. Cicuttini FM, Wluka A, Bailey M, et al. Factors affecting knee cartilage volume in healthy men. Rheumatology (Oxford) 2003;42:258–62.

152. Teichtahl AJ, Wluka AE, Wang Y, et al. Obesity and adiposity are associated with the rate of patella cartilage volume loss over 2 years in adults without knee osteoarthritis. Ann Rheum Dis 2009;68:909–13.

153. Davies-Tuck ML, Martel-Pelletier J, Wluka AE, et al. Meniscal tear and increased tibial plateau bone area in healthy post-menopausal women. Osteoarthritis Cartilage 2008;16:268–71.

154. Cicuttini F, Wluka A, Hankin J, et al. Longitudinal study of the relationship between knee angle and tibiofemoral cartilage volume in subjects with knee osteoarthritis. Rheumatology (Oxford) 2004;43:321–4.

155. Teichtahl AJ, Davies-Tuck ML, Wluka AE, et al. Change in knee angle influences the rate of medial tibial cartilage volume loss in knee osteoarthritis. Osteoarthritis Cartilage 2009;17:8–11.

156. Teichtahl AJ, Wluka AE, Cicuttini FM. Frontal plane knee alignment is associated with a longitudinal reduction in patella cartilage volume in people with knee osteoarthritis. Osteoarthritis Cartilage 2008;16:851–4.

157. Zhai G, Ding C, Cicuttini F, et al. A longitudinal study of the association between knee alignment and change in cartilage volume and chondral defects in a largely nonosteoarthritic population. J Rheumatol 2007;34:181–6.

158. Eckstein F, Benichou O, Wirth W, et al. Magnetic resonance imaging-based cartilage loss in painful contralateral knees with and without radiographic joint space narrowing: Data from the Osteoarthritis Initiative (OAI). Arthritis Rheum, in press.

159. Wluka AE, Hanna F, Davies-Tuck M, et al. Bone marrow lesions predict increase in knee cartilage defects and loss of cartilage volume in middle-aged women without knee pain over 2 years. Ann Rheum Dis 2009;68:850–5.

160. Wluka AE, Wang Y, Davies-Tuck M, et al. Bone marrow lesions predict progression of cartilage defects and loss of cartilage volume in healthy middle-aged adults without knee pain over 2 yrs. Rheumatology (Oxford) 2008;47:1392–6.

161. Ding C, Cicuttini F, Scott F, et al. Association of prevalent and incident knee cartilage defects with loss of tibial and patellar cartilage: a longitudinal study. Arthritis Rheum 2005;52:3918–27.

162. Wluka AE, Ding C, Jones G, et al. The clinical correlates of articular cartilage defects in symptomatic knee osteoarthritis: a prospective study. Rheumatology (Oxford) 2005;44:1311–6.

163. Cicuttini F, Ding C, Wluka A, et al. Association of cartilage defects with loss of knee cartilage in healthy, middle-age adults: a prospective study. Arthritis Rheum 2005;52:2033–9.

164. Ding C, Martel-Pelletier J, Pelletier JP, et al. Two-year prospective longitudinal study exploring the factors associated with change in femoral cartilage volume in a cohort largely without knee radiographic osteoarthritis. Osteoarthritis Cartilage 2008;16:443–9.

165. Moisio KC, Eckstein F, Song J, et al. The relationship of denuded subchondral bone area to knee pain severity and incident frequent knee pain [abstract]. Osteoarthritis Cartilage 2008;16(Suppl 4):S31.

166. Moisio K, Eckstein F, Chmiel JS, et al. Denuded subchondral bone and knee pain in persons with knee osteoarthritis. Arthritis Rheum, in press.

167. Hunter DJ, Niu JB, Zhang Y, et al. Premorbid knee osteoarthritis is not characterised by diffuse thinness: the Framingham Osteoarthritis Study. Ann Rheum Dis 2008;67:1545–9.

Magnetic Resonance Imaging Assessment of Subchondral Bone and Soft Tissues in Knee Osteoarthritis

Michel D. Crema, MD[a,b,c,d,*], Frank W. Roemer, MD[a,b,e],
Monica D. Marra, MD[a,b,c], Ali Guermazi, MD[a,b]

KEYWORDS

- Knee • Osteoarthritis • Magnetic Resonance Imaging
- Bone marrow lesions • Synovitis

Knee osteoarthritis (OA) is a disease of the whole joint including not only the hyaline articular cartilage, but also the subchondral bone, synovium, menisci, and ligaments.[1] For decades, radiography has been the main imaging tool to assess osteoarthritic knees.[2,3] Conventional radiography, however, is only able to depict the osseous joint structures. With magnetic resonance imaging (MRI) now widely available, a major paradigm shift has occurred in highlighting the importance of other tissues than bone. Furthermore, hyaline cartilage has no innervation,[4] and sources of pain in patients with knee OA may include the intrinsic joint structures mentioned already, and periarticular structures such as bursae.[5] This article discusses the role of MRI assessment of the subchondral bone, synovium, ligaments, and other soft tissues in patients with knee OA, focusing on available information on semiquantitative assessment of pathology of these tissues using MRI. Additionally, the role of these alterations in predicting pain and structural progression is discussed.

A version of this article originally appeared in the 47:4 issue of Radiologic Clinics of North America.

[a] Department of Radiology, Quantitative Imaging Center, Boston University School of Medicine, 820 Harrison Avenue, FGH Building, 3rd Floor, Boston, MA 02118, USA

[b] Boston Imaging Core Lab (BICL), 580 Harrison Avenue, 4th Floor, Boston, MA 02118, USA

[c] Institute of Diagnostic Imaging (IDI), 456 Avenida Saudade, Ribeirão Preto, SP 14085-000, Brazil

[d] Division of Radiology, Department of Internal Medicine, Ribeirão Preto School of Medicine, University of São Paulo, 3900 Avenida Bandeirantes, Ribeirão Preto, SP 14049-900, Brazil

[e] Department of Radiology, Klinikum Augsburg, 2 Steglinstrasse, Augsburg 86156, Germany

* Corresponding author. Department of Radiology, Quantitative Imaging Center, Boston University School of Medicine, 820 Harrison Avenue, FGH Building, 3rd Floor, Boston, MA 02118, USA

E-mail address: michelcrema@gmail.com (M.D. Crema).

Rheum Dis Clin N Am 35 (2009) 557–577
doi:10.1016/j.rdc.2009.08.003
0889-857X/09/$ – see front matter © 2009 Elsevier Inc. All rights reserved.

rheumatic.theclinics.com

SUBCHONDRAL BONE ALTERATIONS
Bone Marrow Edema-like Lesions

Bone marrow edema-like lesions (BMLs) are defined on MRI as noncystic subchondral areas of ill-defined hyperintensity on proton density-weighted, intermediate-weighted, T2-weighted or short tau inversion recovery (STIR) sequences and hypointensity on T1-weighted spin echo images (**Fig. 1**).[6–9] MRI assessment of BMLs should be performed only on such sequences, as gradient recalled echo (GRE)-type sequences such as spoiled gradient echo at a steady state (SPGR), fast low angle shot (FLASH), 3-point Dixon, double echo steady state (DESS) and others are insensitive to marrow abnormality, and may lead to underestimation of size of BMLs (**Fig. 2**).[9–11] BMLs may be accurately assessed and quantified using appropriate MRI sequences.[12,13] It is important to distinguish degenerative BMLs from other marrow alterations of traumatic or nontraumatic origin.[14] These degenerative lesions frequently are detected in conjunction with cartilage damage in the same region.[15,16] BMLs play an important role in predicting structural progression and pain incidence and fluctuation of symptoms.[17–22] Histologically, edema appears to be only a minor constituent of these abnormalities, mainly represented by bone marrow necrosis, fibrosis, and trabecular abnormalities.[6,23]

BMLs represent a highly variable feature in patients with or at risk for development of knee OA, as their size may increase or decrease over time.[18–20,24] Mechanical limb alignment is thought to directly affect location, prevalence, and change in BMLs.[21] Furthermore, these lesions are associated with concomitant increased local bone density, suggesting that they may be secondary to long-term excess loading.[25]

Many studies have evaluated the role of BMLs in the progression of knee OA. Felson and colleagues[21] demonstrated that BMLs are powerful predictors of risk of local structural deterioration with radiographic evaluation. The fluctuation of BML size over time seems to have a direct effect on progression of disease assessed on

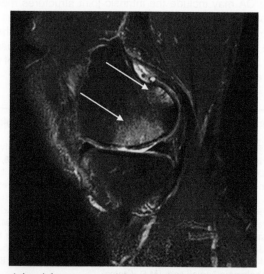

Fig. 1. Sagittal T2-weighted fat-suppressed (T2wFS) MRI shows a typical BML: subchondral ill-defined areas of high signal intensity located in the medial femoral condyle (*arrows*). Note adjacent irregular thinning of the articular cartilage in the weight-bearing region of the femur.

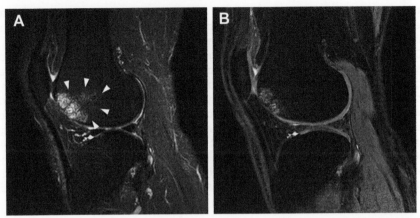

Fig. 2. Subchondral BML located in the lateral femoral trochlea. (*A*) T2wFS MRI demonstrates the full extension of the lesion (*arrowheads*). (*B*) Three-dimensional water excitation DESS MRI at the same level clearly underestimates the size of this lesion, but shows clearly the cystic parts of the lesion.

a subregional basis. Roemer and colleagues[19] showed that subregions with incident and progressive BMLs demonstrate a higher risk of cartilage loss. Hunter and colleagues[20] demonstrated that, compared with stable BMLs, enlarging lesions were strongly associated with cartilage loss at follow-up. Another type of BML includes those localized in areas uncovered by articular cartilage, such as the interspinous region at the tibia and the femoral notch. These lesions, known as traction or insertional BMLs, are highly associated with anterior cruciate ligament tears, and may be a consequence of tensile stress on these ligaments (**Fig. 3**).[26] No relationship

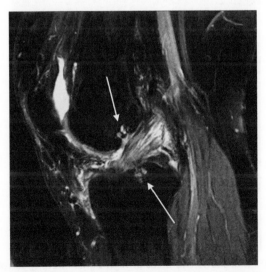

Fig. 3. Sagittal T2wFS MRI depicts a partially ruptured anterior cruciate ligament (ACL). Note associated traction BMLs adjacent to the ligament's insertions at the femur and tibia (*arrows*).

between lesions at the interspinous region and femoral notch and cartilage loss has been demonstrated so far.[26] Lesions extending to the subchondral bone of the medial tibial plateau, however, are associated with regional cartilage loss.

Data about the role of BMLs in predicting pain in patients with knee OA are controversial. In a cross-sectional study, Felson and colleagues[17] demonstrated that subjects with radiographic knee OA and pain were more likely to have BMLs than subjects without pain. In a longitudinal study evaluating the relationship between fluctuation of BMLs and knee pain, Felson and colleagues[18] found that individuals without frequent knee pain who developed knee pain at follow-up were more likely to show an increase in BML size. In contrast, Kornaat and colleagues[24] found in a longitudinal study that changes in BMLs did not correlate with severity of pain measured using the Western Ontario and McMaster Universities (WOMAC) score. Sowers and colleagues[27] found that frequency of BMLs was similar in both painful and painless knee OA, but larger BMLs were seen more frequently in subjects with pain.

Subchondral Cyst-like Lesions

Subchondral cyst-like lesions have a characteristic appearance on MRI, demonstrating well-defined rounded areas of fluid-like signal intensity on nonenhanced imaging (**Fig. 4**).[6,28]

The term "subchondral cyst-like lesion" is probably more appropriate than "subchondral cyst," as no evidence of epithelial lining was detected in several histologic studies.[28–31] The etiology of subchondral cyst-like lesions is unknown. Two principal theories have been proposed, the synovial fluid intrusion and the bony contusion theories. The synovial fluid intrusion theory suggests that elevated intra-articular pressure may lead to the intrusion of joint fluid into the subchondral bone via fissured or ulcerated cartilage.[29,32] The bony contusion theory suggests that subchondral cyst-like

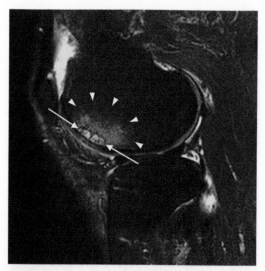

Fig. 4. Sagittal T2wFS MRI shows two areas of high signal intensity surrounded by a well-demarcated hypointense rim (*arrows*), representing subchondral cyst-like signal alterations. These are located directly subchondrally and are part of an ill-defined larger BML (*arrowheads*) in the lateral trochlea. Note intact adjacent cartilage.

lesions are a consequence of traumatic bone necrosis following impact of two opposing articular surfaces.[30,33]

A recent cross-sectional study reported that subchondral cyst-like lesions were present in subregions without full thickness cartilage defects in about half of the cases, a finding that does not support the synovial fluid intrusion theory.[34] Subchondral cysts are strongly associated with BMLs in the same subregion, and may develop within areas of noncystic BMLs.[34,35] This favors the bony contusion theory.

Two studies have found no association between the presence of subchondral cyst-like lesions and pain in subjects with knee OA.[36,37]

Subchondral Bone Attrition

Subchondral bone attrition is defined as depression or flattening of the subchondral bony surface unrelated to gross fracture. It can be assessed on radiographs or semi-quantitatively on MRI (**Fig. 5**).[12,38] Although attrition usually is observed in advanced knee OA, it also may appear in knees with mild OA that do not exhibit joint space narrowing on radiographs.[39]

The pathogenesis of subchondral bone attrition in knee OA is unknown. Subchondral microfracturing and remodeling caused by alterations in mechanical loading, which are reflected as subchondral BMLs, may explain the presence and development of bone attrition in OA. A strong association between prevalent subchondral bone attrition and subchondral BMLs in the same subregion has been reported, and the association increased with BML size.[40] Furthermore, the risk of incident subchondral bone attrition was elevated for subregions presenting baseline BMLs. Neogi and

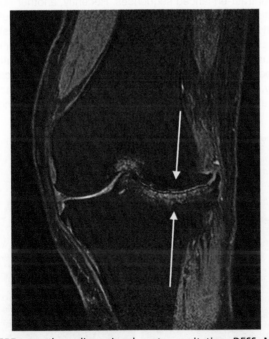

Fig. 5. Coronal GRE-type three-dimensional water excitation DESS MRI shows severe subchondral bone attrition in the lateral tibiofemoral compartment with flattening of the lateral femoral articular surface and depression of the lateral tibial plateau (*arrows*). Note also adjacent osteophytes.

colleagues[41] showed that both prevalence and incidence of subchondral bone attrition are associated with knee malalignment, suggesting that attrition is a reflection of compartment-specific mechanical load. The same group[42] found that subchondral bone attrition is a good predictor of cartilage loss.

Attrition seems to play a role in predicting knee pain. In a recent cross-sectional study, Hernandez-Molina and colleagues[43] demonstrated that bone attrition is associated with knee pain. Other studies have also suggested that subchondral bone attrition predicts knee pain.[37,38]

SYNOVITIS

Although synovitis in OA is thought to be a secondary phenomenon related to cartilage deterioration, its importance in the OA process is recognized.[44–49] Degenerative joints usually demonstrate signs of synovitis, even in the early phase of disease.[50–52]

Several methods for detecting and quantifying synovitis with nonenhanced and contrast-enhanced MRI are available. In a pathologic study conducted by Fernandez-Madrid and colleagues[51] signal alterations in the Hoffa's fat pad correlated with mild chronic synovitis. This work led to the assumption that synovitis may be assessed on nonenhanced images, mainly on proton density- or T2-weighted sequences, using signal alterations in the Hoffa's fat pad as a surrogate for whole-knee synovitis (**Fig. 6**).[45,46] Signal alterations in Hoffa's fat pad are a common finding on MRI of the knee and present a multitude of possible diagnoses (**Fig. 7**).[53] Roemer and colleagues[54] found that signal alterations in Hoffa's fat pad seen on noncontrast-enhanced sequences were a sensitive but not a specific sign of peripatellar synovitis, compared with contrast-enhanced sequences. Recently, another scoring system for assessing synovitis using nonenhanced scans was introduced,[55] but it has not been tested against an established reference standard such as contrast-enhanced MRI or histology.[56] In a recent study comparing three scoring systems for evaluating synovitis and joint effusion on MRI, Loeuille and colleagues[57] found that only scoring of contrast-enhanced T1-weighted images correlated with microscopically proven synovitis. Thus, ideally, synovitis should be assessed on contrast-enhanced T1-weighted MRI sequences, allowing evaluation of enhancement and thickening of the synovial

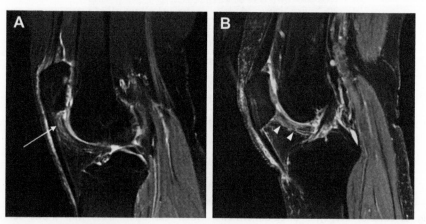

Fig. 6. Sagittal T2wFS MRIs depict signal alterations in the infrapatellar (*arrow—A*) and intercondylar (*arrowheads—B*) regions of Hoffa's fat pad. These are used as a surrogate for peripatellar synovitis in osteoarthritis trials.

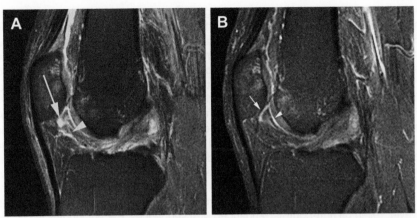

Fig. 7. Example of overestimation using signal changes in Hoffa's fat pad on nonenhanced images as a surrogate for synovitis. (*A*) Sagittal proton density-weighted fat-suppressed (PDwFS) image. Grade 2 infrapatellar signal change (*large arrow*) and grade 2 intercondylar signal change (*large arrowhead*). (*B*) Sagittal contrast-enhanced T1-weighted fat-suppressed (CE T1wFS) image. Discrete grade 1 infrapatellar signal change (*enhancement—small arrow*) and discrete grade 1 intercondylar signal change (*enhancement—small arrowhead*).

membrane (**Fig. 8**).[58–60] A new scoring system that uses contrast-enhanced T1-weighted sequences to assess synovitis at multiple sites in patients with knee OA was presented recently.[49] The reliability of the reading was good to excellent for the 11 different synovitis locations.

There is evidence that synovitis is not only a secondary phenomenon in patients with knee OA but that it also plays a role in progression of cartilage loss. In a longitudinal

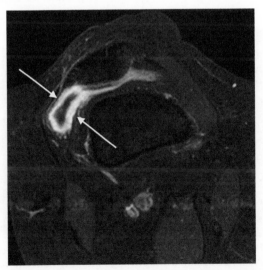

Fig. 8. CE T1wFS MRI demonstrates marked thickening and enhancement of the synovial membrane in the lateral parapatellar region. Note the adjacent low signal intensity of the joint fluid well distinguished from the thickened synovium (*arrows*).

study with 422 subjects, Ayral and colleagues[47] assessed the medial perimeniscal synovium and the medial tibiofemoral cartilage using arthroscopy, and found that 123 subjects (29%) had a reactive aspect, and 89 (21%) had an inflammatory aspect of the synovium. Interestingly, only the inflammatory synovitis group showed an association with cartilage loss at follow-up. Although histologic evaluation was not performed, previous studies have demonstrated a good correlation between arthroscopic and microscopic findings of synovitis.[61,62]

Synovial inflammation is believed to contribute to pain in patients with knee OA, even though nociceptive fibers are inconsistently present within the synovial membrane.[4] Hill and colleagues[46] showed that alterations in Hoffa's fat pad signal changes over time were modestly and directly correlated with changes in knee pain, but not with cartilage loss. In another cross-sectional study, the same group found that these alterations were far more common in subjects with knee pain and radiographic OA than those with radiographic OA and no pain.[45] Both studies, however, relied on non-contrast-enhanced MRI sequences. Recent studies assessing synovitis on contrast-enhanced MRI in subjects with or at risk for knee OA demonstrated that high-grade synovitis (graded from 0 to 2) was associated with knee pain compared with no or low-grade synovitis.[48,49]

EFFUSION

Joint effusion is detected commonly in patients with moderate-to-advanced knee OA,[45,63] and it reflects synovial activation secondary to ligament injury, loose bodies, hyaline cartilage deterioration, and meniscal damage.[64] Joint effusion ideally is assessed and quantified on proton density-weighted, T2-weighted and STIR MRI sequences.[12,13] Synovial thickening as seen in synovitis, however, increases the total synovial volume in such sequences, and differentiating synovium and effusion on nonenhanced MRI sequences is difficult (**Fig. 9**). The prevalence of joint effusion has a direct relationship with radiographic severity in the knee joint.[63] In a cohort of 1368 knees without radiographic knee OA, the prevalence of joint effusion was

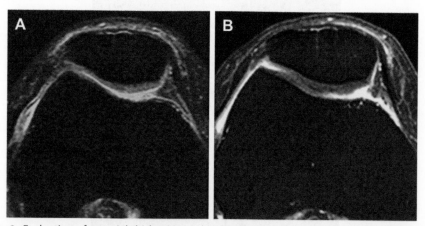

Fig. 9. Evaluation of synovial thickening and joint effusion on nonenhanced PDwFS (A) and CE T1wFS MRI (B). Axial PDwFS MRI (A) shows high-intensity fluid-equivalent signal in the patellofemoral joint space. The axial CE T1wFS MRI (B) demonstrates marked synovial thickening and enhancement in the same region. Apparently the nonenhanced scan was not adequate for assessment.

33.7%, and most effusions were small.[64] Hill and colleagues[45] reported a high prevalence of joint effusion in individuals with radiographic knee OA, and it was demonstrated that moderate and large effusions (graded from 0 to 3) were significantly more common among those with knee pain. A significant association between grades of effusion (graded in conjunction with synovitis on nonenhanced MRI) with knee pain severity was found by Torres and colleagues[37] in a cohort of 143 subjects with knee OA. The joint capsule contains pain fibers, and capsule distension associated with joint effusions may contribute to knee pain in OA.

CRUCIATE AND COLLATERAL LIGAMENTS

It is recognized that traumatic complete anterior cruciate ligament (ACL) tears may lead to premature degeneration of the knee joint.[65–68] The role of traumatic incomplete ACL tears in predicting knee OA, however, is unclear.[69] ACL disruption inevitably will cause alterations in knee kinematics, as the ACL is the primary restraint against anterior tibial translation.[70] Furthermore, ACL failure increases the external adduction moment and consequently medial loading, increasing the risk of medial knee OA.[71] ACL tears frequently are associated with other relevant traumatic lesions in the knee such as meniscal tears and chondral/osteochondral lesions, making the assessment of its role in knee degeneration more difficult.[72]

Incidental ACL tears are common among patients with knee OA, with a reported prevalence ranging from 20% to 35%.[71,73,74] Degeneration within the ligament fibers, alterations in the notch width and depth, and the presence of notch osteophytes (**Fig. 10**) may predispose to ACL tears in patients with knee OA.[75–78] Scoring methods to assess cruciate ligament tears in patients with knee OA are available.[12,13] Hernandez-Molina and colleagues[26] showed that traction BMLs, detected on MRI at the femoral and tibial insertions of the ACL, were strongly related to ACL pathology.

The role of ACL tears in predicting structural progression in patients with knee OA remains unclear. In a recent longitudinal study, Amin and colleagues[79] found that the presence of an ACL tear at baseline increased the risk for cartilage loss in the medial compartment at 30-month follow-up. When adjustment for medial meniscal

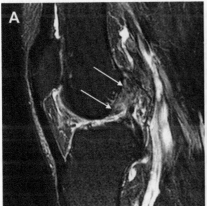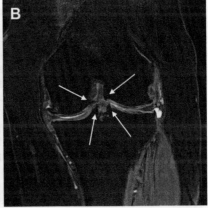

Fig. 10. (*A*) Sagittal T2wFS MRI shows a complete disruption of the ACL (*arrows*). (*B*) Coronal three-dimensional water excitation DESS MRI exhibits osteophytic formation around the femoral notch and the tibial spines (*arrows*), believed to be a risk factor for incidental nontraumatic ACL failure in patients with knee OA.

damage was performed, however, this effect was diluted. In another cohort of 245 elderly individuals (aged 70 to 79 years), a good correlation between any ligament tear in the knee and cartilage loss was found.[80]

The contribution of ACL tears to pain severity in patients with knee OA is also unclear. Hill and colleagues[71] showed that complete ACL tears were common (22.8%) in a population with symptomatic knee OA and poor recall of knee trauma, and rare (2.7%) among those without knee symptoms. Another group reported that subjects with a complete ACL tear tended to have greater knee pain at baseline, but no overall differences in pain severity were found after adjustment for potential confounders.[79]

The posterior cruciate ligament (PCL) plays a role in the kinematics of the knee, mainly for the medial compartment, and a tear with a subsequent deficiency may increase the incidence of knee OA.[81,82] In a long follow-up study of 58 patients with isolated partial or complete PCL tears treated conservatively and evaluated after 2 to 19.3 years (mean 6.9 years), Patel and colleagues[83] found that 10 (17.2%) developed medial tibiofemoral radiographic OA. Incidental complete PCL tears are rare among patients with knee OA.

Incidental collateral ligaments tears are infrequent among patients with knee OA.[37] The WORMS scoring system allows assessment of collateral ligament tears in patients with knee OA.[12] Collateral ligaments are scored as normal, thickened but continuous, and ruptured. In a small cohort of 30 patients with medial compartment knee OA without history of trauma and 30 age-matched patients with atraumatic knee pain but without OA, signal changes in or around the medial collateral ligament (MCL) (grade 1 and 2 lesions) were seen in 27 patients (90%) in the first group, but in only 2 patients (6.6%) in the control group,[84] suggesting that grade 1 and 2 MCL lesions may be related to medial knee OA in patients without history of trauma. The role of collateral ligament abnormalities in predicting structural progression and pain in patients with OA is unknown.

PERIARTICULAR CYSTS AND BURSAE

A wide spectrum of periarticular cystic lesions may be encountered in knee OA.[85] Most cystic lesions around the knee are encapsulated fluid collections exhibiting low signal intensity on T1-weighted images and high signal intensity on T2-weighted images.[85,86]

Popliteal (Baker's) cysts are not true cysts, but fluid in the semimembranosus-medial gastrocnemius bursa (**Fig. 11**), mainly caused by the extravasation of joint fluid through the posteromedial capsule, which seems to occur because of increased intra-articular pressure caused by joint effusions or altered biomechanics within the knee, as seen in meniscal tears or degenerative joint disease. Complications such as rupture of cysts and the presence of intracystic hemorrhage or loose bodies may occur. Popliteal cysts are detected commonly in patients with knee OA.[45,63,87] Hill and colleagues[45] found that the prevalence of these lesions was 43.2% in knees with moderate or larger effusions, compared with 22.7% in those with little or no effusion. In this study, presence of popliteal cysts was not associated with pain. Different grades of synovitis, however, may be present around popliteal cysts (**Fig. 12**).[49] Moderate-to-large popliteal cysts are associated with incident radiographic knee OA.[88]

A spectrum of bursitis may occur in patients with knee OA.[85] Prepatellar bursitis (**Fig. 13**) may be seen in conjunction with knee OA, but its pathogenesis is thought not to be linked directly to degeneration. A less common site of bursitis is the

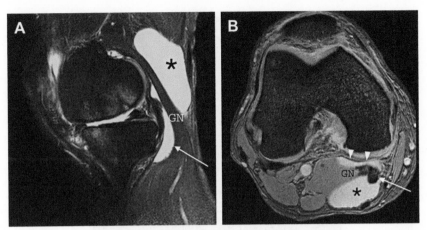

Fig. 11. Popliteal (Baker's) cyst in a patient with knee OA. Sagittal T2wFS spin echo (A) and axial T2wFS gradient echo (B) MRI show a fluid collection within the semimembranosus-gastrocnemius bursa (Baker's cyst, *), extending posteriorly between the semimembranosus tendon (arrow—B) and the medial head of the gastrocnemius (GN). This bursa communicates with the knee joint via the subgastrocnemius bursa (arrow—A; arrowheads—B).

superficial infrapatellar bursa, appearing on MRI as a fluid collection anterior to the tibial tubercle. A tiny amount of fluid within the deep infrapatellar bursa frequently is detected on MRI of the knee, including patients with OA.[5] It may be considered a normal finding without clinical significance, however, because of its high prevalence in asymptomatic subjects (**Fig. 14**).[5,89] Anserine bursitis (**Fig. 15**) may be detected in conjunction with knee OA, but its association with degeneration is controversial. Chronic anserine bursitis is thought to be most common in elderly patients with degenerative disease or rheumatoid arthritis.[90] A recent case–control study, however, found no association between prevalent anserine bursitis and radiographic knee OA.[91]

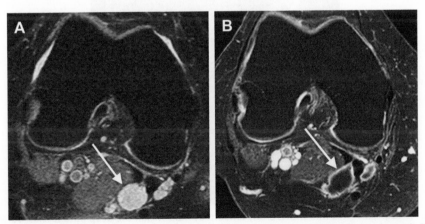

Fig. 12. Popliteal cyst. (A) Axial PDwFS MRI shows a typical popliteal (Baker's) cyst (arrow). (B) Axial CE T1wFS MRI demonstrates enhancement and thickening of the synovial membrane surrounding the popliteal cyst (arrow).

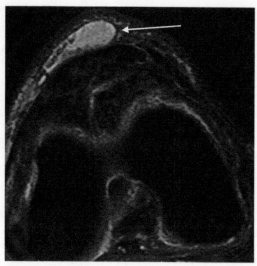

Fig. 13. Axial PDwFS image depicts fluid collection in the subcutaneous fat anteriorly to the proximal patellar tendon, consistent with prepatellar bursitis (*arrow*).

Furthermore, anserine bursitis shows no significant association with incident knee pain or incident radiographic OA.[88]

Parameniscal cysts are thought to be formed by fluid extravasation through a meniscal tear into the parameniscal soft tissue.[89] Most of these cysts result from horizontal tears, which are thought to be of degenerative origin and are a common finding in knee OA (**Fig. 16**).[92–94] Lateral meniscal cysts are associated with incident knee pain

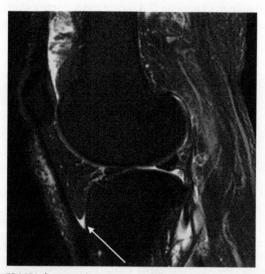

Fig. 14. Sagittal T2wFS MRI shows a tiny amount of fluid within the deep infrapatellar bursa (*arrow*), which is located between the distal patellar tendon and the anterior tibial surface. This finding is observed regularly in asymptomatic individuals, and should not be mistaken for bursitis.

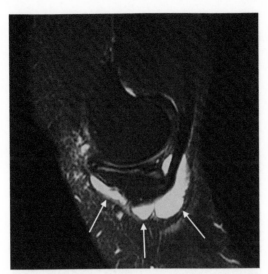

Fig. 15. On the sagittal T2wFS MRI, fluid collection adjacent to the tibial insertion of the pes anserinus tendons is visualized, a finding consistent with anserine bursitis (*arrows*).

longitudinally.[88] Ganglion cysts (**Fig. 17**) around the knee routinely are detected on MRI examinations.[85] They may be seen in conjunction with OA, but accepted theories for ganglia formation are not related directly to OA.[95–97] Tibiofibular synovial cysts (**Fig. 18**) are more prevalent in patients with knee effusion, as in 10% of adults the proximal tibiofibular joint communicates with the knee joint. The probable pathogenesis is increased pressure in the knee joint leading to dilatation of the tibiofibular joint capsule.[98] The reported prevalence in patients with knee OA is low.[5]

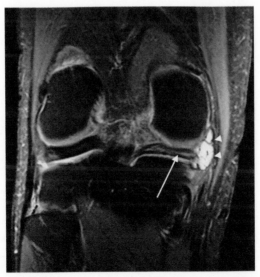

Fig. 16. Coronal T2wFS MRI shows a horizontal meniscal tear (*arrow*) and an adjacent parameniscal cyst originating from the posterior horn of the medial meniscus (*arrowheads*).

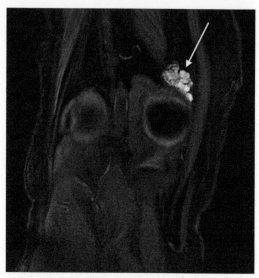

Fig. 17. Coronal three-dimensional water excitation DESS MRI sequence demonstrates an extra-articular multiloculated fluid collection adjacent to the posterior medial femoral condyle, consistent with an extra-articular ganglion cyst (*arrow*).

LOOSE BODIES

Loose bodies are seen regularly in conjunction with knee OA, especially in severe cases. Chondral fragments, detached osteophytes, and meniscal fragments, for example, may originate loose bodies in knee OA. Synovial osteochondromatosis has to be considered also.[99] The presence of loose bodies is related to internal knee derangement in patients with OA.[100,101] They may trigger synovial inflammation

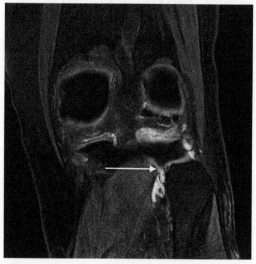

Fig. 18. Coronal three-dimensional water excitation DESS MRI shows a fusiform synovial cyst with its neck originating from the proximal tibiofibular joint (*arrow*).

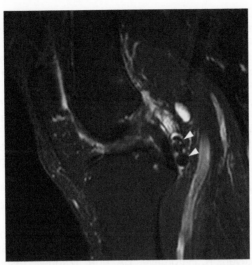

Fig. 19. Sagittal T2wFS MRI illustrates two intra-articular loose bodies (*arrowheads*) located between the posterior cruciate ligament and the posterior joint capsule.

as demonstrated by a recent study using contrast-enhanced MRI,[49] and they are a common indication for arthroscopic treatment.[100,101] On MRI, loose bodies are visualized best in joints with prevalent effusion and may be delineated as solitary or multiple low signal intensity abnormalities within the joint (**Fig. 19**).

SUMMARY

Knee OA is considered a disease of the whole joint. MRI has added much to the understanding of all the joint tissues involved in the disease process such as the subchondral bone, synovium, ligaments, and periarticular soft tissues and their significance in explaining pain and structural progression. The use of appropriate MRI pulse sequences is crucial, allowing accurate semiquantitative assessment of these alterations. Reliable semiquantitative scoring systems are available to assess the subchondral bone, synovium, ligaments, and periarticular alterations. Contrast-enhanced MRI should be considered in the assessment of whole knee synovitis, as it enables accurate evaluation and quantification of synovial thickness.

REFERENCES

1. Felson DT. An update on the pathogenesis and epidemiology of osteoarthritis. Radiol Clin North Am 2004;42:1–9, v.
2. Kellgren JH, Lawrence JS. Radiological assessment of osteoarthrosis. Ann Rheum Dis 1957;16:494–502.
3. Emrani PS, Katz JN, Kessler CL, et al. Joint space narrowing and Kellgren-Lawrence progression in knee osteoarthritis: an analytic literature synthesis. Osteoarthritis Cartilage 2008;16:873–82.
4. Dye SF, Vaupel GL, Dye CC. Conscious neurosensory mapping of the internal structures of the human knee without intra-articular anesthesia. Am J Sports Med 1998;26:773–7.

5. Hill CL, Gale DR, Chaisson CE, et al. Periarticular lesions detected on magnetic resonance imaging: prevalence in knees with and without symptoms. Arthritis Rheum 2003;48:2836–44.

6. Zanetti M, Bruder E, Romero J, et al. Bone marrow edema pattern in osteoarthritic knees: correlation between MR imaging and histologic findings. Radiology 2000;215:835–40.

7. Bergman AG, Willen HK, Lindstrand AL, et al. Osteoarthritis of the knee: correlation of subchondral MR signal abnormalities with histopathologic and radiographic features. Skeletal Radiol 1994;23:445–8.

8. Yu JS, Cook PA. Magnetic resonance imaging (MRI) of the knee: a pattern approach for evaluating bone marrow edema. Crit Rev Diagn Imaging 1996; 37:261–303.

9. Roemer FW, Hunter DJ, Guermazi A. MRI-based semiquantitative assessment of subchondral bone marrow lesions in osteoarthritis research. Osteoarthritis Cartilage 2009;17:414–5.

10. Peterfy CG, Gold G, Eckstein F, et al. MRI protocols for whole-organ assessment of the knee in osteoarthritis. Osteoarthritis Cartilage 2006;14(Suppl A):A95–111.

11. Yoshioka H, Stevens K, Hargreaves BA, et al. Magnetic resonance imaging of articular cartilage of the knee: comparison between fat-suppressed three-dimensional SPGR imaging, fat-suppressed FSE imaging, and fat-suppressed three-dimensional DEFT imaging, and correlation with arthroscopy. J Magn Reson Imaging 2004;20:857–64.

12. Peterfy CG, Guermazi A, Zaim S, et al. Whole-Organ Magnetic Resonance Imaging Score (WORMS) of the knee in osteoarthritis. Osteoarthritis Cartilage 2004;12:177–90.

13. Hunter DJ, Lo GH, Gale D, et al. The reliability of a new scoring system for knee osteoarthritis MRI and the validity of bone marrow lesion assessment: BLOKS (Boston Leeds Osteoarthritis Knee Score). Ann Rheum Dis 2008;67:206–11.

14. Roemer FW, Frobell R, Hunter DJ, et al. MRI-detected subchondral bone marrow signal alterations of the knee joint: terminology, imaging appearance, relevance, and radiological differential diagnosis. Osteoarthritis Cartilage 2009;17:1115–31.

15. Baranyay FJ, Wang Y, Wluka AE, et al. Association of bone marrow lesions with knee structures and risk factors for bone marrow lesions in the knees of clinically healthy, community-based adults. Semin Arthritis Rheum 2007;37:112–8.

16. Guymer E, Baranyay F, Wluka AE, et al. A study of the prevalence and associations of subchondral bone marrow lesions in the knees of healthy, middle-aged women. Osteoarthritis Cartilage 2007;15:1437–42.

17. Felson DT, Chaisson CE, Hill CL, et al. The association of bone marrow lesions with pain in knee osteoarthritis. Ann Intern Med 2001;134:541–9.

18. Felson DT, Niu J, Guermazi A, et al. Correlation of the development of knee pain with enlarging bone marrow lesions on magnetic resonance imaging. Arthritis Rheum 2007;56:2986–92.

19. Roemer FW, Guermazi A, Javaid MK, et al. Change in MRI-detected subchondral bone marrow lesions is associated with cartilage loss—the MOST study. A longitudinal multicenter study of knee osteoarthritis. Ann Rheum Dis 2009;68:1461–5.

20. Hunter DJ, Zhang Y, Niu J, et al. Increase in bone marrow lesions associated with cartilage loss: a longitudinal magnetic resonance imaging study of knee osteoarthritis. Arthritis Rheum 2006;54:1529–35.

21. Felson DT, McLaughlin S, Goggins J, et al. Bone marrow edema and its relation to progression of knee osteoarthritis. Ann Intern Med 2003;139:330–6.

22. Zhang Y, Nevitt M, Niu J, et al. Reversible MRI features and knee pain fluctuation: the MOST study. Osteoarthritis Cartilage 2007;15(Suppl 3):C17.

23. Taljanovic MS, Graham AR, Benjamin JB, et al. Bone marrow edema pattern in advanced hip osteoarthritis: quantitative assessment with magnetic resonance imaging and correlation with clinical examination, radiographic findings, and histopathology. Skeletal Radiol 2008;37:423–31.

24. Kornaat PR, Kloppenburg M, Sharma R, et al. Bone marrow edema-like lesions change in volume in the majority of patients with osteoarthritis; associations with clinical features. Eur Radiol 2007;17:3073–8.

25. Lo GH, Hunter DJ, Zhang Y, et al. Bone marrow lesions in the knee are associated with increased local bone density. Arthritis Rheum 2005;52:2814–21.

26. Hernandez-Molina G, Guermazi A, Niu J, et al. Central bone marrow lesions in symptomatic knee osteoarthritis and their relationship to anterior cruciate ligament tears and cartilage loss. Arthritis Rheum 2008;58:130–6.

27. Sowers MF, Hayes C, Jamadar D, et al. Magnetic resonance-detected subchondral bone marrow and cartilage defect characteristics associated with pain and X-ray defined knee osteoarthritis. Osteoarthritis Cartilage 2003;11:387–93.

28. Pouders C, De Maeseneer M, Van Roy P, et al. Prevalence and MRI-anatomic correlation of bone cysts in osteoarthritic knees. AJR Am J Roentgenol 2008; 190:17–21.

29. Landells JW. The bone cysts of osteoarthritis. J Bone Joint Surg Br 1953;35-B: 643–9.

30. Rhaney K, Lamb DW. The cysts of osteoarthritis of the hip: a radiological and pathological study. J Bone Joint Surg Br 1955;37-B:663–75.

31. Resnick D, Niwayama G, Coutts RD. Subchondral cysts (geodes) in arthritic disorders: pathologic and radiographic appearance of the hip joint. AJR Am J Roentgenol 1977;128:799–806.

32. Freund E. The pathological significance of intra-articular pressure. Edinb Med J 1940;47:192–203.

33. Ferguson AB Jr. The pathological changes in degenerative arthritis of the hip and treatment by rotational osteotomy. J Bone Joint Surg Am 1964;46:1337–52.

34. Crema MD, Roemer FW, Marra MD, et al. MRI-detected bone marrow edema-like lesions are strongly associated with subchondral cysts in patients with or at risk for knee osteoarthritis: the MOST study. Osteoarthritis Cartilage 2008;16(Suppl 4):S160.

35. Carrino JA, Blum J, Parellada JA, et al. MRI of bone marrow edema-like signal in the pathogenesis of subchondral cysts. Osteoarthritis Cartilage 2006;14:1081–5.

36. Kornaat PR, Bloem JL, Ceulemans RY, et al. Osteoarthritis of the knee: association between clinical features and MR imaging findings. Radiology 2006;239:811–7.

37. Torres L, Dunlop DD, Peterfy C, et al. The relationship between specific tissue lesions and pain severity in persons with knee osteoarthritis. Osteoarthritis Cartilage 2006;14:1033–40.

38. Dieppe PA, Reichenbach S, Williams S, et al. Assessing bone loss on radiographs of the knee in osteoarthritis: a cross-sectional study. Arthritis Rheum 2005;52:3536–41.

39. Reichenbach S, Guermazi A, Niu J, et al. Prevalence of bone attrition on knee radiographs and MRI in a community-based cohort. Osteoarthritis Cartilage 2008;16:1005–10.

40. Roemer FW, Guermazi A, Neogi T, et al. Tibiofemoral bone marrow lesions and their association with prevalent and incident subchondral bone attrition: the MOST study. Osteoarthritis Cartilage 2008;16(Suppl 4):S160–1.

41. Neogi T, Nevitt M, Niu J, et al. Subchondral bone attrition is a reflection of compartment-specific mechanical load: the MOST study. Osteoarthritis Cartilage 2008;16(Suppl 4):S140–1.

42. Neogi T, Zhang Y, Niu J, et al. Cartilage loss occurs in the same subregions as subchondral bone attrition: the MOST study. Osteoarthritis Cartilage 2008; 16(Suppl 4):S172–3.

43. Hernandez-Molina G, Neogi T, Hunter DJ, et al. The association of bone attrition with knee pain and other MRI features of osteoarthritis. Ann Rheum Dis 2008;67: 43–7.

44. Pelletier JP, Martel-Pelletier J, Abramson SB. Osteoarthritis, an inflammatory disease: potential implication for the selection of new therapeutic targets. Arthritis Rheum 2001;44:1237–47.

45. Hill CL, Gale DG, Chaisson CE, et al. Knee effusions, popliteal cysts, and synovial thickening: association with knee pain in osteoarthritis. J Rheumatol 2001; 28:1330–7.

46. Hill CL, Hunter DJ, Niu J, et al. Synovitis detected on magnetic resonance imaging and its relation to pain and cartilage loss in knee osteoarthritis. Ann Rheum Dis 2007;66:1599–603.

47. Ayral X, Pickering EH, Woodworth TG, et al. Synovitis: a potential predictive factor of structural progression of medial tibiofemoral knee osteoarthritis—results of a 1-year longitudinal arthroscopic study in 422 patients. Osteoarthritis Cartilage 2005;13:361–7.

48. Marra MD, Roemer FW, Crema MD, et al. Peripatellar synovitis in osteoarthritis: comparison of non-enhanced and enhanced magnetic resonance imaging (MRI) and its association with peripatellar knee pain: the MOST study. Osteoarthritis Cartilage 2008;16(Suppl 4):S167.

49. Guermazi A, Roemer FW, Crema MD, et al. Assessment of synovitis in knee osteoarthritis on contrast-enhanced MRI using a novel comprehensive semiquantitative scoring system. Arthritis Rheum 2008;58:S696–7.

50. Loeuille D, Chary-Valckenaere I, Champigneulle J, et al. Macroscopic and microscopic features of synovial membrane inflammation in the osteoarthritic knee: correlating magnetic resonance imaging findings with disease severity. Arthritis Rheum 2005;52:3492–501.

51. Fernandez-Madrid F, Karvonen RL, Teitge RA, et al. Synovial thickening detected by MR imaging in osteoarthritis of the knee confirmed by biopsy as synovitis. Magn Reson Imaging 1995;13:177–83.

52. Lindblad S, Hedfors E. Arthroscopic and immunohistologic characterization of knee joint synovitis in osteoarthritis. Arthritis Rheum 1987;30:1081–8.

53. Saddik D, McNally EG, Richardson M. MRI of Hoffa's fat pad. Skeletal Radiol 2004;33:433–44.

54. Roemer FW, Guermazi A, Zhang Y, et al. Evaluation of Hoffa's fat pad findings on noncontrast enhanced MR imaging as a measure of patellofemoral knee synovitis in osteoarthritis. AJR Am J Roentgenol 2009;192:1696–700.

55. Pelletier JP, Raynauld JP, Abram F, et al. A new noninvasive method to assess synovitis severity in relation to symptoms and cartilage volume loss in knee osteoarthritis patients using MRI. Osteoarthritis Cartilage 2008;16(Suppl 3):S8–13.

56. Roemer FW, Hunter DJ, Guermazi A. Semiquantitative assessment of synovitis in osteoarthritis on non contrast-enhanced MRI. Osteoarthritis Cartilage 2009;17: 820–1.

57. Loeuille D, Saulière N, Champigneulle J, et al. What is the most accurate MRI approach to assess synovitis and/or effusion in knee OA? Osteoarthritis Cartilage 2008;16(Suppl 4):176.

58. Ostergaard M, Hansen M, Stoltenberg M, et al. Magnetic resonance imaging-determined synovial membrane volume as a marker of disease activity and a predictor of progressive joint destruction in the wrists of patients with rheumatoid arthritis. Arthritis Rheum 1999;42:918–29.

59. Rhodes LA, Grainger AJ, Keenan AM, et al. The validation of simple scoring methods for evaluating compartment-specific synovitis detected by MRI in knee osteoarthritis. Rheumatology (Oxford) 2005;44:1569–73.

60. Clunie G, Hall-Craggs MA, Paley MN, et al. Measurement of synovial lining volume by magnetic resonance imaging of the knee in chronic synovitis. Ann Rheum Dis 1997;56:526–34.

61. Lindblad S, Hedfors E. Intra-articular variation in synovitis. Local macroscopic and microscopic signs of inflammatory activity are significantly correlated. Arthritis Rheum 1985;28:977–86.

62. Kurosaka M, Ohno O, Hirohata K. Arthroscopic evaluation of synovitis in the knee joints. Arthroscopy 1991;7:162–70.

63. Fernandez-Madrid F, Karvonen RL, Teitge RA, et al. MR features of osteoarthritis of the knee. Magn Reson Imaging 1994;12:703–9.

64. Roemer FW, Guermazi A, Hunter DJ, et al. The association of meniscal damage with joint effusion in persons without radiographic osteoarthritis: the Framingham and MOST osteoarthritis studies. Osteoarthritis Cartilage 2008.

65. von Porat A, Roos EM, Roos H. High prevalence of osteoarthritis 14 years after an anterior cruciate ligament tear in male soccer players: a study of radiographic and patient-relevant outcomes. Ann Rheum Dis 2004;63:269–73.

66. Maletius W, Messner K. Eighteen- to twenty-four-year follow-up after complete rupture of the anterior cruciate ligament. Am J Sports Med 1999;27:711–7.

67. Kannus P, Jarvinen M. Post-traumatic anterior cruciate ligament insufficiency as a cause of osteoarthritis in a knee joint. Clin Rheumatol 1989;8:251–60.

68. Nebelung W, Wuschech H. Thirty-five years of follow-up of anterior cruciate ligament-deficient knees in high-level athletes. Arthroscopy 2005;21:696–702.

69. Messner K, Maletius W. Eighteen- to twenty-five-year follow-up after acute partial anterior cruciate ligament rupture. Am J Sports Med 1999;27:455–9.

70. Dargel J, Gotter M, Mader K, et al. Biomechanics of the anterior cruciate ligament and implications for surgical reconstruction. Strategies Trauma Limb Reconstr 2007;2:1–12.

71. Hill CL, Seo GS, Gale D, et al. Cruciate ligament integrity in osteoarthritis of the knee. Arthritis Rheum 2005;52:794–9.

72. Crema MD, Marra MD, Guermazi A, et al. Relevant traumatic injury of the knee joint-MRI follow-up after 7–10 years. Eur J Radiol 2008; Sep 19 [Epub ahead of print].

73. Chan WP, Lang P, Stevens MP, et al. Osteoarthritis of the knee: comparison of radiography, CT, and MR imaging to assess extent and severity. AJR Am J Roentgenol 1991;157:799–806.

74. Link TM, Steinbach LS, Ghosh S, et al. Osteoarthritis: MR imaging findings in different stages of disease and correlation with clinical findings. Radiology 2003;226:373–81.

75. Cushner FD, La Rosa DF, Vigorita VJ, et al. A quantitative histologic comparison: ACL degeneration in the osteoarthritic knee. J Arthroplasty 2003;18:687–92.

76. Lee GC, Cushner FD, Vigoritta V, et al. Evaluation of the anterior cruciate ligament integrity and degenerative arthritic patterns in patients undergoing total knee arthroplasty. J Arthroplasty 2005;20:59–65.

77. Wada M, Tatsuo H, Baba H, et al. Femoral intercondylar notch measurements in osteoarthritic knees. Rheumatology (Oxford) 1999;38:554–8.

78. Mullaji AB, Marawar SV, Simha M, et al. Cruciate ligaments in arthritic knees: a histologic study with radiologic correlation. J Arthroplasty 2008;23:567–72.

79. Amin S, Guermazi A, Lavalley MP, et al. Complete anterior cruciate ligament tear and the risk for cartilage loss and progression of symptoms in men and women with knee osteoarthritis. Osteoarthritis Cartilage 2008;16:897–902.

80. Guermazi A, Taouli B, Lynch JA, et al. Prevalence of meniscus and ligament tears and their correlation with cartilage morphology and other MRI features in knee osteoarthritis (OA) in the elderly. The Health ABC Study. Arthritis Rheum 2002;46(Suppl):S567.

81. Logan M, Williams A, Lavelle J, et al. The effect of posterior cruciate ligament deficiency on knee kinematics. Am J Sports Med 2004;32:1915–22.

82. Dejour H, Walch G, Peyrot J, et al. The natural history of rupture of the posterior cruciate ligament. Rev Chir Orthop Reparatrice Appar Mot 1988;74:35–43 [in French].

83. Patel DV, Allen AA, Warren RF, et al. The nonoperative treatment of acute, isolated (partial or complete) posterior cruciate ligament-deficient knees: an intermediate-term follow-up study. HSS J 2007;3:137–46.

84. Bergin D, Keogh C, O'Connell M, et al. Atraumatic medial collateral ligament oedema in medial compartment knee osteoarthritis. Skeletal Radiol 2002;31:14–8.

85. Marra MD, Crema MD, Chung M, et al. MRI features of cystic lesions around the knee. Knee 2008;15:423–38.

86. Guermazi A, Zaim S, Taouli B, et al. MR findings in knee osteoarthritis. Eur Radiol 2003;13:1370–86.

87. Fam AG, Wilson SR, Holmberg S. Ultrasound evaluation of popliteal cysts on osteoarthritis of the knee. J Rheumatol 1982;9:428–34.

88. Guermazi A, Roemer FW, Niu J, et al. Periarticular cysts and their relation to symptoms in osteoarthritis: the MOST study. Osteoarthritis Cartilage 2007;15 (Suppl 3):C170–1.

89. Tschirch FT, Schmid MR, Pfirrmann CW, et al. Prevalence and size of meniscal cysts, ganglionic cysts, synovial cysts of the popliteal space, fluid-filled bursae, and other fluid collections in asymptomatic knees on MR imaging. AJR Am J Roentgenol 2003;180:1431–6.

90. McCarthy CL, McNally EG. The MRI appearance of cystic lesions around the knee. Skeletal Radiol 2004;33:187–209.

91. Alvarez-Nemegyei J. Risk factors for pes anserinus tendinitis/bursitis syndrome: a case–control study. J Clin Rheumatol 2007;13:63–5.

92. Noble J, Hamblen DL. The pathology of the degenerate meniscus lesion. J Bone Joint Surg Br 1975;57:180–6.

93. De Maeseneer M, Shahabpour M, Vanderdood K, et al. MR imaging of meniscal cysts: evaluation of location and extension using a three-layer approach. Eur J Radiol 2001;39:117–24.

94. Tyson LL, Daughters TC Jr, Ryu RK, et al. MRI appearance of meniscal cysts. Skeletal Radiol 1995;24:421–4.

95. Feldman F, Johnston A. Intraosseous ganglion. Am J Roentgenol Radium Ther Nucl Med 1973;118:328–43.

96. Kim JY, Jung SA, Sung MS, et al. Extra-articular soft tissue ganglion cyst around the knee: focus on the associated findings. Eur Radiol 2004;14:106–11.
97. Bui-Mansfield LT, Youngberg RA. Intra-articular ganglia of the knee: prevalence, presentation, etiology, and management. AJR Am J Roentgenol 1997;168: 123–7.
98. Jerome D, McKendry R. Synovial cyst of the proximal tibiofibular joint. J Rheumatol 2000;27:1096–8.
99. El Andaloussi Y, Fnini S, Hachimi K, et al. Osteochondromatosis of the popliteal bursa. Joint Bone Spine 2006;73:219–20.
100. Steadman JR, Ramappa AJ, Maxwell RB, et al. An arthroscopic treatment regimen for osteoarthritis of the knee. Arthroscopy 2007;23:948–55.
101. Stuart MJ, Lubowitz JH. What, if any, are the indications for arthroscopic debridement of the osteoarthritic knee? Arthroscopy 2006;22:238–9.

The Meniscus in Knee Osteoarthritis

Martin Englund, MD, PhD[a,b,*], Ali Guermazi, MD[c],
L. Stefan Lohmander, MD, PhD[a]

KEYWORDS

- Osteoarthritis • Knee • Meniscus • Menisci • Pain
- Symptoms • MRI • Radiography

The loss of joint cartilage is considered the structural hallmark of osteoarthritis (OA). However, the last decades of research have shown OA to be a whole-joint disorder involving additional tissues such as subchondral bone, ligaments, synovial membrane, muscle, and the menisci. All of these can be evaluated by modern imaging techniques as MRI. This article reviews recent advances in the understanding of the role of the meniscus and meniscus pathology in OA. The meniscus plays a critical protective role in each tibiofemoral compartment through its shock absorbing and load distributing properties. The authors describe typical meniscal lesions found in the osteoarthritic knee and their causes and significance, and review past and current treatment concepts of importance for the practicing rheumatologist.

ANATOMY, HISTOLOGY, AND FUNCTIONS OF THE NORMAL MENISCI IN BRIEF

The menisci are two semi-circular fibrocartilage structures positioned between the joint surfaces of the femur and tibia in the medial and lateral knee joint compartments. Each meniscus covers approximately two-thirds of the corresponding articular surface of the tibia. In cross section, both menisci are wedge-shaped with a thick peripheral base infiltrated by capillaries and nerves that penetrate 10% to 30% of the meniscus width.[1,2] The medial meniscus is firmly attached to the joint capsule, whereas the lateral meniscus is more mobile. Both of the menisci are attached to

A version of this article originally appeared in the 47:4 issue of Radiologic Clinics of North America.

[a] Musculoskeletal Sciences, Department of Orthopedics, Klinikgatan 22, Lund University Hospital, SE-221 85 Lund, Sweden
[b] Clinical Epidemiology Research & Training Unit, Boston University School of Medicine, Boston, MA, USA
[c] Department of Radiology, Boston University School of Medicine, 820 Harrison Avenue, FGH Building, 3rd Floor, Boston, MA 02118, USA
* Corresponding author. Musculoskeletal Sciences, Department of Orthopedics, Klinikgatan 22, Lund University Hospital, SE-221 85 Lund, Sweden.
E-mail address: martin.englund@med.lu.se (M. Englund).

the tibia through the anterior and posterior horns. Here, circumferential matrix fibers continue as ligaments attached to the intercondylar bone.

A sparse population of fibrochondrocytes produces and maintains the meniscal matrix. In contrast to articular cartilage, which contains principally type II collagen and an abundance of proteoglycan, meniscal matrix collagen is approximately 98% type I, and the meniscus contains much less proteoglycan (<1%).[3] The tightly woven collagen fibers are arranged predominantly in a circumferential pattern. This main fiber orientation is important in providing strength and holding the meniscus in place when loaded.

The main functions of the menisci are shock absorption and load transmission in knee joint movement and static loading.[4–6] When the knee is loaded, the tensile strength of the meniscal matrix (hoop tension) counteracts extrusion of the meniscus, and the meniscus distributes stress over a large area of the articular cartilage; the healthy meniscus mainly responds to load with compression. Removal of all or part of the meniscus leads to focally increased joint cartilage strain under static loading, and to increased dynamic deformation in knee joint areas known to develop OA.[7,8] The meniscus has also been reported to contribute to joint stability, proprioception, and joint lubrication.[9–11]

DIFFERENT TYPES OF MENISCAL LESIONS IN KNEE OA

MRI is the preferred imaging modality for evaluating the menisci, and the procedure is an increasingly popular diagnostic procedure of meniscal lesions (**Fig. 1**). The sensitivity and specificity is in the range of 82% to 96% based on patients undergoing arthroscopy (using arthroscopy as the gold standard), but in subjects with prior meniscal repair the evaluation is more complex.[12–15]

A number of typical morphologic tear patterns of the meniscus can be distinguished not only at direct visual inspection and probing at arthroscopy but also on MRI.[16,17] The tear patterns can be classified into two main types of lesions: traumatic and degenerative.[18–21] Traumatic lesions usually occur in younger active individuals due to a distinct knee trauma to a previously healthy joint when the meniscus is trapped between the femoral condyle and the tibial plateau under excessive forces. The

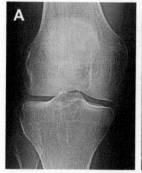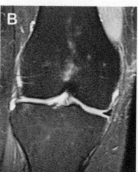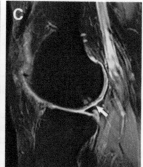

Fig. 1. A 38-year old woman underwent subtotal lateral meniscectomy in her right knee 16 years earlier. For the last year she has experienced aching related to joint use, relieved by rest. The frontal knee radiograph (A) shows normal findings, whereas a coronal T2-weighted MRI (B) reveals status after subtotal lateral meniscectomy, and sagittal image (C) shows reduced cartilage thickness and bone marrow edema (arrow). Findings are compatible with early-stage knee OA. (Reproduced from Englund, et al. Meniscal tear—a feature of osteoarthritis. Acta Orthop Scand Suppl 2004 Apr;75(312):1–45; with permission.)

meniscus often splits vertically and parallel to the circumferentially oriented collagen fibers (longitudinal tear) or, occasionally, perpendicular to the circumferential fibers (radial tear) (**Fig. 2**). Such tears are usually symptomatic, often lead to meniscal surgery, and are associated with increased risk of knee OA.[22,23]

Degenerative lesions—described as horizontal cleavages (**Fig. 3**), flap (oblique), or complex (**Fig. 4**) tears, meniscal maceration (**Fig. 5**), or destruction (**Fig. 6**)—are, in contrast, often associated with older age and preexisting or incipient osteoarthritic disease.[18–21] In a report using a sample from the general population of middle-aged and elderly in Framingham, Massachusetts, unselected for knee joint symptoms, investigators found meniscal damage (tear, maceration, previous resection, or destruction) in 35% of knees (95% CI 32 to 38).[24] The prevalence of meniscal damage in the right knee, as detected on MRI, ranged from 19% among women 50 to 59 years of age to 56% among men 70 to 90 years of age (**Fig. 7**). The vast majority of the tears were classified as degenerative. Prevalences were not materially lower when subjects who had had previous knee surgery were excluded. In the Framingham study sample, 82% of knees with radiographic OA had meniscal damage. In another report including asymptomatic subjects with a mean age of 65 years, a tear was found in 67% using MRI, whereas in patients with symptomatic knee OA a meniscal tear was found in 91%.[25] Other MRI studies support these findings of a high frequency of meniscal pathology in the middle-aged and elderly,[26] and similar findings have also been made in necropsy cases, where 60% of the subjects had a horizontal cleavage lesion.[19] The most frequent location is the posterior horn of the medial meniscus.[24] Even if a meniscal tear is not present on MRI, intrameniscal signal change (not classified as meniscal tear) is a frequent finding in the middle-aged and elderly. Such linear or globular signal changes (**Fig. 8**) have been reported to represent mucoid degeneration and may represent a precursor to degenerative tears.[27,28]

Degenerative meniscal tears may be associated with knee joint symptoms, but most lesions are actually not.[25] In the Framingham sample the majority of subjects with a meniscal tear were without symptoms.[24] However, in some a meniscal tear may cause severe discomfort or even locking of the knee owing to a dislocated fragment, and surgical treatment may become necessary.

MENISCAL DAMAGE—A CAUSE TO OR A CONSEQUENCE OF KNEE OA?

Normally configured menisci are rarely found in knees with OA. Instead they are often torn, macerated, or even totally destructed, which suggests a strong association

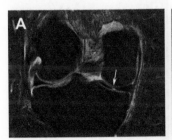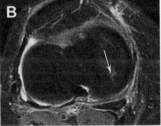

Fig. 2. Radial tear of the meniscus in a 52-year-old woman. (*A*) Coronal fat-suppressed proton density (PD)-weighted MRI shows absence of the inner point of the medial meniscal triangle, typical for radial tear (*arrow*). There is a slight extrusion of the meniscus. (*B*) Axial fat-suppressed PD-weighted MRI shows the radial tear (*arrow*) starts at the free edge of the medial meniscus and extends peripherally.

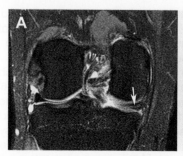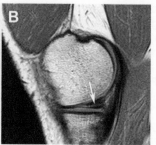

Fig. 3. Horizontal tear of the medial meniscus in a 47-year-old woman. (*A*) Coronal fat-suppressed proton density- and (*B*) sagittal T1-weighted MRIs show almost horizontal tear (*arrow*) of the posterior horn of the medial meniscus with extension to meniscal undersurface.

between the disorder and the meniscus.[24,25,29] However, the relationship between meniscal damage and knee OA is complex. A meniscal lesion in a healthy knee may eventually lead to knee OA due to the loss of meniscal function. However, knee OA may also lead to meniscal tears that, in turn, may further accelerate the disease process.[30] The menisci and articular cartilage share many similar components and properties, and are exposed to similar stresses. The pathologic processes active in the early-stage OA joint that eventually lead to the cartilage destruction characteristic of OA are not limited to the joint cartilage only, but would be expected to affect meniscus and ligament integrity as well. A tear in a meniscus with degenerative changes is often associated with preexisting structural changes in the articular cartilage that may represent early-stage OA.[19] Patients with "meniscal" symptoms due to a degenerative tear may constitute a subpopulation increased with individuals with incipient OA.

In middle-aged or elderly persons, knees with meniscal lesions, but without cartilage lesions, are at much higher risk of radiographic knee OA than knees with intact menisci. This suggests that, in many instances, MRI-visible meniscal damage comes before visible cartilage changes.[31] Shear stress and early proteolytic degradation of the meniscal matrix may result in decreased tensile strength. A meniscal tear could be the result of decreased ability the compromised meniscus to withstand loads and force transmissions during normal knee joint loads. A lesion may develop

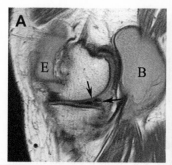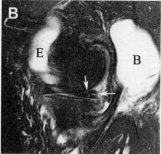

Fig. 4. Complex tear of the medial meniscus in a 53-year-old woman. Sagittal (*A*) proton density- and (*B*) fat-suppressed T2-weighted MRIs show a complex tear (*arrows*) of the posterior horn of medial meniscus with longitudinal and horizontal cleavages. There are also a moderate joint effusion (E) and large partially ruptured Baker cyst (B).

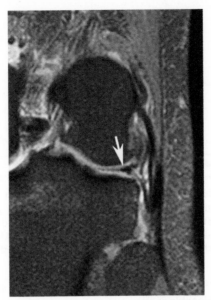

Fig. 5. Partial maceration of the lateral meniscus in a 61-year-old woman with no history of knee surgery. Coronal fat-suppressed proton density-weighted MRI shows small body of the lateral meniscus (*arrow*) with loss of the normal triangular shape.

spontaneously or in conjunction with minor knee trauma. Depending on how much functionality of the meniscus was lost because of the tear and any surgical resection, the OA development may be further accelerated through increased biomechanical loading of the joint cartilage. Many patients may develop knee symptoms and be referred to an orthopedic surgeon, perhaps because a meniscal tear was found during a knee MRI examination. However, a meniscal tear in this age category is only weakly associated with knee symptoms, whereas other features of OA, visible or not, may

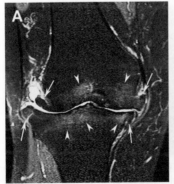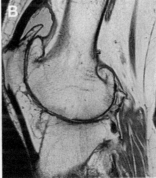

Fig. 6. Destruction of medial and lateral menisci in a 70-year-old woman with severe knee OA and no history of knee surgery. (*A*) Coronal fat-suppressed and (*B*) sagittal proton density-weighted MRIs show absence of both medial and lateral menisci. There is an extensive femoral and tibial osteophytosis (*arrows*), bone marrow lesions (*arrowheads*), cartilage loss, and bone attrition.

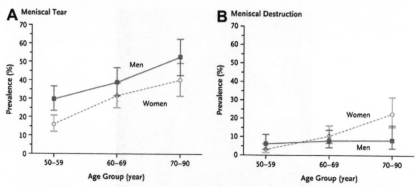

Fig. 7. Prevalence of meniscal tear (*A*) and meniscal destruction (not classified as tear) (*B*) in the right knee among the 426 men and 565 women from the general population of Framingham, Massachusetts. (*Reproduced from* Englund, et al. Incidental meniscal findings on knee MRI in middle-aged and elderly persons. New Engl J Med 2008; 359:1108–15. Copyright © 2008 Massachusetts Medical Society. All rights reserved; with permission.)

cause the symptoms.[24,32] Therefore, based on MRI findings, in such cases the indication for surgery is questionable.[33–35]

Meniscal extrusion is also common among the middle-aged and elderly, and is often another sign of a degraded or torn meniscus and existing OA (**Fig. 9**).[36,37] Meniscal tears predispose to meniscal extrusion, probably by interrupting the circumferential hoop collagen fiber orientation. Meniscal extrusion may also contribute to increased joint-space narrowing seen on radiographs, and meniscal tear and displacement are strong determinants of the rate of cartilage loss in knee OA.[29,38,39]

GENES AND ENVIRONMENT INTERACT

A degenerative meniscal lesion was more frequently found in patients with radiographic hand OA, and subjects with bilateral knee OA had radiographic hand OA

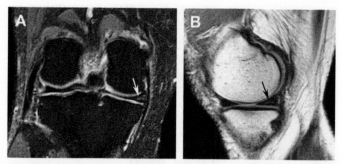

Fig. 8. Mucoid degeneration of meniscus. (*A*) Coronal fat-suppressed proton density-weighted MRI shows an intrameniscal globular hypersignal (*arrow*) of the posterior horn of medial meniscus, which does not communicate with the articular surface. This corresponds to grade 1 mucoid meniscal degeneration. (*B*) Sagittal T1-weighted MRI shows primarily linear intrameniscal hypersignal (*arrow*) of the posterior horn of the medial meniscus, which does not communicate with the articular surface. This corresponds to grade 2 mucoid meniscal degeneration.

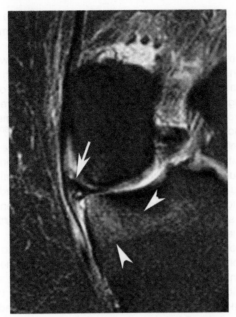

Fig. 9. Meniscal extrusion in a 57-year-woman. Coronal fat-suppressed proton density-weighted MRI shows subluxation of the body of the medial meniscus (*arrow*). There is also a grade 1 meniscal mucoid degeneration and important cartilage loss of the outer aspect of the medial tibiofemoral joint and bone marrow lesion of the medial tibial plateau (*arrowheads*).

more frequently than did subjects with unilateral knee OA.[40] These findings provided additional support for an interaction between genetic and environmental risk factors in OA, although metabolic effects cannot be excluded. Worse outcome after lateral meniscectomy compared with medial has been shown in several studies. The lateral meniscus carries higher loads in the knee compared with the medial meniscus. Consequently, if removed, the slightly convex lateral tibial plateau will be exposed to relatively more cartilage contact stress,[4,5] which may further facilitate the OA process, compared with the more concave medial tibial plateau after removal of the medial meniscus.[22,41–45] This may provide another example of the interaction of local environmental factors with the inherent risk of the individual.

PAST, PRESENT, AND FUTURE TREATMENT STRATEGIES OF A TORN MENISCUS

The first report known was of a meniscal repair: in 1883 a British surgeon successfully sutured a torn medial meniscus.[46] However, 4 years later, he published another report in which he justified total removal of the meniscus rather than repair, and that view prevailed for over 80 years.[47] In the late 1940s, Fairbank[23] speculated that frequent radiographic changes found after total meniscectomy were due to the loss of the load-protective function of the menisci, resulting in remodeling of the joint. However, total removal of the menisci was considered a mostly benign procedure for at least another 20 years. From the late 1960s to the 1980s an increasing number of follow-up reports of meniscectomy were published, all indicating a high frequency of radiographic OA and reduced knee function.[41,44,45,48–53] However, lack of standardized radiographic assessment and outcome measures precluded consistent quantification of the OA risk.[54] In 1998, a study showed a 6-fold increase in the risk of radiographic OA 21 years after total meniscectomy, compared with controls matched for age and sex.[55]

It was not until the 1970s, when the arthroscopic technique was introduced, that interest increased in excising only the damaged portion of the meniscus. In the same period of time, several biomechanical studies reported on the load-bearing and shock-absorbing functions of the menisci.[4–6,56,57] There are several short-term benefits of the arthroscopic technique of surgery and partial meniscal resection in terms of length of hospital stay, rehabilitation, and so forth.[58–60] With a substantial portion of the circumferentially oriented matrix fibers intact in the residual meniscus, hoop tension may still suffice to counteract meniscal extrusion when the knee is loaded. Therefore, substantial function may remain in the residual meniscus in shock absorption and load transmission, yielding a lower risk of radiographic changes related to OA than total meniscectomy.[22] However, the frequency of symptomatic knee OA was not substantially lowered, suggesting that partial removal of the meniscus was not the final answer.[61]

In consequence, for younger individuals with traumatic injury to the meniscus, meniscal repair is presently advocated when the lesion is located near the vascularized zone (with the potential to heal). So, we are back to where it all started in 1883. However, rehabilitation after repair is much more demanding than after meniscal resection, and the long-term outcome of meniscal repair compared with partial meniscectomy with respect to OA is unknown and randomized controlled studies lacking.[62,63] Meniscal resection remains the most frequently performed procedure by orthopedic surgeons in the United States.[64]

Meniscal replacement using allogeneic, xenogeneic, or artificial materials has been tried in younger individuals who have undergone total meniscectomy. However, transplant survival is variable and long-term results using standardized outcomes are lacking.[61,65] Even so, as there is evidence that meniscal damage without surgery would otherwise lead to radiographic OA, it is conceivable that treatments aimed at restoring meniscal function may lower this risk.[66] This remains to be shown in randomized, appropriately controlled trials. Such treatments appear attractive, in particular for younger individuals with a severely torn meniscus, but are hardly the answer to the one-third of middle-aged older adult knees with meniscal damage in the general population.[24,25]

The middle-aged and older patients with knee pain and meniscal lesions represent a great challenge for the health professional. Incidental meniscal findings on MRI are frequent,[24] and it is difficult to discriminate between symptoms caused by a meniscal tear and symptoms of early-stage knee OA.[67] The weak evidence base for many of the current treatments suggests that this therapeutic area is in great need of well-designed, randomized, controlled clinical trials to assess the true effects of arthroscopic meniscal resection, meniscal repair or transplant, or nonsurgical treatments compared with placebo or sham treatment.[33–35] Based on the best evidence, for many patients in this category, medical treatment and structured exercise programs are as effective as arthroscopic surgery. Stratification with regard to lesion type, age, activity level, and other variables will provide a challenge in trial design, but there is no shortage of patients. Blinding of patient and assessor represent additional challenges.

SUMMARY

The menisci play a critical protective role for the knee joint through shock absorption and load distribution. Meniscal lesions are regular findings on MRI, especially in the osteoarthritic knee and in the form of horizontal, flap, and (or) complex tears; maceration; or destruction. However, asymptomatic lesions are common and frequent incidental findings on knee MRI of the middle-aged or older patient. This challenges the health professional in choosing the best treatment in the short- and long-term. A meniscal tear can lead to knee OA, but knee OA can also lead to a meniscal tear. Therefore, a degenerative meniscal lesion, in the middle-aged or older patient, could suggest early-stage knee OA and should be treated accordingly. Referral to an orthopedic surgeon for removal of nonobstructive degenerate lesions may only lead to removal of evidence of the disorder while the OA and associated symptoms proceed.

REFERENCES

1. Day B, Mackenzie WG, Shim SS, et al. The vascular and nerve supply of the human meniscus. Arthroscopy 1985;1(1):58–62.
2. Arnoczky SP, Warren RF. Microvasculature of the human meniscus. Am J Sports Med 1982;10(2):90–5.
3. Eyre DR, Wu JJ. Collagen of fibrocartilage: a distinctive molecular phenotype in bovine meniscus. FEBS Lett 1983;158(2):265–70.
4. Seedhom BB, Hargreaves DJ. Transmission of the load in the knee joint with special reference to the role of the meniscus (part I + II). Eng Med 1979;4:207–28.
5. Walker PS, Erkman MJ. The role of the menisci in force transmission across the Knee. Clin Orthop Relat Res 1975;(109):184–92.
6. Kurosawa H, Fukubayashi T, Nakajima H. Load-bearing mode of the knee joint: physical behavior of the knee joint with or without menisci. Clin Orthop 1980;(149):283–90.
7. Song Y, Greve JM, Carter DR, et al. Meniscectomy alters the dynamic deformational behavior and cumulative strain of tibial articular cartilage in knee joints subjected to cyclic loads. Osteoarthr Cartil 2008;16(12):1545–54.
8. Song Y, Greve JM, Carter DR, et al. Articular cartilage MR imaging and thickness mapping of a loaded knee joint before and after meniscectomy. Osteoarthr Cartil 2006;14(8):728–37.
9. Levy IM, Torzilli PA, Warren RF. The effect of medial meniscectomy on anterior-posterior motion of the Knee. J Bone Joint Surg Am 1982;64(6):883–8.
10. Levy IM, Torzilli PA, Gould JD, et al. The effect of lateral meniscectomy on motion of the Knee. J Bone Joint Surg Am 1989;71(3):401–6.
11. Assimakopoulos AP, Katonis PG, Agapitos MV, et al. The innervation of the human meniscus. Clin Orthop 1992;275:232–6.
12. Cheung LP, Li KC, Hollett MD, et al. Meniscal tears of the knee: accuracy of detection with fast spin-echo MR imaging and arthroscopic correlation in 293 patients. Radiology 1997;203(2):508–12.
13. De Smet AA, Tuite MJ. Use of the "two-slice-touch" rule for the MRI diagnosis of meniscal tears. AJR Am J Roentgenol 2006;187(4):911–4.
14. Escobedo EM, Hunter JC, Zink-Brody GC, et al. Usefulness of turbo spin-echo MR imaging in the evaluation of meniscal tears: comparison with a conventional spin-echo sequence. AJR Am J Roentgenol 1996;167(5):1223–7.
15. Vande Berg BC, Malghem J, Poilvache P, et al. Meniscal tears with fragments displaced in notch and recesses of knee: MR imaging with arthroscopic comparison. Radiology 2005;234(3):842–50.
16. Jee WH, McCauley TR, Kim JM, et al. Meniscal tear configurations: categorization with MR imaging. AJR Am J Roentgenol 2003;180(1):93–7.

17. Newman AP, Daniels AU, Burks RT. Principles and decision making in meniscal surgery. Arthroscopy 1993;9(1):33–51.
18. Poehling GG, Ruch DS, Chabon SJ. The landscape of meniscal injuries. Clin Sports Med 1990;9(3):539–49.
19. Noble J, Hamblen DL. The pathology of the degenerate meniscus lesion. J Bone Joint Surg Br 1975;57(2):180–6.
20. Noble J. Lesions of the menisci. Autopsy incidence in adults less than fifty-five years old. J Bone Joint Surg Am 1977;59(4):480–3.
21. Smillie IS. Surgical pathology of the menisci. Injuries of the knee joint. 3rd edition. Baltimore (MD): The Williams and Wilkins Co; 1962. p. 51–90.
22. Englund M, Lohmander LS. Risk factors for symptomatic knee osteoarthritis fifteen to twenty-two years after meniscectomy. Arthritis Rheum 2004;50(9):2811–9.
23. Fairbank TJ. Knee joint changes after meniscectomy. J Bone Joint Surg Br 1948; 30:164–70.
24. Englund M, Guermazi A, Gale D, et al. Incidental meniscal findings on knee MRI in middle-aged and elderly persons. N Engl J Med 2008;359(11):1108–15.
25. Bhattacharyya T, Gale D, Dewire P, et al. The clinical importance of meniscal tears demonstrated by magnetic resonance imaging in osteoarthritis of the Knee. J Bone Joint Surg Am 2003;85(1):4–9.
26. Ding C, Martel-Pelletier J, Pelletier JP, et al. Meniscal tear as an osteoarthritis risk factor in a largely non-osteoarthritic cohort: a cross-sectional study. J Rheumatol 2007;34(4):776–84.
27. Stoller DW, Martin C, Crues JV 3rd, et al. Meniscal tears: pathologic correlation with MR imaging. Radiology 1987;163(3):731–5.
28. Hodler J, Haghighi P, Pathria MN, et al. Meniscal changes in the elderly: correlation of MR imaging and histologic findings. Radiology 1992;184(1):221–5.
29. Hunter DJ, Zhang YQ, Niu JB, et al. The association of meniscal pathologic changes with cartilage loss in symptomatic knee osteoarthritis. Arthritis Rheum 2006;54(3):795–801.
30. Roos H, Adalberth T, Dahlberg L, et al. Osteoarthritis of the knee after injury to the anterior cruciate ligament or meniscus: the influence of time and age. Osteoarthr Cartil 1995;3(4):261–7.
31. Englund M, Guermazi A, Roemer FW, et al. Meniscal tear in knees without surgery and the development of radiographic osteoarthritis among middle-aged and elderly persons: The multicenter osteoarthritis study. Arthritis Rheum 2009; 60(3):831–9.
32. Englund M, Niu J, Guermazi A, et al. Effect of meniscal damage on the development of frequent knee pain, aching, or stiffness. Arthritis Rheum 2007;56(12): 4048–54.
33. Herrlin S, Hallander M, Wange P, et al. Arthroscopic or conservative treatment of degenerative medial meniscal tears: a prospective randomised trial. Knee Surg Sports Traumatol Arthrosc 2007;15(4):393–401.
34. Kirkley A, Birmingham TB, Litchfield RB, et al. A randomized trial of arthroscopic surgery for osteoarthritis of the Knee. N Engl J Med 2008;359(11):1097–107.
35. Moseley JB, O'Malley K, Petersen NJ, et al. A controlled trial of arthroscopic surgery for osteoarthritis of the Knee. N Engl J Med 2002;347(2):81–8.
36. Adams JG, McAlindon T, Dimasi M, et al. Contribution of meniscal extrusion and cartilage loss to joint space narrowing in osteoarthritis. Clin Radiol 1999;54(8): 502–6.
37. Gale DR, Chaisson CE, Totterman SM, et al. Meniscal subluxation: association with osteoarthritis and joint space narrowing. Osteoarthr Cartil 1999;7(6):526–32.

38. Berthiaume MJ, Raynauld JP, Martel-Pelletier J, et al. Meniscal tear and extrusion are strongly associated with progression of symptomatic knee osteoarthritis as assessed by quantitative magnetic resonance imaging. Ann Rheum Dis 2005; 64(4):556–63.
39. Ding C, Martel-Pelletier J, Pelletier JP, et al. Knee meniscal extrusion in a largely non-osteoarthritic cohort: association with greater loss of cartilage volume. Arthritis Res Ther 2007;9(2):R21.
40. Englund M, Paradowski PT, Lohmander LS. Association of radiographic hand osteoarthritis with radiographic knee osteoarthritis after meniscectomy. Arthritis Rheum 2004;50(2):469–75.
41. Allen PR, Denham RA, Swan AV. Late degenerative changes after meniscectomy. Factors affecting the knee after operation. J Bone Joint Surg Br 1984;66(5): 666–71.
42. Chatain F, Adeleine P, Chambat P, et al. A comparative study of medial versus lateral arthroscopic partial meniscectomy on stable knees: 10-year minimum follow-up. Arthroscopy 2003;19(8):842–9.
43. Hede A, Larsen E, Sandberg H. The long term outcome of open total and partial meniscectomy related to the quantity and site of the meniscus removed. Int Orthop 1992;16(2):122–5.
44. Johnson RJ, Kettelkamp DB, Clark W, et al. Factors effecting late results after meniscectomy. J Bone Joint Surg Am 1974;56(4):719–29.
45. Jørgensen U, Sonne-Holm S, Lauridsen F, et al. Long-term follow-up of meniscectomy in athletes. A prospective longitudinal study. J Bone Joint Surg Br 1987; 69(1):80–3.
46. Annandale T. An operation for displaced semilunar cartilage. Br Med J 1885;1: 779.
47. Annandale T. Excision of the internal semilunar cartilage, resulting in perfect restoration of the joint-movements. Br Med J 1889;1:291–2.
48. Gear MW. The late results of meniscectomy. Br J Surg 1967;54(4):270–2.
49. Tapper EM, Hoover NW. Late results after meniscectomy. J Bone Joint Surg Am 1969;51(3):517–26.
50. Noble J. Clinical features of the degenerate meniscus with the results of meniscectomy. Br J Surg 1975;62(12):977–81.
51. Noble J, Erat K. In defence of the meniscus. A prospective study of 200 meniscectomy patients. J Bone Joint Surg Br 1980;62(1):7–11.
52. Sonne-Holm S, Fledelius I, Ahn NC. Results after meniscectomy in 147 athletes. Acta Orthop Scand 1980;51(2):303–9.
53. Doherty M, Watt I, Dieppe P. Influence of primary generalised osteoarthritis on development of secondary osteoarthritis. Lancet 1983;2(8340):8–11.
54. Lohmander LS, Roos H. Knee ligament injury, surgery and osteoarthrosis. Truth or consequences? Acta Orthop Scand 1994;65(6):605–9.
55. Roos H, Lauren M, Adalberth T, et al. Knee osteoarthritis after meniscectomy: prevalence of radiographic changes after twenty-one years, compared with matched controls. Arthritis Rheum 1998;41(4):687–93.
56. Shrive NG, O'Connor JJ, Goodfellow JW. Load-bearing in the knee joint. Clin Orthop 1978;131:279–87.
57. Fukubayashi T, Kurosawa H. The contact area and pressure distribution pattern of the Knee A study of normal and osteoarthrotic knee joints. Acta Orthop Scand 1980;51(6):871–9.
58. Dandy DJ. Early results of closed partial meniscectomy. Br Med J 1978;1(6120): 1099–100.

59. Oretorp N, Gillquist J. Transcutaneous meniscectomy under arthroscopic control. Int Orthop 1979;3(1):19–25.
60. Northmore-Ball MD, Dandy DJ, Jackson RW. Arthroscopic, open partial, and total meniscectomy. A comparative study. J Bone Joint Surg Br 1983;65(4):400–4.
61. Lohmander LS, Englund PM, Dahl LL, et al. The long-term consequence of anterior cruciate ligament and meniscus injuries: osteoarthritis. Am J Sports Med 2007;35(10):1756–69.
62. Steenbrugge F, Verdonk R, Verstraete K, et al. Long-term assessment of arthroscopic meniscus repair: a 13-year follow-up study. Knee 2002;9(3):181–7.
63. Rockborn P, Messner K. Long-term results of meniscus repair and meniscectomy: a 13-year functional and radiographic follow-up study. Knee Surg Sports Traumatol Arthrosc 2000;8(1):2–10.
64. Hall MJ, Lawrence L. Ambulatory surgery in the United States, 1996. Adv Data 1998;12(300):1–16.
65. Noyes FR, Barber-Westin SD, Rankin M. Meniscal transplantation in symptomatic patients less than fifty years old. J Bone Joint Surg Am 2005;87(Suppl 1 Pt 2): 149–65.
66. Englund M, Guermazi A, Roemer FW, et al. Meniscal tear in knees without surgery and the development of radiographic osteoarthritis. A nested case-control study within the prospective Multicenter Osteoarthritis (MOST) Study. Arthritis Rheum 2009;60(3):831–9.
67. Dervin GF, Stiell IG, Wells GA, et al. Physicians' accuracy and interrator reliability for the diagnosis of unstable meniscal tears in patients having osteoarthritis of the Knee. Can J Surg 2001;44(4):267–74.

Hip MRI and Its Implications for Surgery in Osteoarthritis Patients

Tallal C. Mamisch, MD[a,b,]*, Christoph Zilkens, MD[c,d],
Klaus A. Siebenrock, MD, PhD[a], Bernd Bittersohl, MD[a,c],
Young-Jo Kim, MD, PhD[d], Stefan Werlen, MD[b]

KEYWORDS

- Osteoarthritis • Hip • Femoroacetabular impingement
- MRI • dGEMRIC • Surgery

Osteoarthritis (OA) of the hip stems from a combination of intrinsic factors, such as joint anatomy, and extrinsic factors, such as body weight, injuries, diseases, and load.[1] Possible risk factors for OA are especially instability and impingement. Different surgical techniques, such as osteotomies of the pelvis and the femur,[2] surgical dislocation[3] and hip arthroscopy,[4,5] are being performed to delay or halt OA. Success of salvage hip procedures depends on the existing cartilage and joint damage before surgery; the likelihood of therapy failure rises with advanced OA.[6–8]

For imaging of intra-articular pathology, MRI represents the best technique because it enables clinicians to directly visualize cartilage, it provides superior soft tissue contrast, and it offers the prospect of multidimensional imaging. However, opinions differ on the diagnostic efficacy of MRI and on the question of which MRI technique is most appropriate. Many techniques showing similar promising data have been introduced for the knee.[9–12] Conditions within the hip are different and the relatively thin hip

A version of this article originally appeared in the 47:4 issue of Radiologic Clinics of North America.

[a] Department of Orthopedic Surgery, University of Bern, Freiburgstrasse, 3010 Bern, Switzerland
[b] Department of Radiology, Sonnenhof Clinics, Freiburgstrasse, 3010 Bern, Switzerland
[c] Department of Orthopedic Surgery, University of Düsseldorf, Moorenstrasse 5, 40225 Düsseldorf, Germany
[d] Department of Orthopedic Surgery, Children's Hospital, Harvard Medical School, 300 Longwood Avenue, 02115 Boston, MA, USA
* Corresponding author. Department of Orthopedic Surgery, University of Bern, Freiburgstrasse, 3010 Bern, Switzerland.
E-mail address: mamisch@bwh.harvard.edu (T.C. Mamisch).

Rheum Dis Clin N Am 35 (2009) 591–604
doi:10.1016/j.rdc.2009.09.001
0889-857X/09/$ – see front matter © 2009 Elsevier Inc. All rights reserved.

cartilage and the spherical-shaped joint pose difficulties in the diagnosis of cartilage and labral injury. High MRI resolution and contrast-to-noise ratio between bone, cartilage, synovium, and soft tissue, such as labrum and capsule, are required.

Investigations continue in the search for the best MRI technique for imaging of the hip.[13–15] At present, magnetic resonance (MR) arthrography using intra-articular contrast material has been established as the standard method for imaging of labral lesions.[13,16–18] However, the diagnostic reliability of cartilage lesion remains moderate.[19,20] Furthermore, MRI is still unreliable for diagnosing cartilage delamination.[21] The aim of this review is to discuss the current use of MRI in hip OA and its implications for surgery. Because femoroacetabular impingement (FAI) is becoming an increasingly important clinical diagnosis of the hip joint and is recognized as a precursor to the onset of hip OA, we will focus on this entity. Current standards, difficulties, and possible solutions using high-field MRI, as well as future approaches, will be covered.

FEMOROACETABULAR IMPINGEMENT

During the past decade, FAI has gained increasing attention as possible trigger of hip OA. A static form of impingement is an impingement that does not change with movement, such as the incongruency of the hip after Perthes disease. By comparison, dynamic forms of impingement, which stem from more subtle anatomic deformities, are those forms where the incongruency of the hip joint exists only in certain positions during motion.[4,22,23] Depending on the anatomic abnormality, there are two types of FAI: cam and pincer. In cam FAI, the cause of impact is a nonspherical shape of the femoral head coming along with insufficient femoral head-neck offset. With cam FAI, shear forces lead to acetabular cartilage damage (**Fig. 1**), especially through forced flexion and internal rotation of the hip. In pincer FAI, the impact arises from acetabular overcoverage or some other false configuration or shape of the acetabulum. The shape of the femoral head is spherical. However, the proximal femoral neck abuts frontally against the labrum and the acetabular rim. That way, the labrum is damaged primarily through recurrent trauma (**Fig. 2**) before cartilage damage occurs.[24] Further causes for FAI are rotational anomalies with reduced femoral neck antetorsion, reduced acetabular version,[25,26] or an overcorrection after periacetabular osteotomy (PAO), also called Bernese disease.[27]

Untreated FAI can lead to premature OA of the hip.[28] To relieve symptoms, such as limited range of motion and pain, and to further delay or halt the progression of OA, surgical treatment is necessary. In the case of cam FAI, this includes reshaping of nonspherical femoral. In the case of pincer FAI, this includes trimming the acetabular rim or performing a PAO. The outcome of surgery depends on the quantity of preexisting OA with poor results in patients with advanced degenerative changes. Follow-up examinations after open or arthroscopic FAI surgery have shown favorable results, in particular in the subgroup of patients who did not have signs of advanced hip OA.[28] Therefore, to identify patients who could profit from osteo- or chondroplastic types of surgery, it is important to detect early stages of cartilage degeneration.

Diagnosis of Femoroacetabular Impingement

Diagnosis of FAI is based on clinical findings and radiographic analysis, including MR arthrography.[29] Clinical symptoms of FAI include a slow onset of inguinal pain, usually pronounced with physical activities or prolonged sitting.[30] During physical examination, this can be reproduced by the "impingement test," which pinpoints hip pain produced by passive flexion, internal rotation, and adduction.[31] A positive impingement test can be correlated to acetabular labrum lesions.[24] Radiographic assessment

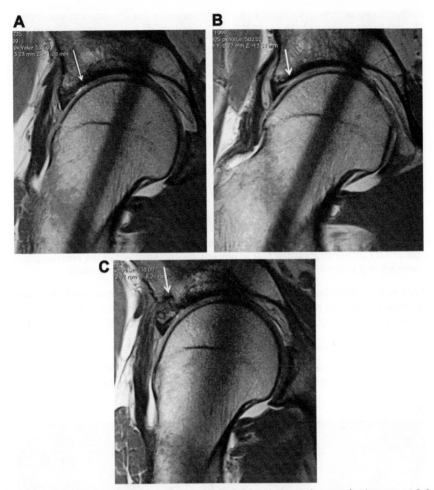

Fig. 1. Radial turbo spin-echo proton density-weighted MR arthrography images at 3.0 T (*A* and *B*) show cartilage damage (*arrow*) at the anterosuperior to superior portion of the acetabular rim due to cam-type impingement. (*C*) Severe cartilage degeneration is associated with intact labrum and cystic deformation (*arrow*) of the acetabular rim.

by means of standard anteroposterior and lateral views[32] is used to assess late stages of hip OA,[33] as well as abnormal femoral head morphology,[34,35] specifically the pistol grip deformity.[36] Additionally, plain radiographic analysis is important in assessing acetabular version and coverage.

However, in FAI, plain radiographs are often inadequate for assessing either femoral head-neck junction morphology or early stage OA.[37] Because of the importance of detecting these hip joint lesions in FAI early on, MRI assessment is quickly becoming the standard tool for diagnostic assessment.[16] Furthermore, it is becoming clear that standard coronal, axial, and sagittal MRI planes are less reliable than radially reconstructed planes perpendicular to the acetabular labrum in detecting early degenerative pathologies of the hip (**Fig. 3**).[16,38] For the assessment of the femoral head-neck morphology, radial reconstructions along the femoral neck axis[35,39,40] improve the understanding of the FAI pathomechanism and correlate well with the prediction of

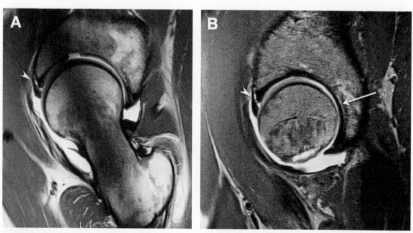

Fig. 2. (A) Radial and (B) sagittal turbo spin-echo proton density-weighted MR arthrography images at 3.0 T demonstrate labral tear in pincer-type impingement at the anterior position (*arrowhead*) and posterior femoroacetabular cartilage degeneration (*arrow*).

an FAI and intraoperative findings.[41] This imaging technique is increasingly recognized as an important tool for morphologic assessment of FAI and is seen as an improvement over alternative techniques for detecting early labral and chondral damage in the hip.[29]

Measurements in Femoroacetabular Impingement

Different MRI parameters have been defined for assessing FAI. These parameters include alpha angle, head-neck offset, acetabular depth, and acetabular version.

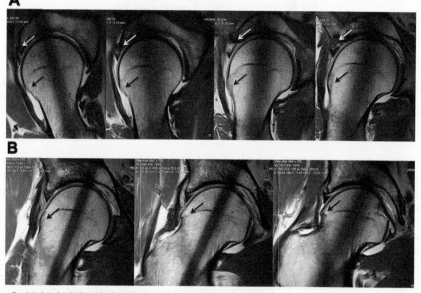

Fig. 3. Multiple (A) radial perpendicular reconstructions around the femoral neck and (B) coronal proton density-weighted MRI show loss of femoral head-neck offset from anterior to superior (*white arrows*). The radial reconstructions (A) also show a labral tear with exact anatomic localization at the anterior-superior position (*black arrows*).

The alpha angle, according to Pfirrmann and colleagues,[21] is the angle between the axis parallel to the femoral neck passing through the narrowest portion of the femoral neck and the axis passing through the point were the head contour passes into the metaphysis (**Fig. 4**). An angle of 55° or more is considered increased and so pathologic. An interval of 30° among the radial reformats should be used to assess alpha angle. The offset can be determined based on the method described by Ito and colleagues.[39] It is the quotient of two lines defining the radius of the femoral head and the extension of the head-neck junction, which is defined by the point where the head contour passes into the metaphysis. Offset is considered reduced when it is ratio of 1.2 or less. In addition, the acetabular coverage can be measured by assessing the acetabular depth within the axial reformat. The depth is expressed as the distance between a line drawn between the anterior and posterior acetabular horns and the center of the femoral head (**Fig. 5**). The acetabular version can be measured using two- or three-dimensional axial T1-weighted MRI through the acetabular roof, as the anterior and posterior rims become apparent. The acetabular version is measured between the distance of the acetabular and posterior rim to the anterior to posterior axis of the pelvis, as shown in **Fig. 6**. **Fig. 7** shows examples of different acetabular versions in patients with cam-type impingement (anteversion), mixed-type impingement (no version), and pincer-type impingement (retroversion).

ASSESSMENT OF THE ACETABULAR LABRUM

For MRI assessment of the acetabular labrum, both noncontrast techniques and arthrographic techniques are used. Based on comparison studies of different techniques in correlation to intraoperative findings, MR arthrography is more reliable in the diagnosis of acetabular labrum lesions. The contrast material, which is administered into the joint under fluoroscopic control, distends the capsule and allows better separation of the labrum and joint capsule. Furthermore, labral tears may be better

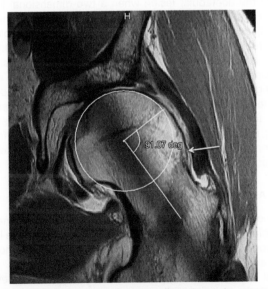

Fig. 4. Radial proton density-weighted reformatted MRI shows the assessment of increased alpha angle (91°) at the anterior-superior position in a cam-type patient (*arrow*).

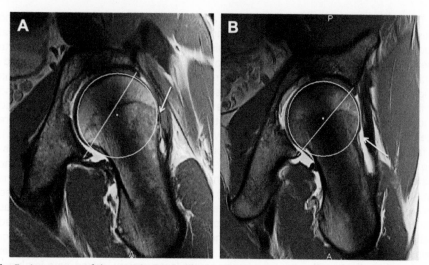

Fig. 5. Assessment of the acetabular depth according to Pfirrmann and colleagues in a radial position. Depth of the acetabulum was defined by the distance between the center of the femoral neck and the line that connect the anterior and posterior acetabular rim. Radial proton density-weighted reformatted MRI show (*A*) the acetabulum is deeper in the patient with pincer FAI and concave head-neck offset (*arrow*) (center of femoral head inside the acetabular fossa; acetabular depth negative) than in (*B*) the patient with cam FAI and loss of head-neck offset (*arrow*) (center of femoral head outside the acetabular fossa; acetabular depth positive).

revealed through contrast filling into the clefts of the labrum. The diagnostic sensitivity of MR arthrography ranges from 90%[13] to 71%.[42] However, the interobserver reliability is only moderate.[20,42] Furthermore, it is not possible to assess the thickness and orientation of the acetabular lesion when a two-dimensional MRI technique is used.[13,42] Also, MR arthrography is an invasive procedure that bears the risk of iatrogenic injury to adjacent neurovascular structures. Regarding staging and grading, most evaluation studies that have been described only determine location (anterior-superior, superior-lateral, and posterior) and whether there is a lesion or not.[42] The added grading classifications of grades 1 through 3 used by Czerny and colleagues[43] depend on the degree of infiltration of the contrast agent into the acetabular labrum, a description of the tear, and changes of signal intensity that don't correlate with structural changes of the acetabular labrum. Other shortcomings, in addition to those related to staging, include a lack of diagnosis for changes of the surface morphology, such as fibrillation, and for changes on the junction between the acetabular cartilage and the acetabular labrum at 1.5 T.

ASSESSMENT OF ACETABULAR CARTILAGE

Compared with the well-established techniques for detecting osteonecrosis[44] and for evaluating the acetabular labrum, techniques for assessing cartilage lesions in the hip have been disappointing.[45] As in acetabular labrum diagnosis, noncontrast techniques and MR arthrography are used. Noncontrast techniques, using two- and three-dimensional sequences, analyze thickness patterns to detect osteoarthritic changes.[46] Reported sensitivity for these measurements is 47% for grade 1 lesions and 49% for grade 2, revealing low diagnostic efficiency and indicating that these

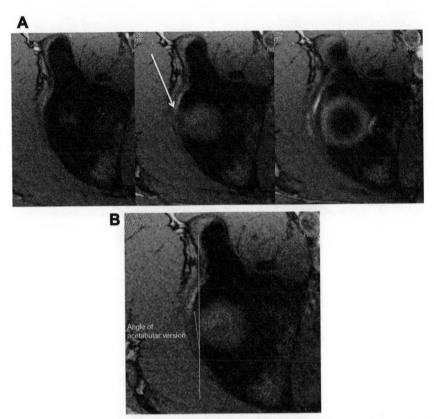

Fig. 6. Assessment of the acetabular version at the acetabular roof on axial three-dimensional fat-suppressed 2-mm slice-thickness T1-weighted MRI show (*A, left to right*) opening of the acetabulum (*arrow*) and (*B*) measurement of the acetabular version.

measurements are more useful in follow-up studies.[46] Mintz and colleagues[47] also tried to classify cartilage based on cartilage thickness and signal intensity changes according to the Outerbridge score,[48] but the results were unreliable. Therefore, they compared only grades 1 through 3 lesions to no lesion (grade 0) for sensitivity and accuracy. Thus, the results are only comparable to thickness measurement studies with the same limitations. With the use of MR arthrography, the detection of cartilage lesions could be improved,[20] but the classification within this study is done without staging or grading, and the accuracy was only moderate (sensitivity of 47%). Additionally, the analysis was limited by low spatial resolution, in particular with regard to separated diagnosis of acetabular and femoral cartilage, restriction to two-dimensional imaging, and low signal-to-noise ratio due to field strength of only 1.0 T or 1.5 T. High interobserver variability was reported. Beaulé and colleagues[45] described cartilage delamination using MR arthrography and its correlation with intraoperative findings in four patients. Using the subdivision of cartilage delamination by Beck and colleagues as a basis,[41] Beaulé and colleagues found that MR arthrography was only able to detect a cleavage (with a frayed edge). Also, MR arthrography did not detect debonding, where the cartilage appears macroscopically sound but is mobile, simulating a carpet phenomenon, which is observed intraoperatively anterior-superior

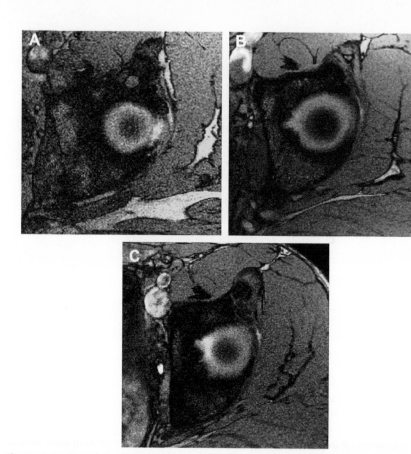

Fig. 7. Examples of acetabular version. Axial three-dimensional fat-suppressed 2-mm slice-thickness T1-weighted MRI show (*A*) cam-type hip with anteversion (12°), (*B*) mixed-type hip with neutral version (0°), and (*C*) pincer-type hip with retroversion (-9°).

in patients with FAI. Overall, the cartilage diagnosis in the hip is limited so far and no reliable staging and grading system has been established. The use of 3.0-T imaging in combination with MR arthrography in the future can overcome these limitations and improve cartilage diagnosis significantly (**Fig. 8**). Nevertheless distinguishing the femoral cartilage layer from the acetabular cartilage layer will remain challenging because the cartilage of the femoroacetabular joint is thin and the cavity is circumferential.

BIOCHEMICAL IMAGING

Articular cartilage is a highly structured tissue made up of chondrocytes and an extracellular matrix composed of water, collagen fibers, negatively charged proteoglycan molecules, and glycosaminoglycans (GAG).[49,50] The collagen fiber network shows a specific arrangement. Indeed, fibers are oriented perpendicularly to the bone-cartilage interface within the radial zone (deepest zone); the orientation is oblique within the intermediate zone; and a parallel orientation is seen within the superficial zone. The layers of cartilage differ not only in orientation of collagen fibers, but also in

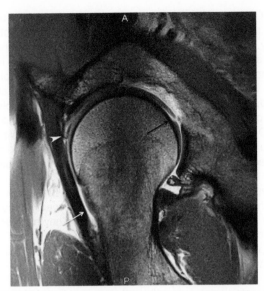

Fig. 8. Radial reformatted turbo spin-echo proton density-weighted MRI at 3.0 T in a patient with a cam-type impingement (*white arrow*) shows femoral cartilage lesion (*black arrow*) and intrasubstance lesion of the labrum (*arrowhead*).

concentration of proteoglycans, which is superior within the intermediate zone, and in amount of water, which is greatest within the superficial zone.

During the progress of OA, the cartilage changes in terms of, for example, water content, collagen orientation, and proteoglycan/GAG content.[51] Biochemical MRI approaches, such as T1 mapping after gadolinium administration, T2 mapping, T2 magnetization transfer, and diffusion-weighted imaging sensitive for cartilage microstructure and biochemical content, may—in addition to morphologic evaluation—provide further insight into the progress of these cartilage alterations. One promising technique recently developed and applied to daily clinical routine is contrast-enhanced MRI, referred to as delayed gadolinium-enhanced MRI of cartilage (dGEMRIC). This technique is based on findings that GAG contributes a strong negative charge to the cartilage matrix. Therefore, if a negatively charged contrast agent, such as $Gd(DTPA)^{2-}$ (gadolinium diethylenetriamine-penta-acetic acid), is given time to penetrate the cartilage, it will distribute in inverse proportion to the GAG content. By means of gadolinium-enhancement within cartilage and subsequent T1 quantification, T1 values can be used as an index for GAG concentration within cartilage. Because GAG seems to be lost early in cartilage degeneration, this technique may improve OA diagnosis at early stages.[12,52] DGEMRIC has been investigated in vitro[53–55] in vivo,[56–60] and for follow-up of cartilage repair procedures.[61]

Kim and colleagues[52] investigated the applicability of dGEMRIC in hip dysplasia. In 68 hips (43 patients), the dGEMRIC index and joint space width were compared with radiographically and clinically relevant factors, such as pain, severity of dysplasia, and age. The dGEMRIC index correlated significantly with pain ($r = -0.50$, $P<.0001$) and with lateral center-edge angle as a measure of severity of dysplasia ($r = 0.52$, $P<.0001$). In contrast, joint space width did not correlate with pain or severity of dysplasia. Furthermore, a statistically significant difference of the dGEMRIC index ($P<.0001$) between mild, moderate, and severe dysplasia could be observed. The average dGEMRIC index ranged from 570 ms (no dysplasia), to 550 ms (mild dysplasia), to 500 ms (moderate dysplasia), to 420 ms (severe dysplasia).

In another study, a cohort of 47 patients who underwent PAO for hip dysplasia was prospectively investigated.[62] Investigators evaluated the dGEMRIC index, in addition to patient age, radiographic severity of OA, and severity of dysplasia. This study showed that PAO is an expedient tool to reduce pain and ameliorate joint function. On the other hand, dGEMRIC was reported as the factor best applicable to identify possible failures of PAO preoperatively. The long-term follow-up of a cohort of patients after PAO with preoperatively low dGEMRIC index showed an increase of the dGEMRIC index postoperatively, implicating that, in defined and reversible stages of cartilage degeneration, OA might be reversible through disease-modifying procedures.[63]

Jessel and colleagues[64] used dGEMRIC to establish a prediction model in 96 hips (74 symptomatic dysplasia patients) and identified age, severity of dysplasia, and labral tear as factors associated with significant hip OA. They showed that dGEMRIC might be able to identify patients who would develop a significant hip OA and who potentially would profit from a salvage procedure like PAO. This was consistent with the other preliminary studies.

Concerning the FAI group, Jessel and colleagues[64] described 30 symptomatic patients (37 hips) treated open-surgically and assessed by dGEMRIC preoperatively. The dGEMRIC index (487 ± 70 ms) was significantly lower than in the control group (570 ± 90 ms). A statistically significant correlation could be established between the dGEMRIC index and the alpha angle ($P<.05$) while there was no correlation between age or gender of patients. They concluded that dGEMRIC index qualifies as a measure for the severity of cartilage damage in patients with FAI and that it reflects the severity of anatomic deformity. Perhaps because of the complex nature

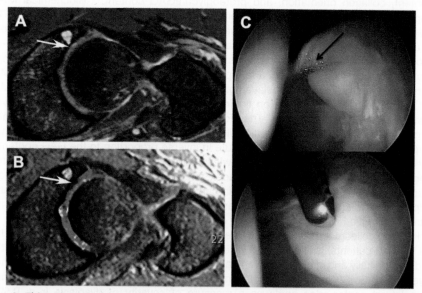

Fig. 9. Thirty-six-year-old patient with cam-type impingement. (*A*) Axial T2-weighted MRI shows possible cartilage damage (*arrow*). (*B*) Axial dGEMRIC clearly shows an area of cartilage damage under the cyst (*arrow*). (*C*) Arthroscopic views demonstrate the cartilage lesion (*arrow*).

of the deformity in FAI, the results in the group of FAI patients are less consistent than those for the group of dysplasia patients.

To reduce acquisition time, a gradient-echo approach for T1 mapping has been developed as an alternative to multi–spin-echo using a dual flip angle technique for obtaining T1 values. This technique has shown promising results in phantom experiments and in vivo for the evaluation of reparative cartilage within the knee after matrix-associated autologous chondrocyte transplantation at 3.0 T.[61] One of the great advantages of this technique, besides a significant reduction of scanning time, is that it offers the possibility of creating three-dimensional maps of the hip cartilage that allow for the assessment of the complex special structure of damage pattern in FAI (**Fig. 9**).

SUMMARY

MRI represents the best available noninvasive tool for hip evaluation in terms of indication and planning for surgical treatment in osteoarthritis. It still has limitations in diagnosing cartilage, especially in the early OA stage. Here, the relatively thin cartilage, the spherical joint shape, and narrowness of tissue structures pose logistical difficulties and demand high MRI technology standards. So far, MR arthrography by means of an intra-articular contrast material in combination with radial reconstructed planes is the method of choice for hip assessment in early OA.

FAI has been identified as a cause of early-onset OA in the hip. Therapeutic strategies do exist but only achieve good results in hips without degenerative changes at the early stage. This emphasizes the need for diagnostic concepts that enable the detection of early cartilage and labral degeneration. Recent developments in high-resolution isotropic imaging, cartilage-specific MRI sequences, local gradient and radio frequency coils, and high field MR systems will improve diagnostic capabilities in terms of signal-to-noise ratio, contrast-to-noise ratio, and shorter acquisition times. In addition to morphologic MRI, biochemical MRI approaches that characterize cartilage microstructure and biochemical content will contribute to a better understanding of cartilage degeneration.

REFERENCES

1. Felson DT. An update on the pathogenesis and epidemiology of osteoarthritis. Radiol Clin North Am 2004;42(1):1–9, v.
2. Jäger M, Westhoff B, Zilkens C, et al. [Indications and results of corrective pelvic osteotomies in developmental dysplasia of the hip]. Orthopade 2008;37(6):556–70 [in German].
3. Ganz R, Gill TJ, Gautier E, et al. Surgical dislocation of the adult hip: a technique with full access to the femoral head and acetabulum without the risk of avascular necrosis. J Bone Joint Surg Br 2001;83(8):1119–24.
4. Ganz R, Parvizi J, Beck M, et al. Femoroacetabular impingement: a cause for osteoarthritis of the hip. Clin Orthop Relat Res 2003;417:112–20.
5. Guanche CA, Bare AA. Arthroscopic treatment of femoroacetabular impingement. Am J Orthop 2006;22(1):95–106.
6. Murphy S, Tannast M, Kim YJ, et al. Debridement of the adult hip for femoroacetabular impingement: indications and preliminary clinical results. Clin Orthop Relat Res 2004;429:178–81.
7. Trousdale RT, Ekkernkamp A, Ganz R, et al. Periacetabular and intertrochanteric osteotomy for the treatment of osteoarthrosis in dysplastic hips. J Bone Joint Surg Am 1995;77(1):73–85.

8. Trumble SJ, Mayo KA, Mast JW. The periacetabular osteotomy. Minimum 2 year followup in more than 100 hips. Clin Orthop Relat Res 1999;363:54–63.
9. Eckstein F. Noninvasive study of human cartilage structure by MRI. Methods Mol Med 2004;101:191–217.
10. Eckstein F, Glaser C. Measuring cartilage morphology with quantitative magnetic resonance imaging. Semin Musculoskelet Radiol 2004;8(4):329–53.
11. Koo S, Gold GE, Andriacchi TP. Considerations in measuring cartilage thickness using MRI: factors influencing reproducibility and accuracy. Osteoarthr Cartil 2005;13(9):782–9.
12. Recht MP, Goodwin DW, Winalski CS, et al. MRI of articular cartilage: revisiting current status and future directions. AJR Am J Roentgenol 2005;185(4):899–914.
13. Czerny C, Hofmann S, Neuhold A, et al. Lesions of the acetabular labrum: accuracy of MR imaging and MR arthrography in detection and staging. Radiology 1996;200(1):225–30.
14. Balkissoon A. MR imaging of cartilage: evaluation and comparison of MR imaging techniques. Top Magn Reson Imaging 1996;8(1):57–67.
15. Plotz GM, Brossmann J, Schunke M, et al. Magnetic resonance arthrography of the acetabular labrum. Macroscopic and histological correlation in 20 cadavers. J Bone Joint Surg Br 2000;82(3):426–32.
16. Locher S, Werlen S, Leunig M, et al. [MR-Arthrography with radial sequences for visualization of early hip pathology not visible on plain radiographs]. Z Orthop Ihre Grenzgeb 2002;140(1):52–7 [in German].
17. Petersilge CA, Haque MA, Petersilge WJ, et al. Acetabular labral tears: evaluation with MR arthrography. Radiology 1996;200(1):231–5.
18. Petersilge CA. MR arthrography for evaluation of the acetabular labrum. Skeletal Radiol 2001;30(8):423–30.
19. Knuesel PR, Pfirrmann CW, Noetzli HP, et al. MR arthrography of the hip: diagnostic performance of a dedicated water-excitation 3D double-echo steady-state sequence to detect cartilage lesions. AJR Am J Roentgenol 2004;183(6):1729–35.
20. Schmid MR, Notzli HP, Zanetti M, et al. Cartilage lesions in the hip: diagnostic effectiveness of MR arthrography. Radiology 2003;226(2):382–6.
21. Pfirrmann CW, Mengiardi B, Dora C, et al. Cam and pincer femoroacetabular impingement: characteristic MR arthrographic findings in 50 patients. Radiology 2006;240(3):778–85.
22. Kim YJ, Bixby S, Mamisch TC, et al. Imaging structural abnormalities in the hip joint: instability and impingement as a cause of osteoarthritis. Semin Musculoskelet Radiol 2008;12(4):334–45.
23. Kim YJ. Nonarthroplasty hip surgery for early osteoarthritis. Rheum Dis Clin North Am 2008;34(3):803–14.
24. Leunig M, Beck M, Dora C, et al. [Femoroacetabular impingement: trigger for the development of osteoarthritis]. Orthopade 2006;35(1):77–84 [in German].
25. Reynolds D, Lucas J, Klaue K. Retroversion of the acetabulum. A cause of hip pain. J Bone Joint Surg Br 1999;81(2):281–8.
26. Dora C, Zurbach J, Hersche O, et al. Pathomorphologic characteristics of post-traumatic acetabular dysplasia. J Orthop Trauma 2000;14(7):483–9.
27. Dora C, Mascard E, Mladenov K, et al. Retroversion of the acetabular dome after Salter and triple pelvic osteotomy for congenital dislocation of the hip. J Pediatr Orthop B 2002;11(1):34–40.

28. Beck M, Kalhor M, Leunig M, et al. Hip morphology influences the pattern of damage to the acetabular cartilage: femoroacetabular impingement as a cause of early osteoarthritis of the hip. J Bone Joint Surg Br 2005;87(7): 1012–8.
29. Kassarjian A, Yoon LS, Belzile E, et al. Triad of MR arthrographic findings in patients with cam-type femoroacetabular impingement. Radiology 2005;236(2): 588–92.
30. Leunig M, Ganz R. [Femoroacetabular impingement. A common cause of hip complaints leading to arthrosis]. Unfallchirurgie 2005;108(1):9–17 [in German].
31. MacDonald S, Garbuz D, Ganz R. Clinical evaluation of the symptomatic young adult hip. Semin Arthroplasty 1997;8:3–9.
32. Siebenrock KA, Schoeniger R, Ganz R. Anterior femoro-acetabular impingement due to acetabular retroversion. Treatment with periacetabular osteotomy. J Bone Joint Surg Am 2003;85(2):278–86.
33. Kellgren JH, Lawrence JS. Radiological assessment of osteo-arthrosis. Ann Rheum Dis 1957;16:494–502.
34. Eijer H, Myers SR, Ganz R. Anterior femoroacetabular impingement after femoral neck fractures. J Orthop Trauma 2001;15(7):475–81.
35. Siebenrock KA, Wahab KH, Werlen S, et al. Abnormal extension of the femoral head epiphysis as a cause of cam impingement. Clin Orthop Relat Res 2004; 418:54–60.
36. Stulberg SD, Cordell LD, Harris WH, et al. Unrecognized childhood hip disease: a major cause of idiopathic osteoarthitis of the hip. In: Proceedings of the Third Open Scientific Meeting of the Hip. CV Mosby Co; 1975. p. 212–28.
37. Locher S, Werlen S, Leunig M, et al. [Inadequate detectability of early stages of coxarthrosis with conventional roentgen images]. Z Orthop Ihre Grenzgeb 2001; 139(1):70–4 [in German].
38. Kubo T, Horii M, Harada Y, et al. Radial-sequence magnetic resonance imaging in evaluation of acetabular labrum. J Orthop Sci 1999;4(5):328–32.
39. Ito K, Minka MA 2nd, Leunig M, et al. Femoroacetabular impingement and the cam-effect. A MRI-based quantitative anatomical study of the femoral head-neck offset. J Bone Joint Surg Br 2001;83(2):171–6.
40. Leunig M, Werlen S, Ungersbock A, et al. Evaluation of the acetabular labrum by MR arthrography. J Bone Joint Surg Br 1997;79(2):230–4.
41. Beck M, Leunig M, Parvizi J, et al. Anterior femoroacetabular impingement: part II. Midterm results of surgical treatment. Clin Orthop Relat Res 2004; 418:67–73.
42. Keeney JA, Peelle MW, Jackson J, et al. Magnetic resonance arthrography versus arthroscopy in the evaluation of articular hip pathology. Clin Orthop Relat Res 2004;429:163–9.
43. Czerny C, Kramer J, Neuhold A, et al. [Magnetic resonance imaging and magnetic resonance arthrography of the acetabular labrum: comparison with surgical findings]. Rofo 2001;173(8):702–7 [in German].
44. Mont MA, Hungerford DS. Non-traumatic avascular necrosis of the femoral head. J Bone Joint Surg Am 1995;77(3):459–74.
45. Beaule PE, Zaragoza E, Copelan N. Magnetic resonance imaging with gadolinium arthrography to assess acetabular cartilage delamination. A report of four cases. J Bone Joint Surg Am 2004;86(10):2294–8.
46. Nishii T, Nakanishi K, Sugano N, et al. Articular cartilage evaluation in osteoarthritis of the hip with MR imaging under continuous leg traction. Magn Reson Imaging 1998;16(8):871–5.

47. Mintz DN, Hooper T, Connell D, et al. Magnetic resonance imaging of the hip: detection of labral and chondral abnormalities using noncontrast imaging. Arthroscopy 2005;21(4):385–93.
48. Outerbridge RE. The etiology of chondromalacia patellae. J Bone Joint Surg Br 1961;43:752–7.
49. Poole AR, Kojima T, Yasuda T, et al. Composition and structure of articular cartilage: a template for tissue repair. Clin Orthop Relat Res 2001;391:S26–33.
50. Cova M, Toffanin R. MR microscopy of hyaline cartilage: current status. Eur Radiol 2002;12(4):814–23.
51. Venn M, Maroudas A. Chemical composition and swelling of normal and osteoarthrotic femoral head cartilage. I. Chemical composition. Ann Rheum Dis 1977; 36(2):121–9.
52. Kim YJ, Jaramillo D, Millis MB, et al. Assessment of early osteoarthritis in hip dysplasia with delayed gadolinium-enhanced magnetic resonance imaging of cartilage. J Bone Joint Surg Am 2003;85(10):1987–92.
53. Woertler K, Buerger H, Moeller J, et al. Patellar articular cartilage lesions: in vitro MR imaging evaluation after placement in gadopentetate dimeglumine solution. Radiology 2004;230(3):768–73.
54. Mlynarik V, Trattnig S, Huber M, et al. The role of relaxation times in monitoring proteoglycan depletion in articular cartilage. J Magn Reson Imaging 1999; 10(4):497–502.
55. Bashir A, Gray ML, Burstein D. Gd-DTPA2- as a measure of cartilage degradation. Magn Reson Med 1996;36(5):665–73.
56. Bashir A, Gray ML, Boutin RD, et al. Glycosaminoglycan in articular cartilage: in vivo assessment with delayed Gd(DTPA) (2-)-enhanced MR imaging. Radiology 1997;205(2):551–8.
57. Burstein D, Velyvis J, Scott KT, et al. Protocol issues for delayed Gd(DTPA) (2-)-enhanced MRI (dGEMRIC) for clinical evaluation of articular cartilage. Magn Reson Med 2001;45(1):36–41.
58. Tiderius C, Olsson L, de Verdier H, et al. Gd-DTPA2- enhanced MRI of femoral knee cartilage: a dose response study in healthy volunteers. Magn Reson Med 2001;46:1067–71.
59. Tiderius CJ, Olsson LE, Leander P, et al. Delayed gadolinium-enhanced MRI of cartilage (dGEMRIC) in early knee osteoarthritis. Magn Reson Med 2003;49(3):488–92.
60. Williams A, Gillis A, McKenzie C, et al. Glycosaminoglycan distribution in cartilage as determined by delayed gadolinium-enhanced MRI of cartilage (dGEMRIC): potential clinical applications. AJR Am J Roentgenol 2004;182(1):167–72.
61. Trattnig S, Marlovits S, Gebetsroither S, et al. Three-dimensional delayed gadolinium-enhanced MRI of cartilage (dGEMRIC) for in vivo evaluation of reparative cartilage after matrix-associated autologous chondrocyte transplantation at 3.0T: preliminary results. J Magn Reson Imaging 2007;26(4):974–82.
62. Cunningham T, Jessel R, Zurakowski D, et al. Delayed gadolinium-enhanced magnetic resonance imaging of cartilage to predict early failure of Bernese periacetabular osteotomy for hip dysplasia. J Bone Joint Surg Am 2006;88(7): 1540–8.
63. Jessel R, Zurakowski D, Zilkens C, et al. Radiographic and patient factors associated with pre-radiographic osteoarthritis in hip dysplasia. J Bone Joint Surg Am 2009;91(5):1120–9.
64. Jessel R, Zilkens C, Tiderius C, et al. Assessment of osteoarthritis in hips with femoroacetabular impingement using delayed gadolinium enhanced MRI of cartilage. JMRM 2009, in press.

Role of Imaging in Spine, Hand, and Wrist Osteoarthritis

Antoine Feydy, MD, PhD*, Etienne Pluot, MD,
Henri Guerini, MD, Jean-Luc Drapé, MD, PhD

KEYWORDS
- Osteoarthritis • Wrist • Hand • Finger
- Spine • Imaging • Grading

OSTEOARTHRITIS OF THE WRIST AND HAND

There is a striking difference between the rarity of osteoarthritis (OA) of the wrist and the high prevalence of OA of the fingers. OA in the fingers usually occurs following a trauma or as a result of ongoing metabolic joint diseases, especially calcium pyrophosphate dehydrate (CPPD) deposition disease, also called chondrocalcinosis. Finger OA is frequent in postmenopausal women, and represents up to one-third of peripheral OA after OA of the knee and hip. Assessing the prevalence of hand OA (HOA) depends on the criteria supporting the diagnosis. The Framingham study has estimated the prevalence to be as high as 26% of women and 12% of men older than 70 years[1]; however, according to Kellgren and Lawrence, radiographic definition HOA is identified in 67% of women and 55% of men in the Rotterdam Study, a population-based cohort (age >55 years).[2] The prevalence of OA in distal interphalangeal and proximal interphalangeal joints after 55 years of age reaches 20% and 5%, respectively. Trapezio-metacarpal joint OA, also called rhizarthrosis, is present in 8% of the population older than 55 years. HOA remains a frequent complaint from patients, the aesthetic harm resulting from deformity being a major concern in some patients. Pain is the main symptom of rhizarthrosis ahead of deformity. Treatment of HOA should be individualized according to: localization of OA; risk factors (age, sex, adverse mechanical factors); type of OA (nodal, erosive, traumatic); presence of inflammation; severity of structural change; level of pain, disability, and restriction of quality of life; comorbidity and comedication (including OA at other sites); and the wishes and expectations of the patient.[3] Management of OA of the wrist and hand

---

A version of this article originally appeared in the 47:4 issue of Radiologic Clinics of North America.
Department of Radiology B, Cochin Hospital, Paris Descartes University, 27 rue du Faubourg Saint Jacques, 75014 Paris, France
* Corresponding author.
E-mail address: antoine.feydy@cch.aphp.fr (A. Feydy).

Rheum Dis Clin N Am 35 (2009) 605–649
doi:10.1016/j.rdc.2009.08.007
0889-857X/09/$ – see front matter © 2009 Elsevier Inc. All rights reserved.

rheumatic.theclinics.com

remains nonsurgical in most cases. Surgery should be discussed in cases of failure of nonsurgical procedures in controlling the symptoms.

Demographics

Age is the main risk factor of developing HOA. The incidence of the condition increases after age 45 years, ranging from 5% at 40 to 65% after 80 years.[4] Degenerative changes tend to be more severe in distal interphalangeal joints, especially of the index finger, than in proximal interphalangeal or carpometacarpal joints. HOA mostly occurs on the dominant hand.[5]

The interphalangeal and trapezio-metacarpal (TMC) joints are the most common localization of HOA in women older than 55 years. Rhizarthrosis is rarely encountered in men younger than 50 years, whereas the condition is present in 8% of women of the same age group. Before 70 years of age, the prevalence of HOA in women exceeds that of men by 50%. The prevalence of finger OA is noticeably higher in women after early or induced menopause. The prevalence of TMC OA is dramatically increased in women after hysterectomy.[6] These differences of prevalence suggest a role of sexual hormones in the pathogenesis of HOA.[7,8]

Genetic factors may also predispose to HOA, especially in women.[9] Mutations of genes that code for collagen II may increase the risk of developing early OA.[10] On the other hand, the role of human leukocyte antigen (HLA) types regarding the risk of OA remains much debated.[11,12]

Trapezio-Metacarpal Joint Osteoarthritis or Rhizarthrosis

Almost constantly bilateral, rhizarthrosis occurs in perimenopausal women and affects the dominant hand more severely. One should probably coin rhizarthrosis "peritrapezial OA" as the degenerative changes extend to the adjacent scapho-trapezial and trapezio-trapezoid joints.

Clinical presentation

Mechanical soreness of the base of the thumb and thenar eminence is the main clinical sign of rhizarthrosis. The pattern of pain can also be inflammatory, and pain appears when sleeping, although this pattern should raise the possibility of associated conditions, especially carpal tunnel syndrome that is present in 40% of cases.[13]

Radiographs

Like in other localizations, there is no correlation between clinical presentation and radiographic findings. Specific posteroanterior (PA) and lateral views of the TMC joint must be obtained (Kapandji's or Robert's views).[14] The radiographic features of rhizarthrosis are characterized by joint space narrowing (JSN) and deformity, osteophytes, and development in the trapezium of subchondral sclerosis and geodes/subchondral cysts. Prominent destruction of the joint cartilage leads to subluxation of M1 laterally and enlargement of the first intermetacarpal space (**Fig. 1**). Secondary loose bodies may also occur. The radiological classifications of Dell and colleagues (**Box 1**) and Eaton and Litter (**Box 2**) are the most commonly used.[15] The Dell classification focuses only on the TMC joint without pre-OA stage. The Eaton and Littler classification includes a pre-OA stage and also the involvement of the scapho-trapezial, trapezio-trapezoid, and TMC joints.

The "trapezial tilt" can be assessed on Kapandji or Robert PA views (**Fig. 2**). The normal values are respectively 125° and 42° ± 4°. Advanced TMC joint OA (Eaton III and IV) is associated with an increased trapezial tilt. Mild trapezio-metacarpal joint arthritis with an increased trapezial tilt may be treated surgically. Dynamic PA views

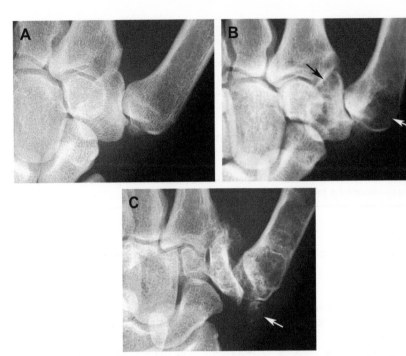

Fig. 1. Rhizarthrosis outcome. (*A*) Posteroanterior radiograph of the wrist at baseline shows lateral trapezio-metacarpal subluxation and slight trapezial osteophytosis with dysplasia. (*B*) Follow-up posteroanterior radiograph 3 years later demonstrates joint space narrowing (JNS) and trapezial subchondral osteosclerosis with large bone cyst of trapezium and M1 (*arrows*). (*C*) Posteroanterior radiograph at 12 years follow-up shows bone loss of trapezium and loose bodies larger than 2 mm (*arrow*).

allow evaluation of the reversibility of the subluxation of M1, and assessment of the increased mobility of the trapezium bone in cases of rhizarthrosis.

Magnetic resonance imaging

MRI may demonstrate an extensive synovitis and bone marrow edema of the TMC joint (**Fig. 3**). Synovial expansions may develop toward the first intermetacarpal space. Bone cyst boundaries are more accurately defined with MRI than with radiographs.

Scapho-Trapezial Osteoarthritis

Scapho-trapezial OA is most commonly associated with rhizarthrosis. Radiographic features of the condition are seen in up to 7% of women and 2% of men.[16]

Box 1
Dell classification of trapezio-metacarpal osteoarthritis

–Stage I: JSN without subluxation or osteophyte

–Stage II: JSN, osteophytes, subtle subluxation

–Stage III: JSN, osteophytes, subluxation or trapezio-metacarpal dislocation

–Stage IV: As stage III, plus geodes

Box 2
Eaton classification of trapezio-metacarpal osteoarthritis

–Stage I: Normal or slightly widened trapezio-metacarpal joint. Normal articular contours. Trapezio-metacarpal subluxation (if present up to one-third of the articular surface).

–Stage II: Decreased trapezio-metacarpal joint space. Trapezio-metacarpal subluxation (if present up to one-third of the articular surface). Osteophytes or loose bodies less than 2 mm in diameter.

–Stage III: Further decrease in trapezio-metacarpal joint space. Subchondral cysts or sclerosis. Osteophytes or loose bodies 2 mm or more in diameter. Trapezio-metacarpal joint subluxation of one-third or more of the articular surface.

–Stage IV: Involvement of the scapho-trapezial joint or, less commonly, the trapezio-trapezoid or trapezio-metacarpal joint to the index finger.

Clinical presentation

In cases of CPPD deposition disease, OA of the scapho-trapezial joint is part of a multi-focal form of OA.

Radiographs

A PA radiograph of the wrist and an oblique view of the semi-pronated wrist should be obtained to visualize the base of the thumb. Comparative studies allow detection of early joint space loss. Radiological features are represented by JSN, subchondral sclerosis, subchondral geodes, osteophytes, and marked cortical irregularities at the distal aspect of the scaphoid, which can simulate erosions (**Fig. 4**). In later stages, the scaphoid bone tilts horizontally, resulting in shortening of the carpus and secondary dorsal intercalated segmental instability (DISI).[17]

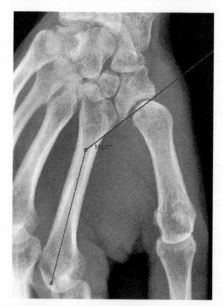

Fig. 2. Trapezial slope assessment. Posteroanterior Kapandji radiograph shows angle between the inferior joint surface of trapezium; the long axis of M2 is significantly increased above 140° and measures 142.7°.

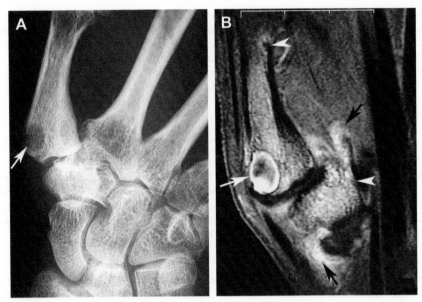

Fig. 3. Rhizarthrosis with extensive bone edema. (*A*) Radiograph shows bone cyst of M1 (*arrow*) and trapezial osteosclerosis. (*B*) Coronal contrast-enhanced fat-suppressed T1-weighted MRI shows peripheral enhancement of the bone cyst (*white arrow*) and extensive bone edema (*arrowheads*) of the whole trapezium and most of the first metacarpal. There are synovial expansions (*black arrows*) superiorly and inferiorly toward the first intermetacarpal space.

Ultrasound

The main ultrasonographic features of tendinopathy of the flexor carpi radialis (FCR) are characterized by enlargement of the tendon and hyporeflective areas replacing the normal fibrillar appearance of the tendon. Areas of tendon necrosis might appear as unreflective areas. In advanced stages of the condition the tendon gradually

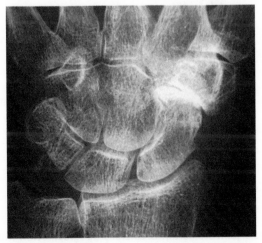

Fig. 4. Isolated severe scapho-trapezial joint osteoarthritis. Posteroanterior radiograph shows complete JSN with subchondral bone sclerosis.

becomes thinner, leading to partial or even full thickness tears. Due to the oblique course of the tendon toward the deeper layers of the hand and its insertion on the base of M2, anisotropy challenges a thorough examination of the distal part of the tendon. In addition, this may also be challenged by a likely hypertrophic tubercle of the scaphoid. A dynamic maneuver with palmar flexion of the wrist allows reduction of the obliquity of the tendon and therefore the associated anisotropy. Ultrasound can also reveal cortical irregularities of the distal aspect of the scaphoid adjacent to the tendon sheath, joint effusion, and scapho-trapezial synovitis.

Arthrography and computed tomographic arthrography

Arthrography obtained following midcarpal opacification may demonstrate an abnormal opacification of the FCR tendon sheath, indicating an abnormal carpal capsular breach near the scapho-trapezial joint (**Fig. 5**). Computed tomographic (CT) arthrography best depicts the topography and severity of chondral lesions. Subchondral geodes are usually partially filled by intra-articular contrast.

Magnetic resonance imaging and magnetic resonance arthrography

MRI can detect early scapho-trapezial OA before radiographic abnormalities in demonstrating a subchondral bone edema (**Fig. 6**). The great advantage of MRI over ultrasound and CT arthrography is the ability to show the scapho-trapezial joint and the adjacent soft tissues. In addition to tenosynovitis of the FCR and midsubstance tendinopathy, MRI is reliable in demonstrating joint effusion, synovitis, and extensive subchondral bone edema within the scapho-trapezial joint (**Fig. 7**). Intra-articular injection of gadolinium does not seem to improve the assessment of this joint and surrounding soft tissues.

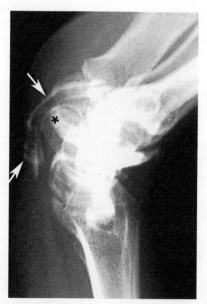

Fig. 5. Scapho-trapezial joint osteoarthritis. Lateral arthrographic view with extension shows leakage of contrast medium toward the tendon sheath of the flexor carpi radialis (*arrows*) in front of the distal tubercle of scaphoid (*asterisk*).

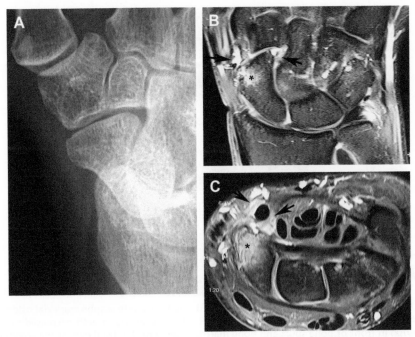

Fig. 6. Early scapho-trapezial osteoarthritis. (*A*) Posteroanterior radiograph shows no discrete abnormality of the scapho-trapezial joint. (*B*) Coronal and (*C*) axial contrast-enhanced fat-suppressed T1-weighted MRI show bone marrow edema of the distal scaphoid (*asterisk*) with cortex irregularities and synovitis of the scapho-trapezio-trapezoid joint (*arrows*). Note on (*C*) the tenosynovitis of the flexor carpi radialis tendon (*arrows*).

Radiocarpal Joint Osteoarthritis

Clinical presentation

Much less frequent than in fingers, radiocarpal OA generally occurs secondary to wrist sprain (scapho-lunate advanced collapse [SLAC] wrist), fracture, or necrosis involving a carpal bone (scaphoid nonunion advanced collapse [SNAC] wrist). The 2 most frequent types of OA in the wrist are the SLAC (55%) and scaphotrapezio-trapezoid (STT) OA (20%).

Radiographs

PA, lateral, and oblique views in neutral position should be obtained to best assess intracarpal instabilities. Findings suggestive of OA are nonspecific, but the distribution of the lesions is stereotyped and classified as follows (**Fig. 8**):

- Grade 1: limited radio-scaphoid OA to the lateral aspect of the joint
- Grade 2: extensive OA of the radio-scaphoid joint
- Grade 3: luno-capitate OA

The scapho-capitate joint may also be severely damaged, leading to impaction of the capitate. The capitate then translates proximally toward the radius, resulting in secondary narrowing of the hamato-lunate joint space (**Fig. 9**). This joint space loss is best diagnosed on PA views obtained with ulnar flexion of the wrist.

Radiographic evidence of CPPD deposition disease should not be overlooked, as the triangular fibrocartilage complex (TFCC), luno-triquetral ligament, and luno-triquetral

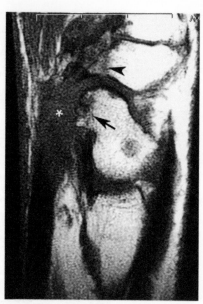

Fig. 7. Tendonitis of the flexor carpi radialis (FCR) due to a severe scapho-trapezial osteoarthritis. Sagittal T1-weighted MRI shows the FCR tendon is enlarged with decreased signal (*asterisk*) in front of bone spurs and bone marrow edema of the distal part of the scaphoid (*arrow*). Note also the degenerative lesions of the tubercle of the trapezium (*arrowhead*).

cartilage are the most common sites of calcification around the wrist. Calcific deposits within hyaline cartilage appear as thin, well defined, and linear, following the contour of the subchondral plate.

Computed tomographic arthrography, magnetic resonance imaging, and magnetic resonance arthrography

Radiographs are usually reliable for the diagnosis of OA. Before any surgical treatment (ie, ligament repair, arthrodesis), a thorough assessment of the cartilage is often required, which is best demonstrated on CT arthrography, MRI or, more accurately, MR arthrography.

Classic features of chondropathy in the wrist are not specific, but the distribution of the chondral lesions is of utmost importance. Some more specific imaging findings of radiocarpal OA should be reported:

- Early subchondral edema of the distal tip of the radius, joint synovitis on MRI and MR arthrography, preceding radiographic abnormalities.
- JSN, subchondral sclerosis and geodes, osteophytes on radiographs and CT arthrography. Osteophytes develop at the junction between the articular and nonarticular surfaces at the lateral edge of the scaphoid, and thinning of the radial styloid process are early signs of SLAC wrist.
- Chondral thinning, deepening of chondral fissures on CT arthrography (**Fig. 10**), MRI, and MR arthrography.
- In later stages, radio-carpal then luno-capitate JSN appears. Once the cartilage surface between the capitate and hamate is worn out, impingement and secondary OA of the luno-hamate joint occurs.
- The radio-lunate joint is usually preserved until late stages of the condition.

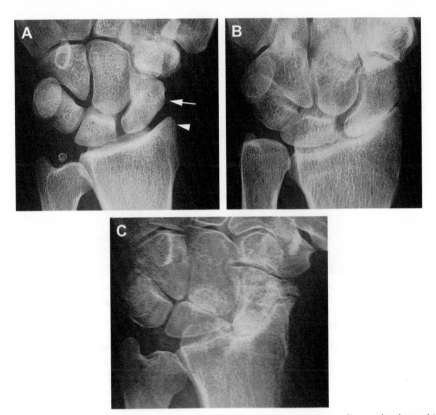

Fig. 8. Scapho-lunate advanced collapse (SLAC) wrist. Posteroanterior radiographs shows (*A*) stage 1 with slight bone sclerosis of the radial styloid (*arrowhead*) and cortex irregularities of the scaphoid (*arrow*), (*B*) stage 2, and (*C*) stage 3. Note the scapholunate diastasis on each view.

To date, there is almost no study in the literature comparing the accuracy of the different imaging modalities in detecting intracarpal chondral lesions. A recent study demonstrates a much better accuracy of CT arthrography, supported by sensitivity and specificity of 100%, compared with an average sensitivity of 10% to 30% and 30% to 40% using MRI and MR arthrography, respectively.[18]

Distal Radio-Ulnar Joint Osteoarthritis

Clinical presentation
Distal radio-ulnar joint (DRUJ) OA usually occurs secondary to various types of trauma (ie, DRUJ dislocation, fracture of both distal radius and ulna).

Radiographs
Oblique views obtained in neutral position show the dorsal displacement of the ulnar head. The pisiform bone should be centrally located between the palmar cortical lines of the scaphoid and capitate bones on oblique views. Other radiographic findings are bone sclerosis and geodes on the ulnar head and the sigmoid notch of the radius.

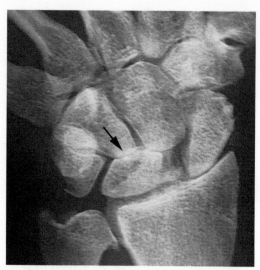

Fig. 9. SLAC wrist. Posteroanterior radiograph with ulnar tilt shows hamato-lunate JSN (*arrow*) and is more sensitive in depicting this joint osteoarthritis than the neutral view.

Ulno-Carpal Joint Osteoarthritis

Ulnar impaction syndrome owing to a relatively long ulna leads to ulno-carpal OA. A relatively long ulna is congenital, or acquired following fractures complicated by vicious callus, and shortening and angulation of the distal radius (Colles fracture).

Radiographs

On PA views of a pronated wrist the ulnar variance is positive, indicating an excessively long ulna. The ulnar variance indicates the level of the distal ulna relative to the distal radius. Normal values range from -2 to 0 mm. Indirect signs of chondropathy

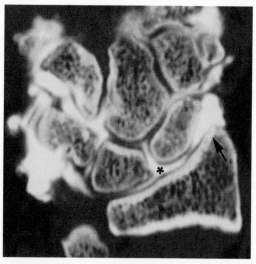

Fig. 10. SLAC wrist stage 1. Coronal CT arthrography view shows cartilage thinning of the radial styloid (*arrow*) and tear of the central part of the scapho-lunate ligament (*asterisk*).

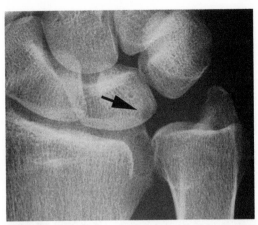

Fig. 11. Ulnocarpal impaction. Posteroanterior radiograph shows positive ulnar index and subchondral bone cyst of the lunate (*arrow*).

(sclerosis, geodes) are demonstrated on the medial part of the proximal aspect of the lunate and ulnar head (**Fig. 11**). Luno-triquetral joint diastasis and disruption of the Gilula first arch related to a tear through the luno-triquetral ligament is also possible.

Arthrography, computed tomographic arthrography, and magnetic resonance imaging

The best imaging modality to reveal an ulnar impaction syndrome is MRI. MRI demonstrates a typical pattern of lesions: medial and proximal chondral defect of the lunate, thinning and perforation of the TFCC associated with excessively long ulna, and luno-triquetral ligament tear. The distribution of subchondral bone edema follows a typical pattern, located at the medial and proximal part of the lunate, adjacent to chondral lesions. The subchondral edema in ulnar impaction syndrome tends to be less extensive than in Kienböck disease, which is also more centrally located. Bone edema can also occur in the ulnar head and at the insertion of the luno-triquetral ligament. There seems to be a strong correlation between subchondral bone edema and the intensity of pain related to ulnar impaction syndrome. Of note, ulnar impaction syndrome can occur without abnormal ulnar variance, and be related to a sole dynamic impingement. In such cases, MRI is therefore of great help in demonstrating associated signs (**Fig. 12**).

Piso-Triquetral Joint Osteoarthritis

Clinical presentation

Diagnosing piso-triquetral joint OA is fairly straightforward, mainly based on clinical examination. Patients present with typical ulnar-sided wrist, pain possibly associated with signs of ulnar nerve entrapment within the Guyon canal.

Radiographs

In addition to PA and oblique views of the wrist, carpal tunnel view and 30° oblique view in supination must be obtained to correctly assess the joint space (**Fig. 13**).[19]

Ultrasound

Joint effusions, distension of the superior and inferior synovial recess, and a potential ganglion developing within the Guyon canal are well demonstrated by ultrasound (**Fig. 14**). Ulnar nerve displacement and likely inflammatory appearance of the synovium are also detected. One may aspirate and inject steroids into the joint under ultrasound guidance. The appearance of the flexor carpi ulnaris enthesis can also be depicted.

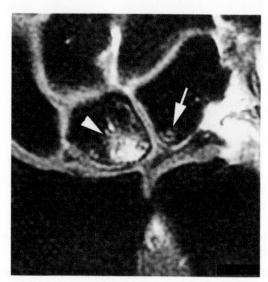

Fig. 12. Occult ulnocarpal impaction. Radiographs are negative with a neutral ulnar index. Coronal short-tau inversion recovery (STIR) MRI shows degenerative thinning of the triangular ligament. There are also cartilage ulceration of the lunate with extensive bone edema (*arrowhead*) and bone edema of radial side of the triquetrum (*arrow*).

Magnetic resonance imaging

MRI provides the same information as ultrasound, but assesses more accurately the joint line and the likely extensive subchondral bone edema (see **Fig. 14**).

Hamato-Lunate Joint Osteoarthritis

Clinical presentation

Hamato-lunate impingement is a recently described uncommon cause of ulnar-sided wrist pain.[20] A normal variant consisting in a joint between the hamate and a medial

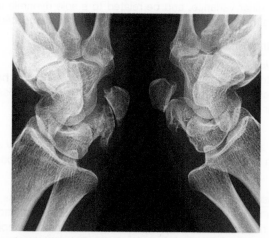

Fig. 13. Piso-triquetral joint osteoarthritis. Comparative ulnar side radiograph shows bilateral piso-triquetral joint osteoarthritis.

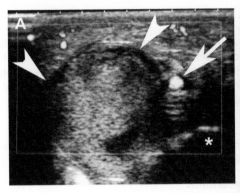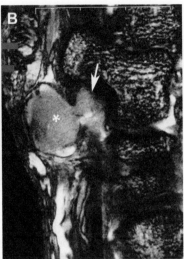

Fig. 14. Hemorrhagic ganglion of the Guyon tunnel. (*A*) Axial ultrasound view shows echoic material within the ganglion cyst due to hemorrhagic pattern (*arrowheads*) with a deep pedicle extending toward the pisiform bone (*asterisk*). Ulnar artery (*arrow*). (*B*) Sagittal T2-weighted MRI shows the ganglion has a relative central low signal due to hemorrhage (*asterisk*). Note the deep pedicle (*arrows*) going to the piso-triquetral joint.

facet of a type II lunate may lead to a significantly high prevalence of chondromalacia (60%–82%).[21–23] In up to 50% of the population, the lunate bears a medial facet separated from the distal facet that articulates with the hamate.[21] This type of chondral lesion may be responsible for ulnar-sided wrist pain, and could be explained by a chronic impingement caused by ulnar flexion of the wrist.[24]

Radiographs
Radiographs may show nothing but a type II lunate at an early stage (**Fig. 15**). Focal areas of demineralization of the proximal hamate or subchondral geodes may also be seen.[25] The hamate facet is visible on plain films in only 64% to 72% of cases.[22]

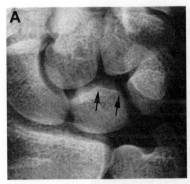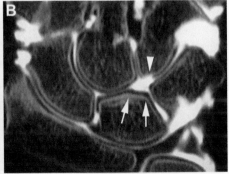

Fig. 15. Early hamato-lunate joint osteoarthritis. (*A*) Posteroanterior radiograph demonstrates type II lunate (*arrows*) without joint space or subchondral abnormality. (*B*) Coronal CT arthrography view shows cartilage ulceration of the proximal part of the hamate (*arrowhead*) and integrity of the lunate facet joint (*arrows*).

Computed tomographic arthrography, magnetic resonance imaging, and magnetic resonance arthrography

Both CT arthrography and MR arthrography clearly demonstrate chondral lesions (see **Fig. 15**).[26] MRI can depict bone marrow edema of the proximal part of the hamate (**Fig. 16**). The association with luno-triquetral ligament tears is debated. Most patients can be treated conservatively. According to the intensity of symptoms, surgical resection of the proximal pole of the hamate infrequently may also be indicated.

Finger Joints Osteoarthritis

Finger joints OA is a complex condition as reflected by the wide and confusing terminology used in the literature to describe it. This terminology is summarized in **Table 1**.

Distal Interphalangeal Joint (DIPJ) Osteoarthritis

Clinical presentation

DIJPs are the sites most commonly affected by finger OA. The condition occurs predominantly in the 40- to 60-year age group, and affects women fourfold more frequently than men. Osteophytes and thickening of the joint capsules and ligaments form 2 dorsolateral swellings separated by a longitudinal groove, named Heberden nodes. Inflammatory changes around the nail are possible, sometimes associated with a mucoid cyst containing a translucent gelatinous fluid developed in the posterior nail fold. The cyst may also develop under the nail[27] and induce a compression of the nail root, leading to a longitudinal fissure of the nail plate.

The erosive form of finger OA was reported in 1961.[28] Metacarpophalangeal, trapezio-metacarpal, and scapho-trapezial joints are less frequently affected than in common OA (**Fig. 17**). The relationship between conventional OA and erosive OA is debated.[29] Erosive OA may represent a separate disease entity,[30] or belong to one end of the spectrum of OA[31] or a particularly aggressive subgroup of generalized OA.[29]

Radiographs

The diagnostic of DIPJ OA is usually confirmed on radiographs that exclude other conditions. Radiographic findings can be very subtle initially: slight JSN, asymmetric hypertrophic appearance of the middle phalanx head. More obvious signs appear later

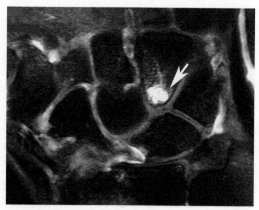

Fig. 16. Hamato-lunate joint osteoarthritis. Coronal contrast-enhanced fat-suppressed T1-weighted MRI shows bone marrow edema of the proximal part of the hamate (*arrow*) with slight cortex irregularities. This is a type II lunate.

Table 1
Terminology used in finger joints osteoarthritis

Term	Definition
Nonnodal OA	Clinical and/or radiographic IPJ OA without nodes
Heberden and Bouchard nodes	Posterolateral firm swellings at distal IPJ (Heberden) and proximal IPJ (Bouchard) Specific hand OA clinical and/or radiological abnormalities may not be present
Nodal OA	Heberden and/or Bouchard nodes with underlying clinical and/or radiological IPJ OA
Generalized OA	Hand OA associated with other OA sites
Thumb base OA	Trapezio-metacarpal joint with or without STTJ OA
Erosive OA	Subchondral bone erosion, cortical destruction, and subsequent reparative change, which may include bony ankylosis

Abbreviations: IPJ, interphalangeal joint; OA, osteoarthritis; STTJ, scapho-trapezio-trapezoid joint.

in the course of DIPJ OA: sclerosis, geodes, and osteophytes. Lateral views are essential, and may demonstrate a dorsal extension of the osteophytes developing from the base of the distal phalanx, bulging under the distal band of the extensor mechanism (**Fig. 18**). Thickening of the posterior nail fold suggests the likely presence of a mucoid cyst. A dorsal cortical bony erosion of the distal phalanx should raise the alternative possibility of a subungueal mucoid cyst (**Fig. 19**). Osteophytes later develop laterally and become therefore more visible on PA views.

In erosive OA the JSN is global, with an impacted appearance of the joint line due to central osteochondral erosions (**Fig. 20**). New bone formation (ie, subchondral bone

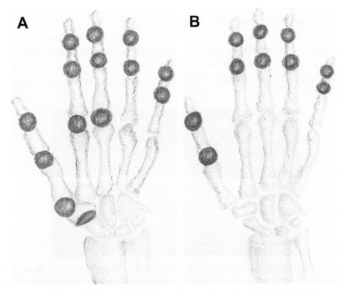

Fig. 17. Target sites of involvement with (*A*) hand osteoarthritis and (*B*) erosive osteoarthritis (blue spots). Less commonly involved joints are indicated with green spots.

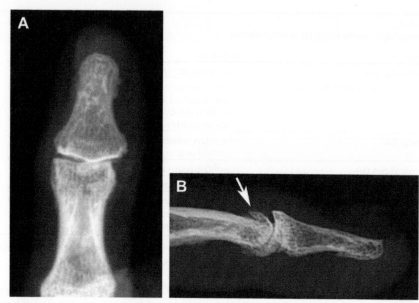

Fig. 18. Interphalangeal joint osteoarthritis of the thumb. (A) Posteroanterior radiograph shows focal JSN, subchondral bone sclerosis, and slight lateral subluxation. (B) Lateral radiograph demonstrates osteophytosis of the proximal phalanx with dorsal preponderance (arrow).

sclerosis and osteophytes) does not differ from common OA. The distal phalanx becomes cup-shaped as the proximal phalanx becomes sharper (**Fig. 21**). The impaction of the joint is usually followed by malalignment. Thin, periarticular, linear opacities are encountered.[32,33]

Ultrasound and magnetic resonance imaging

On MRI, central erosions are seen at sites of cartilage loss, and have more sharply angulated margins than marginal erosions, without evidence of associated synovitis.[34] Cross-sectional imaging can be informative in the case of nail plate fissure to confirm a compressive mass of the nail root. The space-occupying lesion can be an exuberant

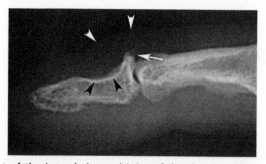

Fig. 19. Mucoid cyst of the interphalangeal joint of the thumb. Lateral radiograph shows osteoarthritis with dorsal osteophytes (white arrow), thickening of the proximal nail fold (white arrowheads), and bone erosion of the dorsal cortex of the distal phalanx (black arrowheads) due to the subungual component of the cyst.

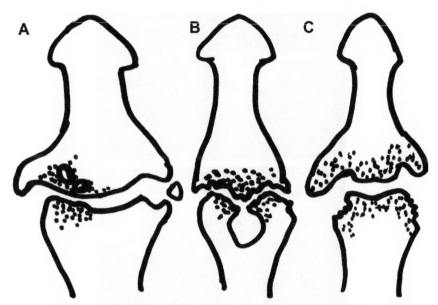

Fig. 20. Differential radiographic diagnosis of distal interphalangeal joints osteoarthritis. (*A*) Osteoarthritis: focal narrowing, marginal osteophyte, bone sclerosis, osteochondral bodies; (*B*) erosive osteoarthritis: subchondral erosion; (*C*) psoriasis: proliferative marginal erosion, retained or increased bone density. (*Modified from* Zhang W, Doherty M, Leeb BF, et al. EULAR evidence-based recommendations for the diagnosis of hand osteoarthritis: report of a task force of ESCISIT. Ann Rheum Dis 2009;68:8–17; with permission.)

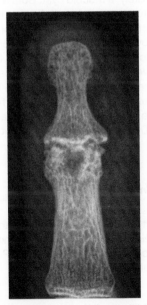

Fig. 21. Erosive osteoarthritis of the distal interphalangeal joint. Posteroanterior radiograph shows subchondral erosion.

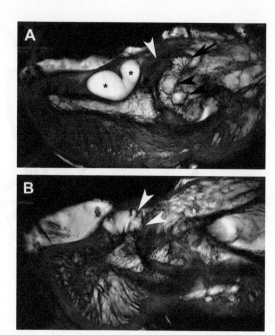

Fig. 22. Mucoid cyst of the distal interphalangeal joint. (A) Midsagittal T2-weighted MRI shows the cyst presents a component in the proximal nail fold and a subungual component (*asterisk*). Dorsal osteophyte (*black arrow*) lifting up the extensor tendon (*white arrowhead*). Subchondral bone cysts (*black arrowheads*). (B) Parasagittal T2-weighted MRI shows lateral pedicle beneath the extensor tendon (*white arrowheads*).

osteophytic growth or, more likely, a mucoid cyst. Both are related, as a cyst generally arises following an injury to the terminal band of the extensor mechanism by osteophytes. One should search for a pedicle tracking along the lateral border of the extensor tendon (**Fig. 22**). A cystic subungueal component is present in 20% of cases and may induce cortical scalloping. Extension of the cyst toward the finger pulp or infiltration of a proper digital nerve is rare. Ultrasound may be a suitable medium to investigate the relationship between erosive and nonerosive OA, although a single study has found ultrasound to be less sensitive to erosions in hand OA than radiographs.[35] Symptomatic joints are more likely to demonstrate ultrasound-detected changes of gray-scale synovitis, power Doppler signal, or osteophytes (**Fig. 23**).[36]

Proximal Interphalangeal Joint Osteoarthritis

Clinical presentation
Proximal interphalangeal joint (PIPJ) OA is less frequent than DIPJ OA, and both localizations are associated in 30% of cases. Similar nodes known as Bouchard nodes also appear around the PIPJs. Compared with DIPJ OA, PIPJ OA is much less disabling and tends to respect range of motion of joints.

Radiographs
Radiographic evidence of PIPJ is usually subtle, and appears late during the course of the disease (**Fig. 24**).

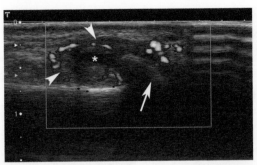

Fig. 23. Distal interphalangeal joint osteoarthritis. Midsagittal ultrasound view shows dorsal osteophyte (*arrow*) with fluid effusion in the dorsal recess (*asterisk*) and thickened synovium with positive power Doppler (*arrowheads*).

Magnetic resonance imaging

Marginal bone erosions are common in PIPJ OA, and are often radiographically occult but well demonstrated with MRI. These erosions are morphologically similar to those of inflammatory arthritides such as rheumatoid and psoriatic arthritis. The erosions commonly occur close to the proximal enthesis site of the collateral ligaments in OA. Synovitis and bone edema are usually present (**Fig. 25**).[34] A recent study compared OA with psoriatic arthritis using MRI, and highlighted involvement of ligaments, tendons, and enthesis sites in both diseases.[37] The collateral ligaments abnormalities influence the expression of the bony changes in the disease. These data are confirmed with histologic correlations in small joint OA and are in favor of a whole organ disease in OA.[38–40] The predictive value of bone edema for joint damage in OA is unknown.

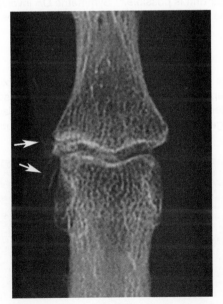

Fig. 24. Proximal interphalangeal joint osteoarthritis. Posteroanterior radiograph shows slight focal JSN with subchondral bone sclerosis, marginal osteophytes, and loose bodies (*arrows*).

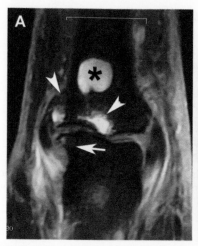 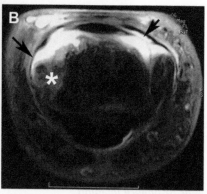

Fig. 25. Proximal interphalangeal joint osteoarthritis. (*A*) Coronal T2-weighted MRI shows both collateral ligaments are thickened with bone erosion at the proximal attachment of the lateral collateral ligament (*arrow*). Bone marrow edema (*arrowheads*) and distant bone cyst (*asterisk*) of the middle phalanx. (*B*) Axial contrast-enhanced fat-suppressed T1-weighted MRI shows thickened lateral collateral ligament (*asterisk*) and synovitis of the dorsal recess (*arrows*).

Metacarpo-Phalangeal Joints Osteoarthritis

Clinical presentation

Metacarpo-phalangeal (MCP) joints OA is rare. MCP joint OA of the thumb is often secondary to traumatic injuries, especially sprains (eg, unhealed Stener lesion). In old MCP joint OA, ulnar drift is possible.[41] Symmetric OA involving index and middle fingers should raise the possibility of crystal-related diseases, especially CPPD deposition disease.

Radiographs

PA and oblique views demonstrate classic findings of OA. Exuberant osteophytes leading to anchor-shaped metacarpal heads may be seen, especially affecting the index and middle fingers. Calcific deposits within hyaline cartilage and intrinsic wrist ligaments should suggest metabolic or crystal-related arthropathies (**Fig. 26**).

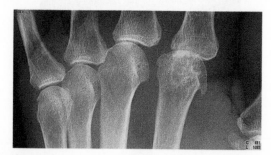

Fig. 26. Metacarpophangeal joint osteoarthritis. Oblique radiograph shows exuberant osteophytes. The disease is limited to the second and third fingers, leading to suspicion of metabolic disease.

Diagnosis and Severity Assessment of Hand Osteoarthritis

The highly variable clinical and radiological natural history of HOA and the large number of joints affected make it difficult to establish strict diagnostic criteria as well as reliable and reproducible tools to evaluate the severity of the disease. Several criteria have been suggested.[42–44] There is no agreed gold standard for diagnosis of HOA. To date, the main reference cited for diagnosis of HOA is the American College of Rheumatology (ACR) criteria for classification of HOA.[42] However, these do not include radiological criteria. The aim of the criteria must be their use in clinical and therapeutic studies. Most studies use the radiographic definition described by Kellgren and Lawrence.[43]

The European League Against Rheumatism (EULAR) OA Task Force developed recommendations for HOA diagnosis using an evidence-based format involving a systematic review of research evidence and expert consensus.[33] Ten propositions were agreed on after 3 anonymous Delphi rounds.

Scoring

HOA represents a valuable model to evaluate structure-modifying treatments in OA. Analysis of clinical data and evaluation of the functional impact of HOA remain difficult. An algofunctional index can be established by adding pain visual analog scale (VAS), consumption of pain killers and nonsteroidal anti-inflammatory drugs, or global evaluation by the patient himself or the physician.[44]

Radiographs

The Osteoarthritis Research Society International (OARSI) group has recently published guidelines for conduct of clinical trials of HOA, recommending conventional radiographs as the standard for assessing structural outcomes.[45] Various methods have been proposed to assess the radiological severity of HOA and to score the progression of damage over time. These criteria are based on radiographs[6,42,46–50] or microfocal radiography.[51] Anteroposterior view of both hands on the same film is usually performed, and 1:1 size of digitized radiographs is recommended. Scoring digitized or plain films does not seem to modify the quality of assessment.[52,53] The JS width may be measured by automatic quantification, and closely reflects semiquantitative scoring of JSN.[54] The Kellgren-Lawrence grading allows a wide range of interpretations for each grade, reducing interobserver reliability.[55,56] The intraobserver reliability is determinant to calculate the smallest detectable difference (SDD) and accounts considerably for the sensitivity to change.[57] Verbruggen and colleagues[58] suggest an easy and reproducible scoring method, using numeric scores for radiographs. The methods proposed differ by the number of hand joints and the radiographic features scored (osteophytes, JSN, subchondral bone sclerosis, bone cysts, erosion, and deformity), the respective importance attributed to each radiological feature in the score, the way of scoring (semiquantitative or global stage of OA), and the summation. None of the proposed radiological scales has proved to be better than others. Maheu and colleagues[59] compared in the same sample of patients the precision and sensitivity to change of 4 radiographic scoring methods proposed to assess the severity and progression of structural changes in HOA. The Verbruggen and Kallman scales perform better regarding reliability, and the Kallman method is slightly more sensitive to change.[59]

Ultrasound

Ultrasound is particularly dedicated to the assessment of small superficial structures like finger joints. The more complex anatomy and deeper structures of the wrist make ultrasound of the wrist less straightforward. The efficiency of ultrasound in the early diagnosis of synovitis and erosions in hands during rheumatoid arthritis has been demonstrated.[60,61] A group of experts in OA, ultrasound, and outcome measures proposed under the auspices of the Disease Characteristics in Hand OA Group (DI-CHOA) a preliminary ultrasound hand scoring system.[62] Fifteen joints of the hand were examined: the first carpometacarpal joint, MCP joints 1 to 5, PIPJs 1 to 5, and DIPJs 2 to 5. Activity and damage criteria were scored: synovial hypertrophy and effusion, gray-scale and power Doppler signal, and osteophytosis (**Fig. 27**).

Chondral defects or JSN cannot be reliably or meaningfully interpreted, despite these being cardinal pathologic features of OA. Erosions are also excluded from the tool, due to perceived problems with the definition and reliability. Erosions can be difficult to detect due to overlying osteophytes. It may also be difficult to determine where focal erosions begin and where osteophytes end when the cortical surface is severely damaged. In a comparative study of symptomatic OA joints and a control group, neither the number of affected joints per individual nor the summative semiquantitative scores for synovitis per individual correlated with symptoms (pain VAS, global VAS, or Australian/Canadian Osteoarthritis Hand Index).[36]

MAGNETIC RESONANCE IMAGING

To date, no scoring method of HOA on MRI is available. Efficiency of MRI in rheumatoid arthritis has been extensively demonstrated by the RAMRIS (rheumatoid arthritis magnetic resonance image scoring) system. A similar approach could be adapted to HOA, as MRI would best reveal subchondral bone edema among other abnormalities.

OSTEOARTHRITIS OF THE SPINE

Low back pain (LBP) is the second most common complaint encountered by primary care physicians. Chronic LBP is a major public health issue. Up to 80% of all individuals will experience LBP at some point in their lives. State-of-the-art imaging provides excellent morphologic details on lumbar spine degenerative changes. With the wide use of MRI, it is now possible to examine the anatomy of the lumbar spine noninvasively, with excellent spatial and contrast resolution in a short time. This improvement has led to a better understanding of the frequency and spectrum of findings that can be present as part of the normal aging process without causing clinical symptoms. It is also now possible to distinguish accurately between mechanical causes of nerve root compression that may result in radicular symptoms and normal imaging findings. The main objective of imaging studies in the context of LBP or radicular pain would be to support the clinical diagnosis by showing objective evidence of any kind of discopathy or facet joint arthropathy in a location consistent with the clinical findings. Abnormal findings have been reported by radiologists in asymptomatic subjects on all imaging modalities including radiographs, myelography, discography, CT, and MRI. The nomenclature used for imaging ideally should correspond to clinical entities and orient the referring physician as to treatment.[63] The results of the studies using MRI in asymptomatic volunteers support the notion that one must be careful before attributing causality to any abnormal finding in a symptomatic patient.[63–66] Finally, there is a trend to develop degenerative disc disease imaging grading systems to further investigate the relationship between morphology, functional parameters, and clinical symptoms. This article now focuses on the most recent and reliable MRI-based grading systems of use in lumbar spine OA.[67]

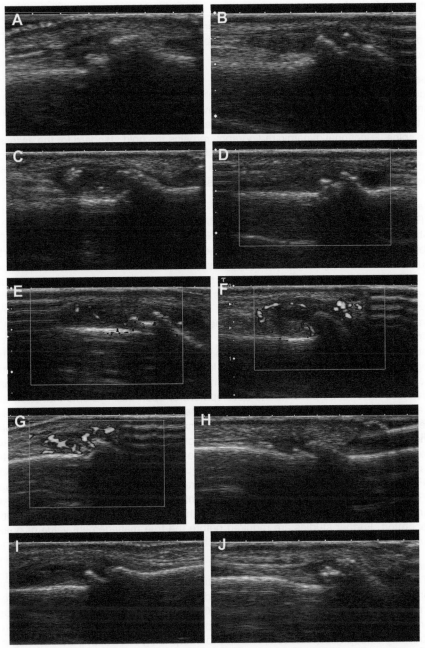

Fig. 27. Ultrasound scoring proposed by DICHOA.[62] Synovial thickening with 3 grades: (A) mild, (B) moderate, and (C) severe. Power Doppler signal with 4 grades: (D) no signal, (E) mild, (F) moderate, and (G) severe. Osteophytes with 3 grades: (H) mild, (I) moderate, and (J) severe.

Imaging Methods

Multiple imaging modalities are available and include radiography, dynamic radiography, multidetector CT (MDCT), MRI, myelography with postmyelographic MDCT, and discography.[68–70]

Radiographs
Radiographs still play an important and preliminary role as an easy screening opportunity. Radiographs are cheap, universally available, and offer a good panoramic view of the lumbar spine, adding meaningful details on bone structures and the stability of the spine. Functional dynamic radiography remains the gold standard for the assessment of lumbar instability. Because of its simplicity, low cost, and availability, functional flexion-extension radiography is the most thoroughly studied and the most widely used method in the imaging diagnosis of lumbar intervertebral instability.[71]

Magnetic resonance imaging
MRI of the lumbar spine has become the initial imaging technique of choice in patients with LBP or radicular pain. Usual clinical MRI has emphasized orthogonal T1- and T2-weighted images for morphologic assessment of the discovertebral complex. Short-tau inversion recovery (STIR) or fat-suppressed T2-weighted images have been added by many groups because they are more sensitive to bone marrow and soft tissue changes. Among the new MRI techniques currently available, only MR neurography and dynamic MRI have expanded beyond the experimental phase and have demonstrated specific clinical utility in selected patients.[72] MR neurography is based on 3D thin-section sequences. MR neurography is capable of depicting a wide variety of pathologic conditions involving the sciatic nerve, including a compression related to degenerative disc disease or extraspinal lesions.[73] MRI is routinely performed with the patients supine and therefore with the spine unloaded. Recent technological advances have made possible the development of open MRI systems that allow an examination in seated or upright position. Dynamic MRI has been used to evaluate the occurrence of occult herniation, which may not be visible or be less visible when the patient is supine, to measure motion between spinal segments, and to measure the canal or foraminal diameter when subjected to axial loading.[74,75] In a study on 30 patients, Weishaupt and colleagues[76] showed that positional (seated) MRI more frequently demonstrated minor neural compromise than did conventional MRI, but no convincing signs of canal or foraminal encroachments were found. The benefit from dynamic MRI seems small for the added machine time and patient discomfort. Further studies are required before the true management value of positional dynamic MRI can be determined, in part due to the various methods used.

Computed tomography
CT provides superior bone detail (**Fig. 28**), but is not as useful in depicting disc lesions compared with multiplanar MRI. With the added value associated with high-quality reformatted sagittal and coronal images, MDCT is useful for depiction of calcification and ossification of the spinal ligaments, spondylosis, facet joint changes with encroaching osteophytes, scoliosis, and also for morphologic evaluation after myelography or discography. However, exposure to radiation dose is an issue of MDCT.

Myelography
Myelography is rarely performed, but is still useful in the case of contraindications to MRI. Myelography is usually combined with postmyelography MDCT. The combined study is complementary to MRI and may be useful in surgical planning. Myelography offers a dynamic view of the lumbar spine with comparison of supine and

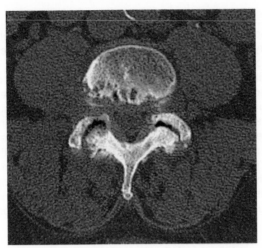

Fig. 28. Axial MDCT scan at L4/5 level shows a marked bilateral facet joint osteoarthritis with erosive lesions, and vacuum phenomenon. Note the erosive changes of the vertebral endplate.

weight-bearing images (**Fig. 29**). However, myelography has the disadvantage of requiring lumbar puncture and intrathecal iodine contrast injection.

Discography
When other studies fail to localize the cause of pain, discography may occasionally be helpful if surgery is planned. Although the images often depict nonspecific aging or degenerative changes, the injection itself may reproduce the patient's pain, which may have a diagnostic value.[77]

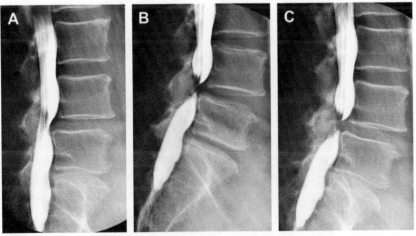

Fig. 29. Lumbar myelography in a 74-year-old man. Lateral radiographs in (*A*) flexion, (*B*) neutral position, and (*C*) extension show degenerative spondylolisthesis at L4/5 level, with a central stenosis. This dynamic stenosis is moderate in flexion, and marked in neutral and extension positions.

Degenerative Disc Disease

MRI is the most accurate anatomic method for assessing intervertebral disc disease. The signal intensity characteristics of the disc on T2-weighted images reflect changes caused by aging or degeneration.[72]

Annular tears, also properly called annular fissures, are probably a critical factor in the process of disc degenerative disease (**Fig. 30**). Annular tears are frequently found in an asymptomatic population.[66] The temporal evolution of annular fissures was studied in 56 patients with an evaluation of the symptoms evolution.[78] In this series, annular tears either did not change or improved spontaneously in a large proportion of cases over a period of time. Furthermore, there was no statistical correlation between annular tears changes and change in patients' symptoms. Annular tears appear in the early stages of disc degeneration, and are often seen in the absence of other identifiable morphologic changes of degeneration in the nucleus pulposus. Discs with annular tears are associated with a faster subsequent nuclear degeneration.[79]

Disc degeneration, and disc herniation reporting and grading

A standardized nomenclature in the assessment of disc abnormalities is a prerequisite for a comparison of data from different investigations. Disc degeneration is a continuum rather than a step-by-step process. As a result, any step-by-step grading system will by design contain ambiguity with respect to whether a disc should be graded as one particular level or another.

Millette[63] proposed a nomenclature and classification based on the expected anatomy and pathology of both the disc and adjacent vertebral bodies. Discs are classified in the categories of normal young disc, normal aging disc, scarred disc, annular tear, and herniated disc. Herniation is defined as a localized displacement of disc material beyond the limits of the intervertebral disc space. The term "localized"

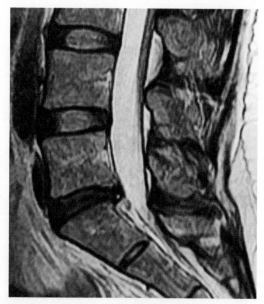

Fig. 30. A 43-year-old man with chronic low back pain (LBP). Sagittal fast spin-echo T2-weighted MRI shows small annular tear of L5/S1 disc space.

contrasts with "generalized," the latter being arbitrarily defined as greater than 50% (180°) of the periphery of the disc.

Localized displacement in the axial (horizontal) plane can be "focal," signifying less than 25% of the disc circumference, or "broad-based," meaning between 25% and 50% of the disc circumference. Presence of disc tissue "circumferentially" (50%–100%) beyond the edges of the ring apophyses may be called "bulging" (**Fig. 31**) and is not considered a form of herniation, nor are diffuse adaptive alterations of disc contour secondary to adjacent deformity as may be present in severe scoliosis or spondylolisthesis.

The nomenclature recommendations of the combined task forces of the North American Spine Society, American Society of Spine Radiology, and American Society of Neuroradiology[80] (http://www.asnr.org/spine_nomenclature/) are the following. Herniated discs may take the form of protrusion or extrusion, based on the shape of the displaced material. Protrusion is present, if the greatest distance, in any plane, between the edges of the disc material beyond the disc space is less than the distance between the edges of the base in the same plane (**Fig. 32**). Extrusion is present when, in at least one plane, any one distance between the edges of the disc material beyond the disc space is greater than the distance between the edges of the base in the same plane, or when no continuity exists between the disc material beyond the disc space and that within the disc space (**Fig. 33**). Extrusion may be further specified as sequestration, if the displaced disc material has lost completely any continuity with the parent disc. The term migration may be used to signify displacement of disc material away from the site of extrusion, regardless of whether sequestrated or not. In the axial plane, disc herniation is classified as central, right-left central, right-left subarticular, right-left foraminal, and right-left extraforaminal.

A specific classification system for lumbar disc degeneration based on routine MRI has been developed by Pfirrmann and colleagues.[81] This comprehensive 5-level

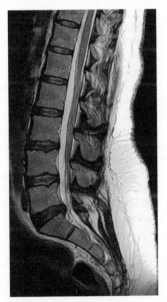

Fig. 31. A 51-year-old woman with chronic LBP. Sagittal fast spin-echo T2-weighted MRI shows degenerative L5/S1 disc with loss of signal intensity and convex posterior bulging.

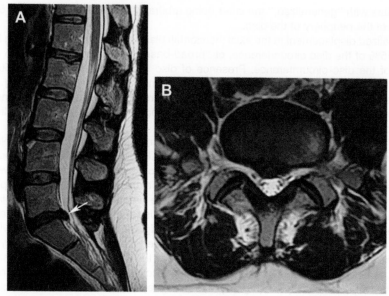

Fig. 32. A 47-year-old man with acute LBP. (*A*) Sagittal and (*B*) axial fast spin-echo T2-weighted sagittal MR images show protruded herniated L5/S1 disc with a convex posterior margin (*arrow*). Protruded disc herniation is characterized by broader base than the extension of disc material beyond the disc space.

grading system was developed from the literature. Pfirrmann classification is based on the following MRI features: structure, distinction of nucleus and annulus, signal intensity, and height of intervertebral disc. Grading is performed on fast spin-echo (FSE) T2-weighted sagittal images of the spine. This grading focuses on the characteristics of disc structure. An algorithm to assess the grading was developed and optimized by reviewing the lumbar MRI. The reliability of the algorithm in depicting intervertebral disc alterations was tested on MRI of 300 lumbar intervertebral discs in 60 patients. In this series, there were 14 Grade I, 82 Grade II, 72 Grade III, 68 Grade IV, and 64 Grade V discs. The kappa coefficients for intra- and interobserver agreement were substantial to excellent. Complete agreement was obtained, on the average, in 83.8% of all the discs. A difference of one grade occurred in 15.9% and a difference of 2 or more grades in 1.3% of all the cases. Pfirrmann and colleagues concluded that this grading system and algorithm allowed a reliable assessment of disc degeneration on routine sagittal T2-weighted MRI. These investigators also suggested combining this grading system with Modic classification for further specification of disc disease in case of concomitant bone marrow changes. This useful 5-point Pfirrmann grading system has been accepted and applied clinically. However, whereas it is discriminatory when applied to younger subjects,[82] it may not distinguish severity of disc degeneration when applied to elderly subjects. A modified Pfirrmann grading system for lumbar intervertebral disc degeneration was therefore proposed recently.[82] This 8-level modified grading system for lumbar disc degeneration was developed to include a description of the changes expected for each grade and a 24-image reference panel. This modified Pfirrmann grading system was useful at discriminating severity of disc degeneration in elderly subjects. The system can be applied with good intra- and interobserver agreement.

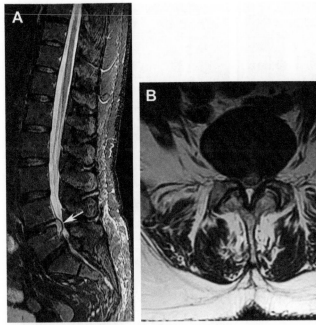

Fig. 33. A 55-year-old woman with acute radicular pain. (*A*) Sagittal and (*B*) axial STIR MRI show extruded herniated L4/5 disc with inferior migration (*arrow*). Extruded disc herniation is characterized by a base that is narrower than the distance of disc material extension beyond the disc space.

Herniation of the disc refers to localized displacement of nucleus, cartilage, fragmented apophyseal bone, or fragmented annular tissue beyond the intervertebral disc space. Disc herniations of the same size may be asymptomatic in one patient and lead to severe nerve root compromise in another patient (**Fig. 34**). MRI reports usually focus on the morphology, location, and size of the herniated disc. The effect of disc herniation depends on the location and extent of the herniation relative to the diameter of the spinal canal. Therefore, a clinically relevant grading system for disc herniation must be based on the spatial relationship between herniated disc material and neural structures.

The system developed by Pfirrmann and colleagues[83] in grading compromise of the intraspinal extradural lumbar nerve root consists of 4-grade categories, summarized as follows.

- Grade 0 (normal): No compromise of the nerve root is seen. There is no evident contact of disc material with the nerve root, and the epidural fat layer between the nerve root and the disc material is preserved.
- Grade 1 (contact): There is visible contact of disc material with the nerve root, and the normal epidural fat layer between the two is not evident. The nerve root has a normal position, and there is no dorsal deviation.
- Grade 2 (deviation): The nerve root is displaced dorsally by disc material.
- Grade 3 (compression): The nerve root is compressed between disc material and the wall of the spinal canal; it may appear flattened or be indistinguishable from disc material.

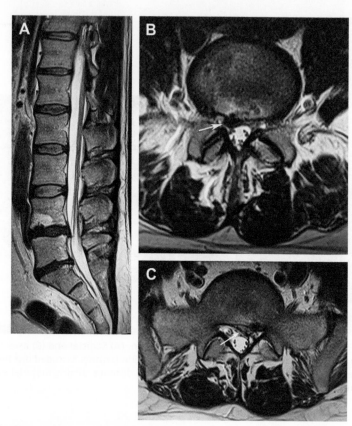

Fig. 34. A 46-year-old man with bilateral chronic radicular pain. (*A*) Sagittal and axial fast spin-echo T2-weighted MRI at (*B*) L4/5 and (*C*) L5/S1 show degenerative disc disease at L4/5 and L5/S1 levels. (*B*) Right herniation at L4/5 level (*arrow*) with contact between disc material and thecal sac. (*C*) Left herniation at L5/S1 level (*arrow*) with extruded disc material and deviation of the left S1 nerve root.

This grading system was tested in the interpretation of routine MRI of 500 lumbar nerve roots in 250 symptomatic patients. Intra- and interobserver reliability was assessed for 3 independent observers. In the 94 nerve roots evaluated at surgery, surgical grading was correlated with image-based grading. Statistics indicated substantial agreement between different readings by the same observer and between different observers. Correlation of image-based grading with surgical grading was high ($r = 0.86$).

Degenerative Bone Marrow Changes of Vertebral Endplates

Signal intensity changes in vertebral body bone marrow adjacent to the endplates of degenerated discs are a common observation on MRI, and appear to take 3 main forms according to Modic classification.[84]

- Type 1 changes demonstrate decreased signal intensity on T1-weighted images and increased signal intensity on T2-weighted images, and have been identified in approximately 4% of patients scanned for lumbar disease (**Fig. 35**). Histopathologic sections of disks with type I changes show disruption and fissuring of the

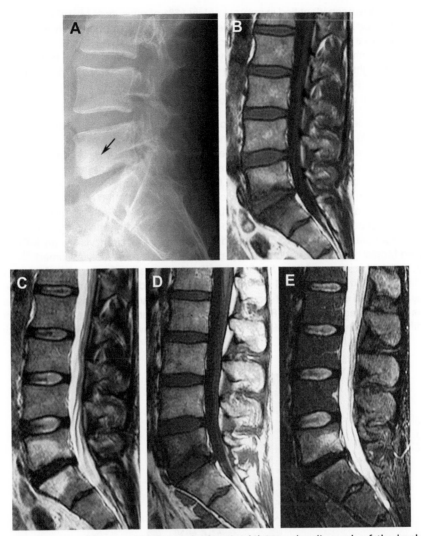

Fig. 35. A 39-year-old man with chronic back pain. (*A*) Lateral radiograph of the lumbar spine shows a moderate narrowing of the L5/S1 disc space with an area of sclerosis of the anterior part of L5 endplate (*arrow*). Initial (*B*) sagittal T1- and (*C*) T2-weighted MRI show extensive type 1 Modic changes at L5/S1 level, with erosive lesions of the L5 inferior endplate. A 6-month follow-up (*D*) sagittal T1-weighted and (*E*) STIR MRI show Modic type 1 changes remain unchanged in the L5 inferior endplate, while they are decreasing in the S1 superior endplate. There is no significant change of the disc signal and morphology.

endplate and vascularized fibrous tissues within the adjacent marrow. Rannou and colleagues[85] have shown that low-grade inflammation indicated by high serum high-sensitivity C-reactive protein level in patients with chronic LBP could point to Modic 1 signal changes. This finding supports the presence of a local inflammation phenomenon occurring at the vertebral endplate level.

• Type 2 changes are represented by increased signal intensity on T1-weighted images and isointense or slightly hyperintense signal on T2-weighted images, and have been identified in approximately 16% of patients at MRI (**Fig. 36**). Discs with type II changes also show evidence of endplate disruption, with yellow (lipid) bone marrow replacement in the adjacent vertebral body.

- Type 3 changes are represented by decreased signal intensity on both T1- and T2-weighted images, and correlate with extensive bony sclerosis on plain radiographs (**Fig. 37**). The lack of signal in the type III change reflects the relative absence of bone marrow in areas of advanced sclerosis.

The absence of Modic changes, a normal anatomic appearance, has often been designated Modic Type 0. Longitudinal studies have shown that Modic Type 2 changes may be less stable than previously assumed.[86] Mixed-type 1 to 2 and 2 to 3 Modic changes have also been reported, suggesting that these changes can convert from one type to another and that they all present different stages of the same pathologic process.[87] Endplate Modic changes most often occur at the anterior aspect of the endplate, particularly at L4/5 and L5/S1 levels. Fatty endplate changes are the most common. Modic changes occur more frequently with aging, evidence of their degenerative etiology.[88] Bony endplate sclerosis is often visible on MDCT in mixed Modic types, and not only in types 3 changes as previously assumed.[89]

A reliability study of the Modic classification was performed by Jones and colleagues[90] on 50 spinal MRI examinations. The individual intraobserver agreement was substantial or excellent. The overall interobserver agreement was excellent. There was complete agreement in 78% of the levels, a difference of one type in 14%, and a difference of 2 or more in 8% of levels. This study showed that Modic classification

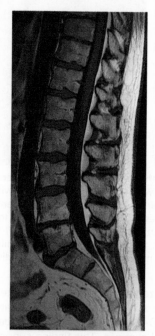

Fig. 36. A 51-year-old woman with moderate chronic LBP. Sagittal T1-weighted MRI shows reduced disc height at L4/5 and L5/S1 levels associated with fatty type 2 Modic changes of the vertebral endplates. At L4/5, the fatty changes involve the whole endplates; at L5/S1, the fatty changes involve only the anterior part of the endplates.

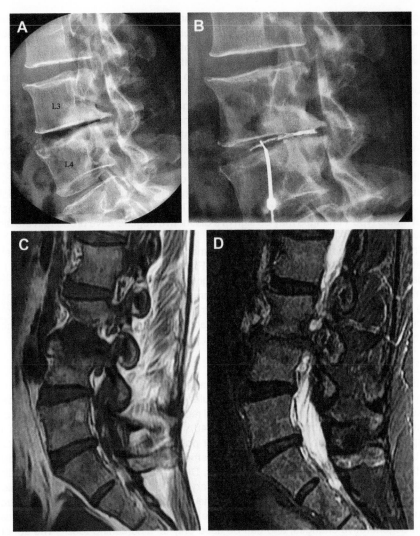

Fig. 37. A 54-year-old woman with chronic back pain. Radiography with oblique view (*A*) before and (*B*) after discography shows severe disc degeneration at L3/4 level with associated sclerosis of the posterior vertebral endplates. (*C*) Sagittal T1-weighted and (*D*) STIR MRI show type 3 Modic changes at L3/4 level.

is both reliable and reproducible. The classification is simple and easy to apply for observers of varying clinical experience. This simplicity and reliability explains the diffusion and extensive use of the original Modic classification in clinical research and practice.

Fayad and colleagues[91] have determined the intra- and interobserver reliability of a modified Modic classification, taking into consideration mixed signals. Pure edema endplate signal changes were classified as Modic type 1, and pure fatty endplate changes as Modic type 2. A mixture of types 1 and 2 but predominantly edema signal changes was classified as Modic 1-2, and a mixture of types 1 and 2 but predominantly fatty changes was classified as Modic 2-1. The intraobserver agreement was excellent. The interobserver agreement was moderate to substantial. Interobserver reliability depended on the experience of the observer, thus highlighting the importance of a learning curve. This study shows that the modified Modic classification is reliable and easy to apply for observers with different clinical experience.

The relationship of Modic type 1 change with disc degeneration has been studied prospectively in 24 chronic LBP patients with a follow-up study lasting for 18 to 74 months.[92] A relatively rapid progression of degenerative changes was found in association with the presence and, in particular, changes in size and intensity of Modic 1. The degenerative changes were already advanced at baseline in most discs with an adjacent Modic type 1, but uncommon in those without. The progressive degenerative changes along with changes in Modic type 1 were deforming to the discovertebral unit, as irregularities and even defects developed in the subchondral bone at the endplate border, while central disc signal intensity changed and disc height strongly decreased as a sign of a collapse of the disc. These results support the hypothesis that Modic type 1 changes may be sign of a distinctive degenerative process in the discovertebral unit.

In summary, Modic changes are dynamic markers of the normal age-related degenerative process affecting the lumbar spine (**Fig. 38**). Type 1 changes are likely to be inflammatory in origin, and seem to be strongly associated with active low back symptoms and segmental instability of the lumbar spine.[93–95] In contrast, type 2 changes are less clearly associated with low back symptoms and seem to indicate a more biomechanically stable state. Finally, the exact nature and pathogenetic significance of type 3 changes remains largely unknown.

Posterior Elements

With disc degeneration and loss of disk space height, there are increased stresses on the facet joints with hypertrophy of the articular process (**Fig. 39**). Facet arthrosis can result in narrowing of the central canal, lateral recesses, and foramina, and is an important component of lumbar stenosis (**Fig. 40**).[72] Degenerative spondylolisthesis is a spreading of a vertebral body anteriorly or posteriorly displaced due to severe OA of the facet joints. Degenerative spondylolisthesis is frequent at the L4/5 level due to the more sagittal orientation of the joints. Degenerative disc disease may predispose to or exacerbate this condition secondary to narrowing of the disc space, which can produce subsequent malalignment of the articular processes and lead to rostro-caudal subluxation (**Fig. 41**). Radiographs are of limited value for the diagnosis of facet joint degenerative changes, and can be used only as a screening tool.[95] The abnormalities associated with OA can be best demonstrated and categorized by MDCT and MRI. There is moderate to good agreement between MRI and MDCT in this setting. If MRI examination is available, MDCT is not required for the assessment of facet joint OA in patients with back pain and no previous surgery.[96]

Friedrich and colleagues[97] have studied and described facet joints bone marrow changes associated with edema of the soft tissue surrounding the facet joints, referred to as "facet joint edema." Lumbar spine MRI with STIR, T1-weighted, and T2-weighted images were performed in 145 consecutive patients with back pain. Facet joint OA was graded using criteria adapted from Pathria and colleagues[98] In summary, the findings of this study support that (a) degenerative changes of the facet joints occur mainly at the level of degenerative disc disease (functional unit) and (b) instability of a discovertebral level is associated with stress and overload for the facet joints. Lakadamyali and colleagues[99] studied the sagittal STIR MRI findings in 372 patients with nonradicular LBP and in 249 controls. All patients were diagnosed with pathologic changes in at least one of the posterior elements stabilizing the

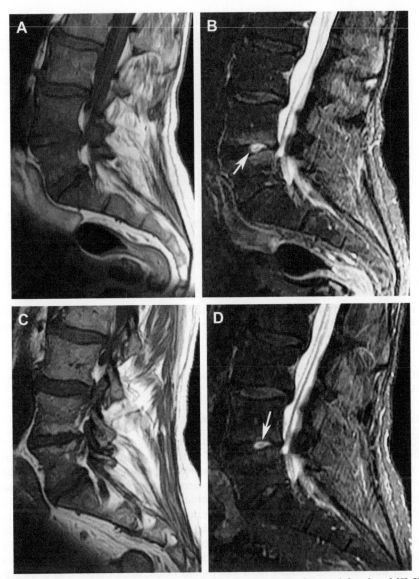

Fig. 38. A 65-year-old man with chronic back pain. Initial sagittal T1-weighted and (*B*) STIR MRI show type 1 Modic changes at L4/5 level, with erosive lesions of the endplates and a bright central disc signal (*arrow*) on STIR image. A 3-month follow-up (*C*) sagittal T1-weighted and (*D*) STIR MRI show change of signal of the endplates to type 2 Modic with a fatty signal of the endplates. There is no significant change of the disc signal (*arrow*) and morphology.

vertebral column. The incidences of facet joint effusion, interspinous ligament edema, neocyst formation, and paraspinal muscle edema were found to be statistically significantly higher in patients with LBP than in controls. The most common finding in these patients was facet joint effusion, which had a frequency of 85.5% versus 45.8% in controls. Because of homogeneous fat suppression and better depiction of soft tissue

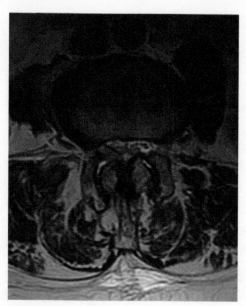

Fig. 39. A 68-year-old man with chronic back pain. Axial T2-weighted MRI at L4/5 level shows a marked bilateral facet joint osteoarthritis with hypertrophy, joint effusion, sagittalization, and stenosis of the spinal canal.

edema, the STIR sequence is warranted for a good detection and visualization of these posterior changes.[99,100]

Reliability of Magnetic Resonance Imaging Findings

Some prior work regarding observer performance in the interpretation of lumbosacral spine MRI data has been done in a variety of settings involving intervertebral disc and other abnormalities.[96,101] Recent imaging studies focus on disc contour and nondisc contour degenerative spine MRI findings. Van Rijn and colleagues[102] assessed observer variation in MRI evaluation (disc contour findings) in patients suspected of lumbar disc herniation. Two experienced neuroradiologists independently evaluated 59 consecutive patients with lumbosacral radicular pain. Per patient, 3 levels (L3/4 through L5/S1) and the accompanying roots were evaluated on both sides. For each segment, the presence of a bulging disc or a herniation and compression of the root was reported. Images were interpreted twice: once before and once after disclosure of clinical information. On average, more than 50% of interobserver variation in MRI evaluation of patients with lumbosacral radicular pain was caused by disagreement on bulging discs. Knowledge of clinical information did not influence the detection of herniation but lowered the threshold for reporting bulging discs.[102] In addition to disc contour abnormalities, many spine MRI-depicted degenerative findings involving the intervertebral discs, bone marrow, neuroforamina, spinal canal, and facet joints exist, and may be overlooked or poorly understood by those treating patients with spine conditions. Results of prior investigations[96,101] suggest that the reliability of characterizing nondisc contour lumbar spine MRI findings is reasonable. Carrino and colleagues[103] were interested in the effectiveness of MRI findings as potential predictors of outcome. Thus, their work attempted to characterize inter- and intraobserver variability of qualitative, nondisc contour degenerative findings of

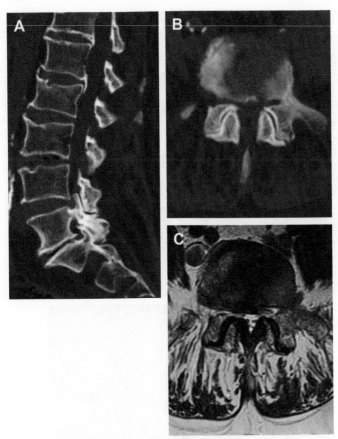

Fig. 40. Multilevel spinal osteoarthritis in a 73-year-old man. (*A*) Sagittal and (*B*) axial MDCT scans show marked osteoarthritis at L5/S1 level with a reduced disc height, disc vacuum phenomenon, and facet joint hypertrophy with bony spurs and foraminal stenosis. (*C*) Axial T2-weighted MRI at L5/S1 level shows marked bilateral facet joint osteoarthritis with hypertrophy and stenosis of the spinal canal. Note the bilateral fatty changes of posterior spinal muscles.

the lumbar spine at MRI. The nondisc contour degenerative spine MRI findings assessed were spondylolisthesis, disc degeneration, marrow endplate abnormality (Modic changes), intervertebral disc posterior annular tears, and facet arthropathy. The 111 baseline MRI examinations were rated by 4 independent readers according to defined criteria for nondisc contour-related degenerative MRI findings, and a subgroup of the 40 MRI examinations were rerated by the same readers. The interobserver agreement was good in rating disc degeneration and moderate in rating spondylolisthesis, Modic-type degenerative changes, facet arthropathy, and annular tears. The intraobserver agreement based on 40 MRI examination cases was good for rating spondylolisthesis, disc degeneration, Modic-type degenerative changes, facet arthropathy, and annular tears. Inter- and intraobserver agreement was moderate for rating the superior anteroposterior, inferior anteroposterior, superior craniocaudal, and inferior craniocaudal extents of Modic-type changes. Thus, some variability existed between readers despite standardized definitions and reader training. Carrino and colleagues concluded that nondisc contour degenerative lumbar spine

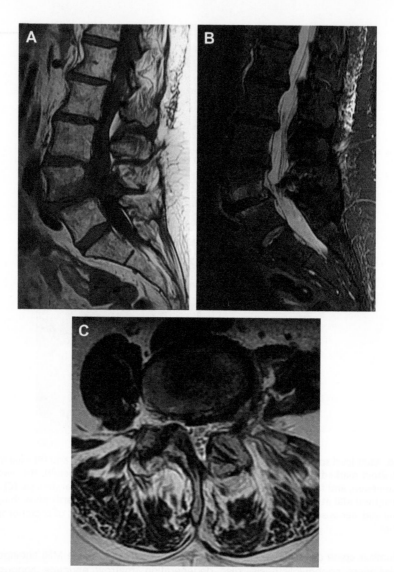

Fig. 41. Spinal osteoarthritis in a 73-year-old woman. (A) Sagittal T1-weighted, and (B) STIR and (C) axial T2-weighted MRI at L4/5 level show multilevel degenerative disc disease. There are also degenerative spondylolisthesis with vertebral endplate Modic mixed 1-2 changes at L4/5 level secondary to facet joint osteoarthritis.

MRI findings have sufficient reliability to potentially be used as predictors of clinical prognoses and outcomes if a rigorous MRI reader training paradigm is used.

Clinical Relevance of Magnetic Resonance Imaging Findings in Spine Osteoarthritis

Any study looking at the natural history of degenerative disc disease, the prognostic value of imaging, or its effect on therapeutic decision making will be confounded by the high prevalence of morphologic changes in the asymptomatic population.[101,104] Jensen and colleagues[64] examined the prevalence of abnormal findings on MRI of the lumbar spine in 98 subjects without back pain. Thirty-six percent of the 98 asymptomatic subjects had normal discs at all levels. Fifty-two percent of the subjects had a bulge at at least one level, 27% had a protrusion, and 1% had an extrusion. Thirty-eight percent had an abnormality of more than one intervertebral disc. The prevalence of bulges, but not of protrusions, increased with age. The most common noninintervertebral disk abnormalities were Schmorl nodes found in 19% of the subjects, annular defects in 14%, and facet arthropathy in 8%. The conclusions were that many people without back pain have disc bulges or protrusions but not extrusions. Given the high prevalence of these findings and of back pain, the discovery by MRI of bulges or protrusions in people with LBP may frequently be coincidental. In an MRI study on 60 asymptomatic volunteers of age 20 to 50 years, Weishaupt and colleagues[65] concluded that disc bulging and protrusion, and annular fissures are common findings in asymptomatic individuals younger than 50 years. However, disc extrusion and sequestration, nerve root compression, end plate abnormalities, and OA of the facet joints were rare and, therefore, may be predictive of LBP in symptomatic patients.[65] Recent studies show that type 1 Modic endplate changes seem to be associated with a higher prevalence of active LBP symptoms.[10,23] Type 1 Modic endplate changes on MRI have positive predictive value in the presence of concordant pain provocation at provocative lumbar discography in a large sample population. However, no individual MRI finding is sufficient to predict pain provocation at discography.[77] The clinical importance of type 2 endplate changes remains unclear and limited.

SUMMARY

Radiographs are a validated imaging technique for the demonstration of morphologic changes in HOA. Diagnosis based on this single imaging modality (JSN or osteophyte) has limited value, whereas detection of associated clinical and radiographic changes dramatically improves diagnostic performance. Other imaging modalities (ultrasound, MRI) are understudied and their indications remain debated. Some imaging modalities are routinely indicated before wrist surgery (CT arthrography, MRI, MR arthrography). Severity scores based on imaging findings mostly rely on plain films. In the future, one may be assured that ultrasound and MRI will provide a better evaluation of established structural damages as well as the level of activity of the condition. All these imaging-based scoring methods should be cross-validated for HOA with clinical status, including disease activity, function and performance, biomarkers, and long-term outcome. In the future, recently developed clinical and radiological tools might help conceive OA of the wrist and hand as a model of OA along with OA of the hip or knee.

MRI is the best imaging technique to demonstrate the morphologic changes of lumbar spine OA, including disc and vertebral endplate changes, facet joint lesions, spinal canal narrowing, and nerve root compromise. Other imaging modalities such as MDCT may be useful in selected cases. The use of a standardized nomenclature and reader training are recommended to reduce the variability in MRI reporting and to improve intra- and interobserver agreement. All validated grading scores based on imaging findings now rely on MRI. In patients with subacute or chronic back pain, the Modic classification is clinically useful, reliable, and relevant.

REFERENCES

1. Zhang Y, Niu J, Kelly-Hayes M, et al. Prevalence of symptomatic hand osteoarthritis and its impact on functional status among the elderly: the Framingham Study. Am J Epidemiol 2002;156:1021–7.

2. Dahaghin S, Bierma-Zeinstra SM, Ginai AZ, et al. Prevalence and pattern of radiographic hand osteoarthritis and association with pain and disability (The Rotterdam Study). Ann Rheum Dis 2005;64:682–7.

3. Zhang W, Doherty M, Leeb F, et al. EULAR evidence based recommendations for the management of hand osteoarthritis: report of a Task Force of the EULAR Standing Committee for International Clinical Studies Including Therapeutics (ESCISIT). Ann Rheum Dis 2007;66:377–88.

4. Hautefeuille P, Delcambre B, Duquesnoy B, et al. Etude clinique et épidémiologique des arthroses de la main. A partir de 500 observations sélectionnées dans un centre d'examen de santé. Rev Rhum Mal Osteoartic 1991;58:35–41 [in French].

5. Acheson RM, Chan YK, Clemet AR. New Haven Survey of joint diseases XII: distribution and symptoms of osteoarthritis in the hands with reference to hand-edness. Ann Rheum Dis 1970;29:275–86.

6. Kallman DA, Wigley FM, Scott WW, et al. New radiographic grading scales for osteoarthritis of the hand. Arthritis Rheum 1989;32:1584–91.

7. Spector TD, Brown GC, Silman AJ. Increased rates of prior hysterectomy and gy-naecological operations in women with osteoarthritis. Br Med J 1988;297:899–900.

8. Felson DT. The epidemiology of knee osteoarthritis: results from the Framingham osteoarthritis study. Semin Arthritis Rheum 1990;20:42–50.

9. Spector TD, Cicuttini F, Baker J, et al. Genetic influences on osteoarthritis in women: a twin study. Br Med J 1996;312:940–3.

10. Patotie A, Vaisanen P, Ott J, et al. Previous predisposition to familial osteoarthritis linked to type II collagen gene. Lancet 1989;1(8644):924–7.

11. Pattrick M, Manhire A, Ward AM, et al. B antigens and alpha 1-antitrypsin pheno-types in nodal and generalized osteoarthritis and erosive osteoarthritis. Ann Rheum Dis 1989;48:470–5.

12. Brodsky A, Appelboom A, Govaerts A, et al. HLA antigenes and Heberden nodes. Acta Rheumatol 1979;3:95–103.

13. Florak TM, Miller RJ, Pellegrini VT, et al. The prevalence of carpal tunnel syndrome in patients with basal joint arthritis of the thumb. J Hand Surg 1992; 17:624–30.

14. Kapandji A, Moatti E, Raab C. La radiographie spécifique de l'articulation trapézométacarpienne. Sa technique, son intérêt. Ann Chir 1980;34:719–26 [in French].

15. Dell PC, Brushart TM, Smith RJ. Treatment of trapeziometacarpal arthritis: results of resection-arthroplasty. J Hand Surg 1978;3:243–9.

16. Forestier J. L'ostéoarthrite sèche trapézométacarpienne (rhizarthrose du pouce). Presse Med 1937;45:315–7 [in French].

17. Allieu Y, Chammas M, Cenac P. L'arthrose scapho-trapézo-trapézoïdienne iso-lée, une entité méconnue. Rhumatol Prat 1991;58:4–6 [in French].

18. Moser T, Dosch JC, Moussaoui A, et al. Wrist ligament tears: evaluation of MRI and combined MDCT and MR arthrography. AJR Am J Roentgenol 2007;188:1278–86.

19. Le Nen D. Arthrose pisotriquétrale. Maîtrise Orthop 1996;156:4–9 [in French].

20. Thurston AJ, Stanley JK. Hamato-lunate impingement: an uncommon cause of ulnar-sided wrist pain. Arthroscopy 2000;16:540–4.

21. Pfirmann CW, Theumann NH, Chung CB, et al. The hamatolunate facet: character-ization and association with cartilage lesions-magnetic resonance arthrography and anatomic correlation in cadaveric wrists. Skeletal Radiol 2002;31:451–6.

22. Sagerman SD, Hauck RM, Palmer AK. Lunate morphology: can it be predicted with routine x-ray films? J Hand Surg 1995;20A:38–41.

23. Viegas SF, Patterson RM, Hokanson JA, et al. Wrist anatomy: incidence, distribution, and correlation of anatomic variations, tears and arthrosis. J Hand Surg Am 1993;18:463–75.
24. Nakamura K, Beppu M, Patterson RM, et al. Motion analysis in two dimensions of radial-ulnar deviation of type I versus type II lunates. J Hand Surg Am 2000;25: 877–88.
25. Viegas SF, Wagner K, Patterson R, et al. Medial (hamate) facet of the lunate. J Hand Surg 1990;15A:564–71.
26. Malik AM, Schweitzer ME, Culp RW, et al. MR imaging of the type II lunate bone: frequency, extent, and associated findings. AJR Am J Roentgenol 1999;173:335–8.
27. Delcambre B, Guyot-Drouot MH. Arthroses digitales et rhizarthrose. Rev Prat 1996;46:2187–91 [in French].
28. Crain DC. Interphalangeal osteoarthritis characterized by painful inflammatory episodes resulting in deformity of the proximal and distal articulations. JAMA 1961;175:1044–53.
29. Punzi L, Ramonda R, Sfriso P. Erosive osteoarthritis. Best Pract Res Clin Rheumatol 2004;18:739–58.
30. Peter JB, Pearson CM, Marmor L. Erosive osteoarthritis of the hands. Arthritis Rheum 1966;9:365–88.
31. Cobby M, Cushnaghan J, Creamer P, et al. Erosive osteoarthritis: is it a separate disease entity? Clin Radiol 1990;42:258–63.
32. Amadio PC, De Silva SP. Comparison of the results of trapeziometacarpal arthrodesis and arthroplasty in men with osteoarthritis of the trapeziometacarpal joint. Ann Chir Main 1990;9:358–63.
33. Zhang W, Doherty M, Leeb BF, et al. EULAR evidence-based recommendations for the diagnosis of hand osteoarthritis: report of a task force of ESCISIT. Ann Rheum Dis 2009;68:8–17.
34. Grainger AJ, Farrant JM, O'Connor PJ, et al. MR imaging of erosions in interphalangeal joint osteoarthritis: is all osteoarthritis erosive? Skeletal Radiol 2007;36:737–45.
35. Iagnocco A, Filippucci E, Ossandon A, et al. High resolution ultrasonography in detection of bone erosions in patients with hand osteoarthritis. J Rheumatol 2005;32:2381–3.
36. Keen HI, Wakefield RJ, Grainger AJ, et al. An ultrasonographic study of osteoarthritis of the hand: synovitis and its relationship to structural pathology and symptoms. Osteoarthr Cartil 2008;16:12–7.
37. Tan AL, Grainger AJ, Tanner SF, et al. A high-resolution magnetic resonance imaging study of distal interphalangeal joint arthropathy in psoriatic arthritis and osteoarthritis: are they the same? Arthritis Rheum 2006;54:1328–33.
38. Tan AL, Grainger AJ, Tanner SF, et al. High-resolution magnetic resonance imaging for the assessment of hand osteoarthritis. Arthritis Rheum 2005;52: 2355–65.
39. Tan AL, Toumi H, Benjamin M, et al. Combined high-resolution magnetic resonance imaging and histology to explore the role of ligaments and tendons in the phenotypic expression of early hand osteoarthritis. Ann Rheum Dis 2006; 65:1267–72.
40. Hunter DJ, Felson DT. Osteoarthritis. BMJ 2006;332:639–42.
41. Williams WV, Cope R. Metacarpophalangeal arthropathy associated with manual labor. Arthritis Rheum 1987;30:1362–71.
42. Altman R, Alarcon G, Appelrouth D, et al. The American College of Rheumatology criteria for the classification and reporting of osteoarthritis of the hand. Arthritis Rheum 1990;33:1601–10.

43. Campion G, Dieppe P, Watt I. Heberden's nodes in osteoarthritis and rheumatoid arthritis. BMJ 1983;287:1512.
44. Hart D, Spector T, Egger P, et al. Defining osteoarthritis of the hand for epidemiological studies: the Chingford study. Ann Rheum Dis 1994;53:220–3.
45. Maheu E, Altman RD, Bloch DA, et al. Design and conduct of clinical trials in patients with osteoarthritis of the hand: recommendations from a task force of the Osteoarthritis Research Society International. Osteoarthr Cartil 2006;14:303–22.
46. Kallman DA, Wigley FM, Scott WW Jr, et al. The longitudinal course of hand osteoarthritis in a male population. Arthritis Rheum 1990;33:1323–32.
47. Dougados M, Nguyen M, Mijiyawa M, et al. Reproducibility of X-ray analysis of hand osteoarthrosis. Rhumatologie 1990;42:287–91.
48. Verbruggen G, Veys EM. Erosive and non erosive hand osteoarthritis. Use and limitations of two scoring systems. Osteoarthr Cartil 2000;8(suppl A):S45–54.
49. Lane NE, Kremer LB. Radiographic indices for osteoarthritis. Rheum Dis Clin North Am 1995;21:379–94.
50. Kessler S, Dieppe P, Fuchs J, et al. Assessing the prevalence of hand osteoarthritis in epidemiological studies. The reliability of a radiological hand scale. Ann Rheum Dis 2000;59:289–92.
51. Buckland-Wright JC, Macfarlane DG, Lynch JA, et al. Quantitative microfocal radiographic assessment of progression in osteoarthritis of the hand. Arthritis Rheum 1990;33:57–65.
52. Richmond BJ, Powers C, Piraino DW, et al. Diagnostic efficacy of digitized images vs plain films: a study of the joints of the fingers. Am J Roentgenol 1992;158:437–41.
53. Swee RG, Gray JE, Beabout JW, et al. Screen film versus computed radiography imaging of the hand: a direct comparison. AJR Am J Roentgenol 1997;168:539–42.
54. van 't Klooster R, Hendriks EA, Watt I, et al. Automatic quantification of osteoarthritis in hand radiographs: validation of a new method to measure joint space width. Osteoarthr Cartil 2008;16:18–25.
55. Spector TD, Cooper C. Radiographic assessment of osteoarthritis in population studies: whither Kellgren and Lawrence? Osteoarthr Cartil 1993;1:203–6.
56. Spector TD, Hochberg M. Methodological problems in the epidemiological study of osteoarthritis. Ann Rheum Dis 1994;53:143–6.
57. Ravaud P, Giraudeau B, Auleley GR, et al. Assessing smallest detectable change over time in continuous structural outcome measures: application to radiological change in knee osteoarthritis. J Clin Epidemiol 1999;52:1225–30.
58. Verbruggen G, Veys EM. Numerical scoring systems for the anatomic evolution of osteoarthritis of the finger joints. Arthritis Rheum 1996;39:308–20.
59. Maheu E, Cadet C, Gueneugues S, et al. Reproducibility and sensitivity to change of four scoring methods for the radiological assessment of osteoarthritis of the hand. Ann Rheum Dis 2007;66:464–9.
60. Lopez-Ben R, Bernreuter WK, Moreland LW, et al. Ultrasound detection of bone erosions in rheumatoid arthritis: a comparison to routine radiographs of the hands and feet. Skeletal Radiol 2004;33:80–4.
61. Szkudlarek M, Court-Payen M, Strandberg C, et al. Power Doppler ultrasonography for assessment of synovitis in the metacarpophalangeal joints of patients with rheumatoid arthritis: a comparison with dynamic magnetic resonance imaging. Arthritis Rheum 2001;44:2018–23.
62. Keen HI, Lavie F, Wakefield RJ, et al. The development of a preliminary ultrasonographic scoring system for features of hand osteoarthritis. Ann Rheum Dis 2008;67:651–5.

63. Millette PC. The proper terminology for reporting lumbar intervertebral disk disorders. AJNR Am J Neuroradiol 1997;18:1859–66.
64. Jensen MC, Brant-Zawadzki MN, Obuchowski N, et al. Magnetic resonance imaging of the lumbar spine in people without back pain. N Engl J Med 1994; 331:69–73.
65. Weishaupt D, Zanetti M, Hodler J, et al. MR imaging of the lumbar spine: prevalence of intervertebral disk extrusion and sequestration, nerve root compression, end plate abnormalities, and osteoarthritis of the facet joints in asymptomatic volunteers. Radiology 1998;209:661–6.
66. Stadnik TW, Lee RR, Coen HL, et al. Annular tears and disk herniation: prevalence and contrast enhancement on MR images in the absence of low back pain or sciatica. Radiology 1998;206:49–55.
67. Kettler A, Wilke HJ. Review of existing grading systems for cervical or lumbar disc and facet joint degeneration. Eur Spine J 2006;15:705–18.
68. Brandt-Zawadzki M, Dennis SC, Gade GF, et al. Low back pain. Radiology 2000; 217:321–30.
69. Gallucci M, Puglielli E, Splendiani A, et al. Degenerative disorders of the spine. Eur Radiol 2005;15:591–8.
70. Bradley WG Jr. Low back pain. AJNR Am J Neuroradiol 2007;28:990–2.
71. Leone A, Guglielmi G, Cassar-Pullicino VN, et al. Lumbar intervertebral instability: a review. Radiology 2007;245:62–77.
72. Modic MT, Ross JS. Lumbar degenerative disk disease. Radiology 2007;245:43–61.
73. Moore KR, Tsuruda JS, Dailey AT. The value of MR neurography for evaluating extraspinal neuropathic leg pain: a pictorial essay. AJNR Am J Neuroradiol 2001;22:786–94.
74. Jinkins JR, Dworkin JS, Damadian RV. Upright, weight-bearing, dynamic-kinetic MRI of the spine: initial results. Eur Radiol 2005;15:1815–25.
75. Hiwatashi A, Danielson B, Moritani T, et al. Axial loading during MR imaging can influence treatment decision for symptomatic spinal stenosis. AJNR Am J Neuroradiol 2004;25:170–4.
76. Weishaupt D, Schmid MR, Zanetti M, et al. Positional MR imaging of the lumbar spine: does it demonstrate nerve root compromise not visible at conventional MR imaging? Radiology 2000;215:247–53.
77. Thompson KJ, Dagher AP, Eckel TS, et al. Modic changes on MR images as studied with provocative discography: clinical relevance—A retrospective study of 2457 disks. Radiology 2009;250:849–55.
78. Mitra D, Cassar-Pullicino VN, McCall IW. Longitudinal study of high intensity zones on MR of lumbar intervertebral discs. Clin Radiol 2004;59:1002–8.
79. Sharma A, Pilgram T, Wippold FJ. Association between annular tears and disk degeneration: a longitudinal study. AJNR Am J Neuroradiol 2009;30:500–6.
80. Fardon DF, Milette PC. Nomenclature and classification of lumbar disk pathology: recommendations of the combined task forces of the North American Spine Society, American Society of Spine Radiology, and American Society of Neuroradiology. Spine 2001;26:E93–113.
81. Pfirrmann CW, Metzdorf A, Zanetti M, et al. Magnetic resonance classification of lumbar intervertebral disc degeneration. Spine 2001;26:1873–8.
82. Griffith JF, Wang YX, Antonio GE, et al. Modified Pfirrmann grading system for lumbar intervertebral disc degeneration. Spine 2007;32:E708–12.
83. Pfirrmann CW, Dora C, Schmid MR, et al. MR image-based grading of lumbar nerve root compromise due to disk herniation: reliability study with surgical correlation. Radiology 2004;230:583–8.

84. Modic MT, Steinberg PM, Ross JS, et al. Degenerative disk disease: assessment of changes in vertebral body marrow with MR imaging. Radiology 1988;166: 193–9.
85. Rannou F, Ouanes W, Boutron I, et al. High-sensitivity C-reactive protein in chronic low back pain with vertebral end-plate Modic signal changes. Arthritis Rheum 2007;57:1311–5.
86. Kuisma M, Karppinen J, Niinimäki J, et al. A three-year follow-up of lumbar spine endplate (Modic) changes. Spine 2006;31:1714–8.
87. Rahme R, Moussa R. The Modic vertebral endplate and marrow changes: pathologic significance and relation to low back pain and segmental instability of the lumbar spine. AJNR Am J Neuroradiol 2008;29:838–42.
88. Karchevsky M, Schweitzer ME, Carrino JA, et al. Reactive endplate marrow changes: a systematic morphologic and epidemiologic evaluation. Skeletal Radiol 2005;34:125–9.
89. Kuisma M, Karppinen J, Haapea M, et al. Modic changes in vertebral endplates: a comparison of MR imaging and multislice CT. Skeletal Radiol 2009; 38:141–7.
90. Jones A, Clarke A, Freeman BJ, et al. The Modic classification: inter- and intraobserver error in clinical practice. Spine 2005;30:1867–9.
91. Fayad F, Lefevre-Colau MM, Drapé JL, et al. Reliability of a modified Modic classification of bone marrow changes in lumbar spine MRI. Joint Bone Spine 2009; 76:286–9.
92. Luoma K, Vehmas T, Grönblad M, et al. Relationship of Modic type 1 change with disc degeneration: a prospective MRI study. Skeletal Radiol 2009;38: 237–44.
93. Mitra D, Cassar-Pullicino VN, McCall IW. Longitudinal study of vertebral type-1 end-plate changes on MR of the lumbar spine. Eur Radiol 2004;14: 1574–81.
94. Fayad F, Lefevre-Colau MM, Rannou F, et al. Relation of inflammatory Modic changes to intradiscal steroid injection outcome in chronic low back pain. Eur Spine J 2007;16:925–31.
95. Wybier M. Imaging of lumbar degenerative changes involving structures other than disk space. Radiol Clin North Am 2001;39:101–14.
96. Weishaupt D, Zanetti M, Boos N, et al. MR imaging and CT in osteoarthritis of the lumbar facet joints. Skeletal Radiol 1999;28:215–9.
97. Friedrich KM, Nemec S, Peloschek P, et al. The prevalence of lumbar facet joint edema in patients with low back pain. Skeletal Radiol 2007;36:755–60.
98. Pathria M, Sartoris DJ, Resnick D. Osteoarthritis of the facet joints: accuracy of oblique radiographic assessment. Radiology 1987;164:227–30.
99. Lakadamyali H, Tarhan NC, Ergun T, et al. STIR sequence for depiction of degenerative changes in posterior stabilizing elements in patients with lower back pain. AJR Am J Roentgenol 2008;191:973–9.
100. D'Aprile P, Tarantino A, Jinkins JR, et al. The value of fat saturation sequences and contrast medium administration in MRI of degenerative disease of the posterior/perispinal elements of the lumbosacral spine. Eur Radiol 2007;17: 523–31.
101. Weishaupt D, Zanetti M, Hodler J, et al. Painful lumbar disk derangement: relevance of endplate abnormalities at MR imaging. Radiology 2001;218:420–7.
102. van Rijn JC, Klemetsö N, Reitsma JB, et al. Observer variation in MRI evaluation of patients suspected of lumbar disk herniation. AJR Am J Roentgenol 2005; 184:299–303.

103. Carrino JA, Lurie JD, Tosteson AN, et al. Lumbar spine: reliability of MR imaging findings. Radiology 2009;250:161–70.
104. Modic MT, Obuchowski NA, Ross JS, et al. Acute low back pain and radiculopathy: MR imaging findings and their prognostic role and effect on outcome. Radiology 2005;237:597–604.

Pre- and Postoperative Assessment in Joint Preserving and Replacing Surgery

Adnan Sheikh, MD*, Mark Schweitzer, MD

KEYWORDS

- Arthroplasty • Cartilage repair • Computed tomography
- Magnetic resonance imaging • High tibial osteotomy

The number of joint replacement surgeries performed throughout the world increases annually. Joint replacements are among the most common surgical procedures in most developed countries. Of these patients, 1% to 5% develop complications that may require revision, such as fracture, particle disease, and infection.[1] Advances in techniques and the type and quality of the metals, polyethylene, and ceramics used in prosthesis have increased longevity. A basic understanding of these surgical procedures and devices is important for imaging evaluation.

The detection of complications can be challenging as these patients usually present with nonspecific and subtle clinical symptoms, such as pain and decreased range of motion. Conventional radiography, arthrography, scintigraphy, ultrasound, computed tomography (CT), and magnetic resonance imaging (MRI) can be used to assess the orthopedic prosthesis and, to some degree, the adjacent osseous and soft-tissue structures. With the transition from salvage to reconstruction techniques the role of imaging in the preoperative assessment will increase further. Knowledge of the usefulness, limitations, and optimization of technique is essential for diagnosing pathology in postoperative patients. This article reviews the radiographic, ultrasound, CT, and MRI appearance of knee and hip joint preserving surgeries.

IMAGING TECHNIQUES
Conventional Radiography

Conventional radiography remains the cornerstone of postoperative musculoskeletal imaging. A minimum of 2 views of the affected joint should be obtained to assess the

A version of this article originally appeared in the 47:4 issue of Radiologic Clinics of North America.

Department of Diagnostic Imaging, The Ottawa Hospital, University of Ottawa, General Campus, 501 Smyth Road, Ottawa, KIH 8L6, Canada

* Corresponding author.

E-mail address: asheikh@ottawahospital.on.ca (A. Sheikh).

Rheum Dis Clin N Am 35 (2009) 651–673

doi:10.1016/j.rdc.2009.08.008

rheumatic.theclinics.com

0889-857X/09/$ – see front matter © 2009 Elsevier Inc. All rights reserved.

orthopedic hardware and adjacent bone. Serial radiographs continue to play a major role in the evaluation of hardware complications.

Fractures and osteolysis can be more easily diagnosed when baseline imaging is available. The radiographic findings of hardware loosening include lucency of greater than 2 mm at the bone-metal or cement-bone interface, increase in the zone of lucency more than a year after surgery, fracture of the cement, or change in the alignment or migration of prosthesis components.[2,3] Well-defined radiolucencies around a hardware component suggest particle disease, especially if these lucencies are close to the joint surface. Most loosening from modern arthroplasties is a sequela of particle disease. Careful attention should be paid to the position of the femoral head within the acetabulum component to assess for polyethylene wear.

Arthrography

Arthrography can be performed concurrently with aspiration to distinguish infection from loosening. The presence of contrast material between the bone-metal or cement-bone interface suggests loosening,[4–6] especially as it goes more distal. This loosening is not diagnostic and the major role of arthrography is a guided and confirmed joint aspiration. The more contrast fills sacculations around the joint, however, the more likely there is to be secondary loosening.

Scintigraphy

Scintigraphy can be used in the assessment of painful arthroplasty. Although Tc-methylene diphosphonate (Tc-MDP) can show increased uptake around the arthroplasty component in the early postoperative period, little imaging is done during that time period. A 3-phase bone scan is more useful when the first 2 phases are normal to exclude infection than it is to diagnose infection. The more unilateral the uptake, the closer it is to the joint line, and the more lateral the uptake, the more likely the changes are related to particle disease. Increased activity after gallium- or indium-labeled leukocyte injection suggests infection.[7,8] However, these studies should usually be combined with sulfur colloid scanning to distinguish this "inflammatory" uptake from displaced marrow. All scintigraphic examinations are more accurate in the hip than the knee, with knee arthroplasties especially prone to false-positive scintigraphies. Currently gallium is infrequently used even for chronically infected arthroplasties.

Ultrasound

Ultrasound can also be used in the assessment of painful arthroplasty as it is an excellent modality to assess soft tissues. Ultrasound can be used in the assessment and therapeutic intervention of periprosthetic collection and bursitis.[9–11] The integrity of the adjacent tendons and ligaments can also be assessed. However, ultrasound more often plays a secondary role to determine if joint fluid is present and to guide the aspiration of this fluid.

In the past, CT was considered to be of limited usefulness in patients with metallic hardware. However, CT is helpful in the evaluation of fracture mapping and assessment of osteolytic lesion.[10] The present generation of multidetector CT along with improved computer software has overcome the attenuation of the radiograph beam by the metal.[9,12] The type of metal also has an effect on these artifacts. The more recent titanium prosthesis has a lower x-ray coefficient compared with steel and cobalt-chrome devices.[10] Radiation dose is drastically increased when an arthroplasty is present. CT is helpful in the evaluation of fracture mapping and assessment of osteolytic lesions.[10] Metal artifact reduction techniques include:

- Positioning the patient in the gantry such that the radiograph beam courses through the smallest diameter of the hardware
- High kilovolt and milliampere with thin overlap slices, thus minimizing noise, which contributes to degradation of image quality
- Reformatting the images in multiple planes with slice thickness greater than originally acquired decreases streak artifact and thereby improves visualization of structures around the hardware
- The use of soft tissue reconstruction kernels rather than bone algorithm and wide windows when viewing images reduce metal artifact.[9–11]

MRI had a limited role in postoperative assessment because of severe susceptibility artifact. The modification of imaging parameters has led to less motion degradation of image quality and improved diagnostic images. MRI is currently widely used in postoperative patients because of its multiplanar imaging capability, better contrast resolution, and lack of ionizing radiation compared with CT.[9,13] The metallic artifact can be reduced by:

- Using a higher bandwidth
- Using fast spin echo instead of spin echo sequences
- Avoiding gradient echo sequence
- Using short tau inversion recovery (STIR) instead of T2-weighted fat-suppressed sequence
- Lowering echo time
- Using large frequency encoding matrix
- Orienting frequency encoding direction along the longitudinal axis of the implant.[9–11,14,15]

ARTHROPLASTY

Arthroplasty is an orthopedic procedure for partially or completely resurfacing, remodeling, rebuilding, or replacing an arthritic, dysfunctional, or necrotic joint. This article focuses on the hip and knee joints. The components of arthroplasty are held in position using a cemented, noncemented, or hybrid procedure, depending on the clinical indication and age of the patient.

In a cemented procedure the components are fixed with polymethyl-methacrylate, which allows the implant to fit to the irregularities of the bone. The advantage is that this type of replacement is stable and immediate full weight bearing is possible. The disadvantage is that if the component becomes loose, some bone will grind away, making revision more difficult.[15] In a noncemented procedure the components have a roughened porous surface that allows bone to grow into it. These implants are press fit against the bone. The advantage is that there is minimal bone loss and preservation of bone stock compared with cemented arthroplasty in component lessening.[15] In the hip few arthroplasties are currently fully cemented.

Knee Arthroplasty

Unicompartmental knee arthroplasty (UKA) is one of several options for the treatment of unicompartmental arthritis in young patients. The advantage of unicompartmental arthroplasty compared with total knee arthroplasty is smaller incision and more rapid recovery, but more importantly loss of less than 75% of bone and cartilage.[2] By retaining all the undamaged parts, the joint bends and functions more naturally. UKA is commonly used to treat medial compartment arthritis. However, it may also be used to treat lateral compartment osteoarthritis (OA) and more recently patellofemoral disease. Indications for medial UKA include medial compartment arthritis, intact anterior and posterior cruciate ligament (ACL and PCL), intact lateral compartment, correctable varus deformity, and less than 10° of fixed flexion.[16,17] Contraindications include inflammatory arthropathy, high tibial osteotomy (HTO), tibial and femoral shaft deformity, and sepsis.[16–18] Clinical trials by Savard and Price[19] and Berger and colleagues[20] have indicated a success rate of 95% and 98%, respectively, for this limited procedure.

Medial compartment OA affects the anteromedial aspect of the tibial plateau and in the lateral compartment the femoral side is usually affected.[20] Preoperative radiographic assessment includes weight-bearing anteroposterior (AP) and tunnel views to evaluate for cartilage narrowing and a lateral radiograph to assess for posterior bone loss. Long leg radiographs to assess for malalignment may also be obtained.[2,18]

Total knee arthroplasty is usually provided for patients with severe OA. The aim is to resurface the damaged tibiofemoral surface with metal components and provide low friction articulation with a polyethylene liner. Patellar resurfacing is also indicated if severe patellofemoral disease is present. There is a recent trend to use 2-component rather than 3-component knee arthroplasties. Preoperative radiological evaluation with standing AP, lateral view, skyline radiograph to assess the patellofemoral joint is obtained. Long leg view to assess for malalignment, Rosenberg view, and standing radiographs in 45° of flexion can also be obtained to assess for cartilage degeneration.[21] Indium 111 scintigraphy can help to rule out infection, but is not usually necessary.[22–24]

Postoperatively, AP views are performed in supine and standing position along with lateral and skyline views of the patella for follow-up of patients and to assess for fracture, loosening, component dislocation, liner wear, and infection in knee arthroplasty.

Complications of knee arthroplasty

Thromboembolism Deep venous thrombosis (DVT) with potential to propagate a pulmonary embolism is the most feared complication of knee arthroplasty. The incidence of DVT without prophylaxis ranges from 40% to 88%, symptomatic pulmonary embolism from 0.5% to 3%, and mortality is 2%. DVT can be easily diagnosed on ultrasound.[21]

Fracture Periprosthetic fractures incurred during surgery or postoperatively can be diagnosed with conventional radiography. Occasionally, a CT may be required for better delineation of the fracture. Most fractures are seen later through areas of particle disease. These fractures are more common in the hip than in the knee.

Joint instability An asymmetric widening of the prosthetic joint space suggests ligamentous imbalance and varus-valgus instability, which accounts for 1% to 2% of primary instability following TKA.[21]

Patellar complications Stress fracture of the patella, loosening, and dislocation of patellar components are the most common complications. Patellar stress fractures are commonly seen in older patients and have been reported in 21% of patients.[3,25] These fractures can be easily detected on radiographs. Fatigue fractures are not uncommonly seen with metal-backed prosthesis, usually at the peg-plate junction.[3,25] Patellar subluxation and tilt can be recognized on tangential view of the patella and is caused by imbalance of soft tissue (tight lateral retinaculum), malpositioning, and malalignment of components. The thin polyethylene liner may wear or become displaced from the metal backing into the Hoffa fat pad. The liner wear causes the femoral metal component to rub against the metal backing of the patellar component, resulting in metallosis, which may be visible radiographically as a line of linear opacity outlining the distended joint effusion (metal line sign).[3] Patellar and quadriceps tendon rupture has also been reported, resulting in abnormal positioning of the patella, which can be seen on radiographs and confirmed with ultrasound. Fibrosis and scarring of the Hoffa fat pad may result in a low-lying patella (patella baja).[21]

Prosthesis loosening Prosthesis loosening can be seen along the tibial and femoral components as a result of stress shielding, infection, and osteolysis.[26] Loosening is more commonly seen with uncemented tibial components along the medial side, resulting in varus angulations. Loosening may be diagnosed when the normal 1- to 2-mm lucency at the bone-cement interface is exceeded, often focally.[2,26] The normal lucency is secondary to cement shrinkage and endothermal injury to the adjacent bone. Widening of greater than 2 mm at the bone-cement, metal-cement, and prosthesis-bone interface or an increase on serial weight-bearing radiographs often indicates loosening (**Fig. 1**).[26] A bone scan can also be used to diagnose loosening. Contrast between the bone-cement and bone-metal interface on arthrography also indicates loosening. Currently loosening is most commonly seen secondary to particle disease.

Prosthesis wear Increased weight and physical activity, irregularities of the surface condylar component articulating with the polyethylene liner, and abnormal alignment of the condylar component contribute to liner wear, which causes shedding of metal or polyethylene, resulting in hypertrophic synovium, which incites a histocytic response and leads to osteolysis.[2,21] Osteolysis can occasionally be appreciated on radiographs, although when it is visible it is usually at an advanced stage. Various studies have shown CT to be more sensitive in detection and quantification of osteolysis. Polyethylene wear is evaluated by measuring from the femoral condyles to the tibial base plate on serial radiographs. Interval narrowing of the joint space suggests polyethylene wear. Ultrasound can also be used to assess the polyethylene linear and osteolysis, but this is difficult in practice. The best way to diagnose particle disease is to be vigilant as its presence is almost invariable over time.

Infection Infection is the most common cause of failure of knee arthroplasty. The prevalence of infection ranges from 0.5% to 2%.[21] The radiographic appearance of

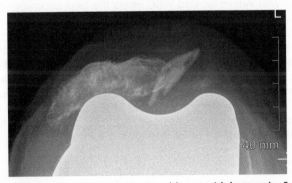

Fig. 1. Polyethylene liner dislocation in a 50-year-old man with knee pain. Sunrise patellofemoral joint view shows liner dislocation and lateral subluxation of the patella.

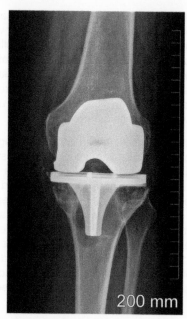

200 mm

Fig. 2. Loosening. Anteroposterior radiograph of the knee shows increased lucency surrounding the tibial stem and under the tibial tray, in keeping with loosening of the hardware.

infection can be variable. In most patients radiographs are normal. Serial radiographs may show periosteal reaction, progressive periprosthetic widening, and osteolysis, but this is rare (**Fig. 2**). Joint aspiration is the most useful confirmatory test. However, false-negative results have been seen and are common, particularly if saline irrigation is required. The sensitivity and specificity of joint aspiration can vary, ranging between 67% and 82% and 91% and 95%, respectively.[21,27] A positive delayed bone scan may be positive for years following arthroplasty. Attention should be paid to the first phases of this test as they are useful in excluding infection, although they may frequently be false positive.

Increased activity following injection of gallium- and indium-labeled leukocytes is suggestive of infection. The latter is more often performed although these infections are more chronic. However, labeled white blood cells (WBC) may be displayed in the marrow, yielding a false-positive result, and because of this, combined sulfur colloid scanning with indium-labeled WBC offers the best accuracy up to 95%.[21,28] When the uptake on both studies is in similar anatomic distribution it represents displaced marrow. Increased indium-WBC activity in a distribution dissimilar to that of sulfur colloid is specific for infection. Fludeoxyglucose-positron emission tomography (FDG-PET) studies have shown sensitivity and specificity of 100% and 86%, respectively, in limited numbers.[28] It should be noted that nearly all hip arthroplasties show uptake about the neck on PET images. Ultrasound can be used to assess for periprosthetic infection for limited indications. CT and MRI can also be used to assess the extent of soft-tissue infection and collections and marrow outside that area and close to the arthroplasty, but usually not for diagnosis of infection.

Hip Arthroplasty

Hip arthroplasty is one of the most frequently performed reconstructive surgeries. It is estimated that 1.5 million procedures are performed annually worldwide,[11] thereby providing pain relief and improvement in the function of patients suffering with OA and inflammatory arthritis (seropositive and seronegative).

Depending on the pathophysiology and age of the patient, different types of prosthesis are used. Unicompartmental arthroplasty is used in elderly patients to treat femoral neck fracture; it involves replacement of the femoral head and neck. A bipolar hemiarthroplasty is used to replace the femoral head and neck with an acetabular component that is not attached to the acetabulum. Normal motion can be seen between the acetabular cup and femoral head and between the acetabular cup and native acetabulum.[2,15] Bipolar arthroplasties are indicated for avascular necrosis (AVN) of the hip and displaced femoral neck fractures, at risk of developing AVN.

A total hip arthroplasty (THA) is recommended when the acetabular and the femoral head are affected, as in OA and rheumatoid arthritis. THA has an acetabular component, ceramic cup, polyethylene liner, and a femoral component. Most current total joint arthroplasties have an acetabular component that is cementless and may be press fit or have a roughened surface for bone in-growth. The femoral component may be fixed with cement or also may be press fit type. An AP view of the pelvis centered over the pubis with a second AP view centered over the replaced hip and a true lateral view are used to assess the hip prosthesis postoperatively.[2]

Component position

The acetabular inclination angle indicates the tilt of the actetabular component compared with a horizontal base line; 40° to 50° is considered neutral, an angle of greater than 40° suggests horizontal orientation, and an angle of less than 50° vertical orientation.[2,29,30]

Anteversion angle is measured on the lateral view; this is the angle between the axis of the acetabular marker wire and a line perpendicular to the base line. There is normally 5° to 25° of anteversion.[31–33] The tip of the femoral component should be ventrally placed on an AP projection or directed centrally to slightly medially (valgus).[2] The anteversion angle can also be measured on CT scan, by measuring the angle of rotation of the femoral neck relative to the femoral condyle.

Complications of hip arthroplasty

Loosening Loosening is the most common complication of cemented prosthesis. Lucency of less than 2 mm at the bone-cement interface outlined by a thin sclerotic demarcation line is usually normal and represents fibrous tissue. Lucency wider than 2 mm or progression of lucencies on serial radiographs suggests loosening. Acetabular loosening is identified better by component migration. A 2-mm continuous lucency suggests impending loosening. Cement fracture and motion of the components on stress views or fluoroscopy also suggest loosening. On arthrography, extension of contrast material along the prosthesis-cement or bone-cement interface below the intertrochanteric line is suggestive of loosening (**Fig. 3**),[2,34] but this test is usually performed for the aspiration of fluid rather than the diagnosis of loosening.

Infection Identification of lucency greater than 2 mm is suggestive of infection/loosening/particle disease. It is usually difficult to distinguish between these 3 entities; the last two are often coexisting conditions, with particle disease leading to loosening. Rapidly developing cement-bone lucency, endosteal scalloping, and periostitis may indicate infection. Joint aspiration and bone scan are recommended for confirmation, as described earlier. Ultrasound, CT scan, and MRI may also be used to assess for other soft-tissue markers for infection-like, soft-tissue collection, bursitis, and joint effusion.[35–39]

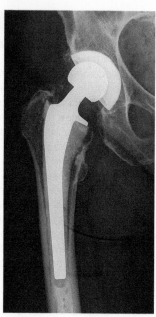

Fig. 3. Loosening. Anteroposterior radiograph of the right hip shows increased widening at the cement-bone interface, in keeping with loosening.

Osteolysis As described in the knee section, osteolysis is related to polyethylene or metal debris that is phagocytosed by macrophages, which accumulate to form foreign body granulomas. These granulomas stimulate osteoclastic activity and cause peri-prosthetic erosions (**Fig. 4**). Because of its multiplanar capabilities, CT has a greater detection rate of 82% compared with radiographs, which have a detection rate of 52%.[2,11,38,40]

On CT, osteolysis is manifest as well-defined lucencies devoid of trabaculae with associated soft-tissue mass of Hounsfield units (HU) ranging between −40 and 100 HU. Following contrast administration they show marked peripheral enhancement (**Figs. 5, 6**).[11,40] On MRI they are typically low signal on T1- and intermediate-to-high signal on T2-weighted sequences[11,41] and enhance if contrast is administered. MRI plays an increasingly significant role in the assessment of the soft tissues adjacent to the prosthesis. Trochanteric bursitis (**Fig. 7**), avulsion of the gluteus tendons (**Fig. 8**) and short external rotators, can easily be identified on MRI.[11] Psoas tendon impingement secondary to friction against the anterior acetabular spur or extruded cement can easily be seen on CT scan. A pseudomass in the iliopsoas tendon sheath caused by polyethylene wear has also been reported.[2,11,42] Lymphadenopathy secondary to dissemination of a large amount of polyethylene and metallic debris can easily be identified with cross-sectional imaging.

Other complications Other complications of hip arthroplasty include periprosthesis fracture, metallosis, acetabular liner wear, prosthetic dislocation, and heterotrophic bone. Each can usually be identified on radiographs (**Figs. 9–14**).

Resurfacing Hip Arthroplasty

Resurfacing hip arthroplasty is a metal-on-metal hip replacement that replaces the arthritic surface of the joint but removes far less bone than a traditional hip

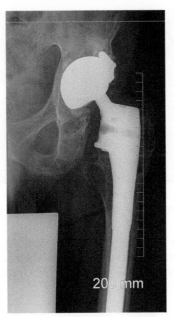

Fig. 4. Aggressive granulomatous disease. Anteroposterior radiograph of the left hip demonstrates loosening of the femoral and acetabular components with well-defined focal areas of endosteal erosions in the proximal femur and ischium indicating granuloma formation. Wear of the polyethylene acetabular cup is also present.

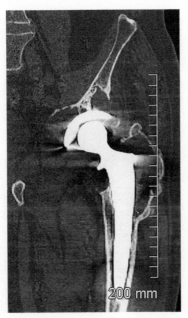

Fig. 5. Extensive granulomatous disease. Coronal CT reformat shows granuloma formation in the proximal femur and acetabulum.

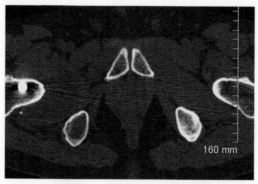

Fig. 6. Iliopsoas pseudomass. Axial CT scan shows complex cystic mass in the right iliopsoas tendon sheath in a patient with metal-on-metal surface replacement.

replacement. The femoral head and neck are retained and thus a femoral stem component of the prosthesis is not necessary. The ideal candidate is a young active adult with degenerative hip disease, congenital hip dysplasia, or Perthes disease, with good bone quality and morphology.[42]

Postoperative assessment
Review of the literature has suggested that there are 6 radiographic features of the component that should be monitored[42–46]:

- Peg femoral angle: the orientation of peg should be parallel to the trabecular bone; progressive change in the angle between the peg and femoral shaft particularly varus suggests loosening or fracture.

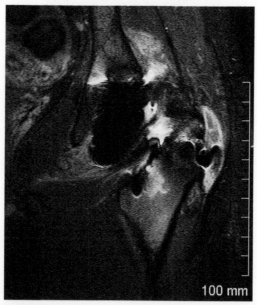

Fig. 7. Trochanteric bursitis. Coronal fat-suppressed T2-weighted MRI shows trochanteric bursitis following resurfacing arthroplasty.

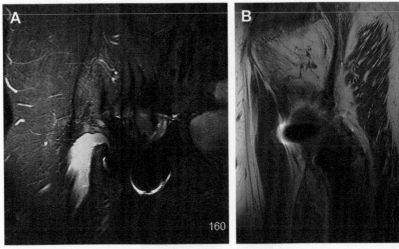

Fig. 8. (*A*) Coronal fat-suppressed T2- and (*B*) sagittal T1-weighted MRI show evidence of rupture of the gluteus medius tendon after THA.

- Implant subsidence: progressive reduction in the distance between the peg and the lateral femoral cortex over time suggests subsidence.
- Femoral neck narrowing: this is commonly seen following hip arthroplasty, and can be seen up to 3 years following the procedure; progressive narrowing of the femoral neck beyond 3 years should be carefully monitored; this may be

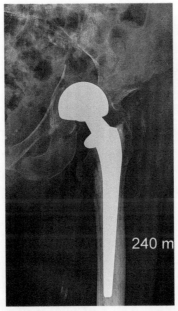

Fig. 9. Bipolar prosthesis with acetabular fracture. The bipolar prosthesis has migrated superomedially.

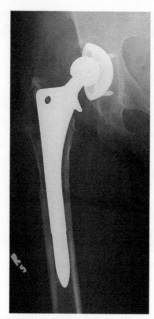

Fig. 10. Acetabular disruption. Anteroposterior radiograph of the right hip shows displacement of the bone in-growth acetabular component from the bone.

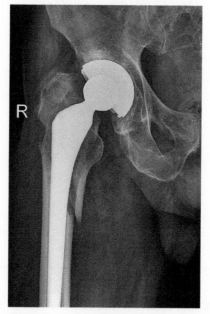

Fig. 11. Anteroposterior radiograph of the right hip shows periprosthetic fracture.

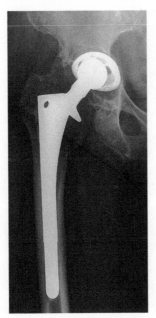

Fig. 12. Liner wear. Anteroposterior radiograph of the right hip demonstrates eccentric position of the femoral head within the acetabular component, in keeping with liner wear.

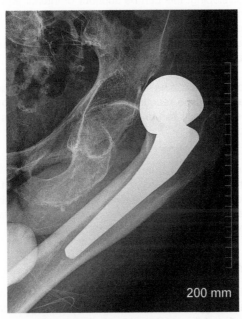

Fig. 13. Dislocation of bipolar prosthesis. Anteroposterior radiograph of the left hip shows superolateral dislocation of the bipolar prosthesis.

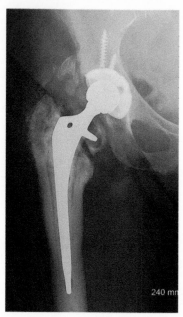

240 mm

Fig. 14. Anteroposterior radiograph of the right hip shows extensive heterotopic bone formation after THA.

secondary to stress shielding, loosening, and femoroacetabular impingement or caused by inflammatory response and metal hypersensitivity.

- Femoral neck scalloping: this can be superior or inferior and is often related to bony remodeling; superior scalloping is secondary to bony resorption or femoroacetabular impingement.
- Radiolucent lines: similar to the femoral stem in total arthroplasty, the peg can be divided into 3 zones; widening of more than 2 mm in any of the zone suggests loosening.
- Periprosthetic osteolysis can be located superior, inferior, or adjacent to the peg; this is secondary to tissue reactions related to liner wear or metal sensitivity; usually osteolysis is close to the joint and tends to be most prominent about the greater trochanter.

Complications

Femoral neck fracture is the most common complication, seen in 12% of resurfacing hip arthroplasties, and is more common in women **(Fig. 15)**.[42–45] It may be related to osteoporosis or suboptimal operative technique, like notching of the superior portion of the femoral neck and varus position of the femoral peg. Component loosening and femoral impingement are the other complications.[46]

IMAGING OF CARTILAGE REPAIR

Cartilage research has assumed increased importance because of better understanding of cartilage biology and function and newer cartilage repair techniques and pharmacologic therapies. Advanced imaging techniques have improved recognition of treatable injuries, hence restoring the function of the joint.

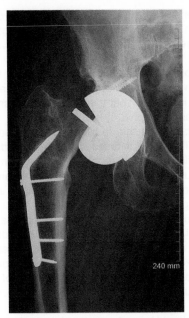

Fig. 15. Anteroposterior radiograph of the right hip shows femoral neck fracture related to resurfacing arthroplasty.

The hyaline cartilage is an avascular and aneural connective tissue composed mainly of water, chondrocytes, collagen, and proteoglycans. The articular cartilage is divided into 4 zones: superficial, intermediate, deep, and calcified zones. The calcified zone attaches to the subchondral bone. The tidemark separates the deep zone from the calcified zone. The composition and organization of the collagen and cells in these zones explain to some degree the differing mechanical properties of the zones. The superficial zone has the maximum water content and resistance to shear force. The intermediate zone is the thickest, with maximum proteoglycan concentration and reasonable resistance to compressive forces. The deep zone, however, best resists compressive forces. The calcified zone is the deepest layer, which contains type X collagen, which is associated with mineralization. Any disruption of the normal articular biochemistry can lead to cartilage degeneration.

Imaging of the cartilage has evolved significantly in recent years. The usefulness of conventional radiographs and CT in the assessment of cartilage is limited. MRI is the standard method for postoperative assessment of success of implantation and cartilage healing as it allows assessment of the repair cartilage morphology, thickness, volume, and subchondral bone. MRI evaluation of cartilage can be performed by using the same acquisition technique as used for native cartilage, as recommended by the International Cartilage Repair Society.[47,48]

The most commonly used sequences are the intermediate-weighted fast spin echo (FSE) and three-dimensional (3D) fat-suppressed gradient echo (GRE). In the FSE sequences, the articular cartilage shows lower signal than fluid, resulting in high contrast between joint fluid and cartilage, and between cartilage and bone marrow. This sequence should be done with a wide bandwidth that accentuates the trilaminar appearance of the cartilage. New 3D isotropic GRE sequences such as true fast imaging with steady state precession (true FISP), vibrational integrated biophotonic energizer (VIBE), and multiple echo data image combination (MEDIC) are promising in cartilage imaging.[49] The advantage of 3D GRE is that it is easy to perform, requires no postprocessing, and allows 3D visualization and volume measurements.[49–53]

Indirect MR-arthrography has been used postoperatively to differentiate between delamination at the base of the graft and normal high signal repair tissue following autologous chondrocyte implants,[53] but this technique is less useful in postoperative assessment than direct arthrography.

The biomechanical changes in the cartilage can be assessed by various tissue parameters. The T1 and T2 relaxation times and apparent diffusion constants change during cultivation of cartilage, suggesting change in the biomechanical properties of the cartilage during maturation.[54,55] Delayed gadolinium-enhanced MRI of cartilage (dGEMRIC) techniques and sodium MRI have been used to assess the proteoglycan content within the cartilage. T2 mapping by assessing the collagen content and $T1\rho$ imaging have also been used to evaluate the status of cartilage repair.

In the dGEMRIC technique, a single or double dose of gadolinium is injected intravenously. Then, after 10 minutes of exercise and 90 minutes of delay, a T1 map is obtained using a specialized inversion recovery spin echo sequence.[47] In T2 mapping, the loss of a structural framework of the collagen and loss of tissue isotropy result in increased T2 value. Sodium MRI, and to a lesser degree $T1\rho$, image the proteoglycan content directly.

MRI of cartilage repair should be performed at high resolution to detect early surface change.[49] To evaluate cartilage on a 1.5-T magnet, the scanner should have high performance gradients and an extremity or phased array coil should be used. A 3-T magnet is more efficient as it can generate images with high resolution and signal-to-noise ratio.[49] The baseline postoperative MRI should be performed at 3 to 6 months postsurgery to assess the volume and integration of repair tissue and at 1 year to assess the maturation of graft and identification of any complication.[49] The best method to evaluate the surface of the repair remains direct MR-arthrography.

The surgical options for cartilage repair are microfracture, chondral abrasionplasty, autologous osteochondral allograft transplantation (OATS or mosaicplasty), autologous chondrocyte implantation, autologous perichondral or periosteal transplantation, and transplantation of bioabsorbable screws.

MRI is a noninvasive technique to assess cartilage repair by evaluating the surface integrity, contour, cartilage thickness, characteristics of graft substance, and underlying bone. The MRI observation of cartilage repair tissue (MOCART) is a widely accepted system for standardization of reports of the imaging feature of cartilage repair, as it has excellent interobserver reproducibility.[56]

BONE MARROW STIMULATION

Microfracture is the most commonly performed cartilage repair procedure.[47] The chondral defect is debrided to a stable articular margin. The base of the defect is debrided through the calcified cartilage layer and 3 to 4 perforations are made per square centimeter.[57,58]

In chondral abrasion, 1 to 3 mm of subchondral bone is removed beneath the cartilage defect, resulting in formation of a fibrin clot. The pluripotent stem cells migrate to the defect from the marrow, thereby promoting formation of fibrocartilaginous repair tissue. On MRI the signal changes can be variable. Early MRI may show bone marrow edema and hyperintense repaired cartilage compared with the native cartilage caused by less organized matrix and increased water mobility. The follow-up MRI shows progressive decrease in subchondral edema and filling of the defect. Persistent edema and incomplete filling of the defect with thin repair tissue are considered signs of failure.[59–62]

In OATS, or mosaicplasty, osteochondral cylinders are harvested from a non–weight-bearing surface and transplanted into an articular defect. This procedure is recommended for chondral lesions between 1.5 and 4.0 cm^2. This technique is most often used to treat osteochondral lesions in the ankle and knee.[63–65] MRI evaluation postoperatively should include evaluation of graft incorporation, cartilage contour, subchondral bone, and the donor site. A well-incorporated plug has uniform fatty signal intensity.[59,66] Bone marrow edema, synovitis, and joint effusion may be seen in the early postoperative period. These imaging findings should show a gradual reduction on the follow-up scans. Persistent bony edema, fluid between the cartilage and bone, incongruity of the articular surface, subchondral cyst, and subsidence of the graft all suggest poor graft integration. Osteonecrosis of the graft can also be detected on MRI, but this is an uncommon complication[59] and evolving grafts may show low signal that can be misleading.

Autologous chondrocyte implantation was first described in 1990 in Sweden by Peterson for treatment of full thickness chondral defects. It consists of 2 stages. First the healthy chondrocytes are harvested from the non–weight-bearing surface and cultured for 4 to 5 weeks. In the second stage, the articular cartilage is debrided and implanted with the cultured chondrocytes. The cartilage is then covered by a periosteal graft. If successful a hyaline-like cartilage similar to native cartilage is formed. This procedure is used to treat defects of 2 to 12 cm^2.[67]

In the early postoperative period, bony edema and subchondral bone plate irregularity can be seen. The bone marrow edema progressively decreases but can last up to 1 year. In the late phase, the repair cartilage should have signal intensity similar to native cartilage. Complete edge integration with native cartilage may take up to 2 years. The presence of fluid between the bone and repaired cartilage is suggestive of delamination, which usually occurs during the first 6 months. Subchondral bone cyst formation, worsening surface defects, loose fragments, and underfilling of the defect are signs of graft incongruity. Intraarticular adhesions and synovitis are less common complications.[59,68–71]

HTO

High tibial osteotomy has been an accepted method of treatment of OA of the knee since 1958, after early studies by Jackson and Waugh. It is a surgical procedure to realign a bone to change the biomechanics of a joint by changing the transmission force through the joint.

This surgery is indicated for relatively young (<60 years) active patients with OA with varus or valgus deformity, and patients with medial compartment OA, medial compartment OA with ACL, PCL or combined deficiency, painful medial knee with either meniscal pathology, cartilage defect or osteochondritis dissecans lesions.[72] Knee replacement is generally offered for similar patients older than 65 years.[73]

The consensus is that osteotomy provides best results in mild-to-moderate unicompartmental OA.[75] Patients with bone attrition (>1 cm), tibiofemoral subluxation, patellofemoral degenerative disease, patella baja, more than 15° of flexion contracture, and moderate-to-severe lateral compartment OA have shown poor results.[74,75] Many patients who were historically offered osteotomy currently undergo unicompartmental arthroplasties.

Surgical Technique

The goal of osteotomy is to reposition the weight-bearing line so that the load distribution is through the knee, thus minimizing stress to the affected compartment.

Medial opening wedge tibial osteotomy

A wedge osteotomy is performed through the proximal tibia just proximal to the tibial tubercle. The space is filled with bone graft and plate and screws are applied.

Lateral closing wedge osteotomy

The bony varus alignment is corrected by removing a lateral wedge of bone and closing the defect. The degree of correction and the amount of bone to be removed are assessed from the preoperative radiographs. As a result of leg shortening a fibular shaft osteotomy or fibular head resection is also performed.

Distal femoral osteotomy

Distal femoral osteotomy is performed when there is valgus deformity associated with OA. Pins are inserted through the femoral condyles and shaft to create an angle that is required for correction of deformity and 1° to 2° of overcorrection. After osteotomy the proximal fragment is impacted to the distal fragment until the pins are parallel. A compression plate is then applied.

Correction with external fixator

Correction with external fixator consists of an external ring fixator for HTO, with the plane of the osteotomy being distal to the tibial tuberosity.

Preoperative Radiographic Assessment

Knee radiographs are an essential component of the preoperative assessment of potential osteotomy patients. Bilateral weight-bearing AP views in extension, bilateral weight-bearing posteroanterior tunnel views in 30° of flexion, true lateral views with superimposition of the medial and lateral condyles, and skyline views must be obtained. In addition to assessing the degree of OA, the presence of joint effusion, loose bodies, and tibiofemoral subluxation should be documented. The patellofemoral and other joint spaces should be evaluated. The following angles should be measured to assess the angle of deformity:

1. The mechanical axis of lower extremity is determined by a line drawn from the center of the femoral head to the center of the talus. Normally this line should pass between the tibial spines.
2. Femorotibial angle (FTA) is the angle between the anatomic axis of the femur and tibia. The medial angle subtended at the point at which these 2 lines meet in the center of the tibial spines is the anatomic angle. Normal FTA is 182° to 184°.
3. Posterior tibial slope angle (PTSA) is measured in the lateral view. It is the angle between the line drawn perpendicular to the tangential line of the posterior tibial cortex and the posterior slope of the tibial plateau. The preoperative mechanical and anatomic axes are measured and are used to calculate the angular correction necessary for restoration of normal mechanical axis with overcorrection of about 3° to 5°. Complications from this procedure are infrequent (**Fig. 16**). Fracture or ischemic necrosis of the proximal tibial fragment may occur but infection and nonunion are rare. The average healing time for HTO is 9 weeks.[2] However, various investigations have shown that by 5 years nearly half of the patients who underwent HTO eventually require total knee replacement.

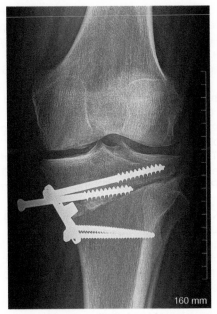

160 mm

Fig.16. Hardware failure. Anteroposterior radiograph of the left hip shows retraction of the screw transfixing the high tibial osteotomy.

SUMMARY

Various imaging modalities can be used in the pre- and postoperative assessment of arthroplasty. Serial plain film radiographs remain the modality of choice for postoperative evaluation of patients with arthroplasty. With proper image modification techniques, CT and MRI with their increased sensitivity can evaluate the joint and surrounding osseous and soft-tissue structures. CT can assess for subtle fractures and the extent of osteolysis better than radiographs. The ability to demonstrate intraosseous and soft-tissue abnormalities has given MRI an advantage compared with other imaging modalities. Ultrasound offers dynamic evaluation and can provide real-time guidance for percutaneous procedures. Injection and aspiration of the joint along with scintigraphy are important for the preoperative diagnosis of infection. In recent years, cartilage imaging has become one of the leading areas of research. With the development of newer surgical therapies and the improved cartilage imaging techniques, MRI plays a pivotal role in the evaluation of cartilage abnormalities and postoperative assessment.

REFERENCES

1. Loone RJ, Boyd A, Totterman S, et al. Volumetric computerized tomography as a measurement of periprosthetic acetabular osteolysis and its correlation with wear. Arthritis Res 2002;4:59–63.
2. Weissman BN. Orthopedic imaging. In: Resnick D, editor. Diagnosis of bone and joint disorders. 4th edition. Philadelphia: Saunders; 2002. p. 595–644.
3. Tigges S, Stiles RG, Roberson JR. Complications of hip arthroplasty causing periprosthetic radiolucency on plain radiographs. AJR Am J Roentgenol 1994;162: 1387–91.

4. Miller TT. Imaging of hip arthroplasty. Semin Musculoskelet Radiol 2006;10:30–46.
5. Weissman BN. Imaging of total hip replacement. Radiology 1997;202:611–23.
6. Weissman BN, Sledge CB. The hip. Orthopedic radiology. Philadelphia: WB Saunders Co; 1991. p. 385–495.
7. Rosenthall L. Radionuclide investigation of osteomyelitis. Curr Opin Radiol 1992; 4:62–9.
8. Kirchner PT, Simon MA. Radioisotopic evaluation of skeletal disease. J Bone Joint Surg Am 1981;63:673.
9. Sofka CM. Optimizing techniques for musculoskeletal imaging of the postoperative patient. Radiol Clin North Am 2006;44:323–9.
10. White LM, Miller T, Schweitzer M, editors. Imaging of joint replacement. Diagnostic musculoskeletal imaging. New York: McGraw-Hill; 2004. p. 417–32.
11. Cahir JG, Toms AP, Marshall TJ, et al. CT and MRI of hip arthroplasty. Clin Radiol 2007;62:1163–71.
12. White LM, Kim JK, Mehta M, et al. Complications of total hip arthroplasty: MR imaging, initial experience. Radiology 2000;215:254–62.
13. Buckwalter KA, Parr JA, Choplin RH, et al. Multichannel CT imaging of orthopedic hardware and implants. Semin Musculoskelet Radiol 2006;10:86–97.
14. Naraghi AM, White LM. Magnetic resonance imaging of joint replacements. Semin Musculoskelet Radiol 2006;10:98–106.
15. Jacobson JA. Hip replacement. Available at: e-medicine.medscape.com/article/ 398669-overview. Accessed May 1, 2008.
16. Ahlback S. Osteoarthrosis of the knee. A radiographic investigation. Acta Radiol Diagn 1968;277(Suppl):7–72.
17. Amin AK, Patton JT, Cook RE, et al. Unicompartmental or total knee arthroplasty: results from a matched study. Clin Orthop Relat Res 2006;451:101–6.
18. White SH, Ludkowski PF, Goodfellow J. Anteromedial osteoarthritis of the knee. J Bone Joint Surg 1991;73:582–6.
19. Savard UC, Price AJ. Oxford medial unicompartmental knee arthroplasty. A survival analysis of an independent series. J Bone Joint Surg 2001;83:191–4.
20. Berger RA, Nedeff DD, Barden RM, et al. Unicompartmental knee arthroplasty. Clinical experience at 6- to 10-year follow-up. Clin Orthop 1999;367:50–60.
21. Feiock DA, Newman JS, Newberg AH, et al. Radiological evaluation of total knee arthroplasty. In: Bono J, Scott RD, editors. Revision total knee arthroplasty. New York: Springer; 2005. p. 36–52.
22. Duus BR, Boeckstyns M, Kjaer L, et al. Radio-nuclide scanning after total knee replacement: correlation with pain and radiolucent lines, a prospective study. Invest Radiol 1987;22:891–904.
23. Kantor SG, Schneider R, Insall JN, et al. Radionuclide imaging of asymptomatic versus symptomatic total knee arthroplasties. Clin Orthop Relat Res 1990;260: 118–23.
24. Schneider R, Soudry M. Radiographic and scintigraphic evaluation of total knee arthroplasty. Clin Orthop 1986;205:108–20.
25. Brick GW, Scott RD. The patellofemoral component of knee arthroplasty. Clin Orthop 1988;231:168–78.
26. Schneider R, Hood RW, Ranawat CS. Radiological evaluation of knee arthroplasty. Orthop Clin North Am 1982;13:225–44.
27. Hanssen AD, Rand JA. Evaluation and treatment of infection at the site of a total hip or knee arthroplasty. J Bone Joint Surg Am 1998;80:1127–39.
28. Love C, Tomas MB, Marwin SE, et al. Role of nuclear medicine in diagnosis of the infected joint replacement. Radiographics 2001;21:1229–38.

29. Herrlin K. Space orientation of total hip prosthesis. Acta Radiol 1986;27:619–27.

30. McLaren RH. Prosthetic hip angulation. Radiology 1973;107:705–6.

31. Fackler CD, Poss R. Dislocation in total hip arthoplasties. Clin Orthop 1980;151: 169–78.

32. Ghelman B. Radiographic localization of the acetabular component of a hip prosthesis. Radiology 1979;130:540–2.

33. Mian SW, Truchly G, Pflum FA, et al. Computed tomography measurement of acetabular cup anteversion and retroversion in total hip arthroplasty. Clin Orthop 1992;276:206–9.

34. Kitamura N, Pappedemos PC, Duffy PR, et al. The value of anteroposterior pelvic radiographs for evaluating pelvic osteolysis. Clin Orthop Relat Res 2006;453: 239–45.

35. Van Holsbeeck MT, Eyler WR, Sherman LS, et al. Detection of infection in loosened hip prostheses: efficacy of sonography. AJR Am J Roentgenol 1994;163: 381–4.

36. Foldis K, Balint P, Gaal M, et al. Ultrasonography after hip arthroplasty. Skeletal Radiol 1992;21:297–9.

37. Graif M, Schwartz E, Strauss S. Occult infection of hip prosthesis: sonographic evaluation. J Am Geriatr Soc 1991;39:203–4.

38. Huo MH, Gilbert NF, Parvizi J. What's new in total hip arthroplasty? J Bone Joint Surg Am 2007;89:1874–85.

39. Tigges S, Stiles RG, Roberson JR. Appearance of septic hip prostheses on plain radiographs. AJR Am J Roentgenol 1994;163:377–80.

40. Claus AM, Totterman SM, Synchterz CJ, et al. Computed tomography to assess pelvis lysis after total hip replacement. Clin Orthop 2004;422:167–74.

41. Mueller PR, Stark DD, Simeone JF, et al. MR-guided aspiration biopsy: needle design and clinical trials. Radiology 1986;161:605–9.

42. Shimmin A, Beaulé PE, Campbell P. Metal-on-metal hip resurfacing arthroplasty. J Bone Joint Surg Am 2008;90:637–54.

43. Wank R, Miller TT, Shapiro JF. Sonographically guided injection of anesthetic for iliopsoas tendinopathy after total hip arthroplasty. J Clin Ultrasound 2004;32: 354–7.

44. Amstutz HC, Beaule PE, Dorey FJ, et al. Metal-on-metal hybrid surface arthroplasty: two to six-year follow-up study. J Bone Joint Surg Am 2004;86: 28–39.

45. Pollard TC, Baker RP, Eastaugh-Waring SJ, et al. Treatment of the young active patient with osteoarthritis of the hip. A five- to seven-year comparison of hybrid total hip arthroplasty and metal-on-metal resurfacing. J Bone Joint Surg Br 2006;88:592–600.

46. Hing CB, Young DA, Dalziel RE, et al. Narrowing of the neck in resurfacing arthroplasty of the hip: a radiological study. J Bone Joint Surg Br 2007;89: 1019–24.

47. Bobic V. ICRS articular cartilage imaging committee. ICRS MR imaging protocol for knee articular cartilage. 2000. p. 12.

48. Recht M, Bobic V, Burstein D, et al. Magnetic resonance imaging of articular cartilage. Clin Orthop Relat Res 2001;391(Suppl):S379–96.

49. Potter HG, Chong le R. Magnetic resonance imaging assessment of chondral lesions and repair. J Bone Joint Surg Am 2009;91(Suppl 1):126–31.

50. Peterfy CG, van Dijke CF, Lu Y, et al. Quantification of the volume of articular cartilage in the metacarpophalangeal joints of the hand: accuracy and precision of three-dimensional MR imaging. AJR Am J Roentgenol 1995;165:371–5.

51. Kawahara Y, Uetani M, Nakahara N, et al. Fast spin-echo MR of the articular cartilage in the osteoarthrotic knee. Correlation of MR and arthroscopic findings. Acta Radiol 1998;39:120–5.

52. Peterfy CG, Majumdar S, Lang P, et al. MR imaging of the arthritic knee: improved discrimination of cartilage, synovium, and effusion with pulsed saturation transfer and fat-suppressed T1-weighted sequences. Radiology 1994;191:413–9.

53. Trattnig S, Huber M, Breitenseher MJ, et al. Imaging articular cartilage defects with 3D fat-suppressed echo planar imaging: comparison with conventional 3D fat-suppressed gradient echo sequence and correlation with histology. J Comput Assist Tomogr 1998;22:8–14.

54. Yao L, Gentili A, Thomas A. Incidental magnetization transfer contrast in fast spin-echo imaging of cartilage. J Magn Reson Imaging 1996;6:180–4.

55. Gillis A, Bashir A, McKeon B, et al. Magnetic resonance imaging of relative glycosaminoglycan distribution in patients with autologous chondrocyte transplants. Invest Radiol 2001;36:743–8.

56. Marlovits S, Singer P, Zeller P, et al. Magnetic resonance observation of cartilage repair tissue (MOCART) for the evaluation of autologous chondrocyte transplantation: determination of interobserver variability and correlation to clinical outcome after 2 years. Eur J Radiol 2006;57:16–23.

57. Bert JM. Abrasion arthroplasty. Tech Orthop 2001;11:90–5.

58. Mithoefer K, Williams RJ 3rd, Warren RF, et al. The microfracture technique for the treatment of articular cartilage lesions in the knee: a prospective cohort study. J Bone Joint Surg Am 2005;87:1911–20.

59. Choi YS, Potter HG, Chun TJ. MR Imaging of cartilage repair in the knee and ankle. Radiographics 2008;28:1043–59.

60. Alparslan L, Winalski CS, Boutin RD, et al. Postoperative magnetic resonance imaging of articular cartilage repair. Semin Musculoskelet Radiol 2001;5:345–63.

61. Fuchsjager MH, Mlynarik V, Marlovits S, et al. High field MR imaging in reconstituted articular cartilage: evaluation of cartilage maturation for determination of optimal transplantation time. Radiology 2004;233:442–8.

62. Potter HG, Linklater JM, Allen AA, et al. Magnetic resonance imaging of articular cartilage in the knee. An evaluation with use of fast-spin-echo imaging. J Bone Joint Surg Am 1998;80:1276–84.

63. Takahashi T, Tins B, McCall IW, et al. MR appearance of autologous chondrocyte implantation in the knee: correlation with the knee features and clinical outcome. Skeletal Radiol 2006;35:16–26.

64. Trattnig S, Millington SA, Szomolanyi P, et al. MR imaging of osteochondral grafts and autologous chondrocyte implantation. Eur Radiol 2007;17:103–18.

65. Potter HG, Foo LF. Magnetic resonance imaging of articular cartilage: trauma, degeneration, and repair. Am J Sports Med 2006;34:661–77.

66. Link TM, Mishung J, Wortler K, et al. Normal and pathological MR findings in osteochondral autografts with longitudinal follow-up. Eur Radiol 2006;16:88–96.

67. Brittberg M, Peterson L, Sjogren-Jansson E, et al. Articular cartilage engineering with autologous chondrocyte transplantation: a review of recent developments. J Bone Joint Surg Am 2003;85-A(Suppl 3):109–15.

68. Peterson L, Minas T, Brittberg M, et al. Two- to 9-year outcome after autologous chondrocyte transplantation of the knee. Clin Orthop Relat Res 2000;374:212–34.

69. Peterson L, Minas T, Brittberg M, et al. Treatment of osteochondritis dissecans of the knee with autologous chondrocyte transplantation: results at two to ten years. J Bone Joint Surg Am 2003;85 A(Suppl 2):17–24.

70. Henderson I, Gui J, Lavigne P. Autologous chondrocyte implantation: natural history of postimplantation periosteal hypertrophy and effects of repair-site debridement on outcome. Arthroscopy 2006;22:1318–24.

71. Alparslan L, Minas T, Winalski CS. Magnetic resonance imaging of autologous chondrocyte implantation. Semin Ultrasound CT MR 2001;22:341–51.

72. Hernigou P, Medevielle D, Debeyre J, et al. Proximal tibial osteotomy for osteoarthritis with varus deformity: a ten to thirteen-year follow-up study. J Bone Joint Surg Am 1987;69:332–54.

73. Magyar G, Ahl TL, Vibe P, et al. Open-wedge osteotomy by hemicallotasis or the closed-wedge technique for osteoarthritis of the knee: a randomised study of 50 operations. J Bone Joint Surg Br 1999;81:444–8.

74. Dugdale TW, Noyes FR, Styer D. Preoperative planning for high tibial osteotomy: the effect of lateral tibiofemoral separation and tibiofemoral length. Clin Orthop 1992;274:248–64.

75. Ogata K, Yoshii I, Kawamura H, et al. Standing radiographs cannot determine the correction in high tibial osteotomy. J Bone Joint Surg Br 1991;73:927–31.

Index

Note: Page numbers of article titles are in **boldface** type.

A

Acetabulum
   cartilage loss in, 596–598
   dysplasia of, 470–471
   labrum of, assessment of, 595–596
Acromioclavicular joint osteoarthritis, ultrasonography for, 504, 511–512
Active shape models, for joint space width measurement, 495
Adduction moments, in gait, 469
Alignment, in knee osteoarthritis, 456, 472–473
Alpha angle, in femoroacetabular impingement, 595
American College of Rheumatology, hand osteoarthritis criteria of, 625
Ankle osteoarthritis, ultrasonography for, 514
Anserine bursitis, 568
Anterior cruciate ligament, injury to, 565–566
Arthrography. *See also* Computed tomography arthrography; Magnetic
       resonance arthrography.
   for joint preserving and replacing surgery, 652, 657
   for scapho-trapezial joint osteoarthritis, 610
   for ulno-carpal joint osteoarthritis, 615
Arthroplasty, 653–664
   hip, 656–664
   knee, 653–656
Arthroscopy, for meniscal lesions, 586
Automated methods, for joint space width measurement, 494–496

B

Baker's (popliteal) cysts, 513, 566
Biomechanics, of osteoarthritis, **465–483**
   alignment measures in, 472–473
   contact area measurement in, 474
   etiopathogenesis and, 466
   ex vivo studies of, 472
   gait analysis in, 473
   hip, 470–471
   imaging assessment of, 471–474
   kinematics of, 472–474
   knee, 466–470
   models for, 472
Biopsychosocial framework, for osteoarthritis, 451
Bone
   attrition of, in knee osteoarthritis, 561–562

Rheum Dis Clin N Am 35 (2009) 675–686
doi:10.1016/S0889-857X(09)00097-0
0889-857X/09/$ – see front matter © 2009 Elsevier Inc. All rights reserved.

rheumatic.theclinics.com

Bone (*continued*)
    cortex of, ultrasonography of, 507–509
    subchondral, symptoms related to, 452–453
Bone marrow, stimulation of, 666–667
Bone marrow lesions
    in facet joint osteoarthritis, 638–640
    in knee osteoarthritis, 558–560
        cartilage loss due to, 544
        imaging evidence of, 457
    in spinal osteoarthritis, 634–638
    subchondral, 452–453
Boston-Leeds Osteoarthritis Knee Score (BLOKS), 523, 526–528, 530, 535
Bouchard nodes, 622–623
Bursitis, in knee osteoarthritis, 566–569

C

Calipers, for joint space width measurement, 493–494
Carpometacarpal joint osteoarthritis, 449
Cartilage
    biochemical changes in, in hip joint, 598–600
    loss of
        clinical correlations of, 543
        in hip osteoarthritis, 471, 596–598
        risk factors for, 544–545
        spatial patterns of, 541–543
        synovitis and, 562–564
    quantitative measurement of, in knee osteoarthritis, 537–545
    rate of change of, 541
    repair of, 664–667
    symptoms related to, 451–452
    ultrasonography of, 509
Chondrocyte implantation, 667
Chondropathy, of wrist, 612–613
Collateral ligaments, injury to, 565–566
Computed tomography
    for joint preserving and replacing surgery
        for cartilage assessment, 665
        hip, 657–658
    knee, 654
    for knee osteoarthritis, 473, 654
    for spinal osteoarthritis, 628
Computed tomography arthrography
    for hamato-lunate joint osteoarthritis, 618
    for radiocarpal joint osteoarthritis, 612–613
    for scapho-trapezial joint osteoarthritis, 610
    for ulno-carpal joint osteoarthritis, 615
Contact area, knee osteoarthritis, 474
Cruciate ligaments, injury to, 565–566
Cyst(s)
    mucoid, in interphalangeal joint osteoarthritis, 618–622

periarticular, in knee osteoarthritis, 566–569
subchondral, in knee osteoarthritis, 560–561

D

Debridement, in cartilage repair, 666–667
Degenerative spondylolisthesis, 638–640
Delayed gadolinium-enhanced MRI of cartilage (dGEMRIC), in hip osteoarthritis, 599–600
Dell classification, of trapezio-metacarpal joint osteoarthritis, 606
Digital analysis, knee images, 495–496
Disc degeneration, spinal osteoarthritis in, 630–634
Discography, for spinal osteoarthritis, 629
Disease Characteristics in Hand OA Group (DICHOA), 626–627
Distal femoral osteotomy, 668
Dorsal intercalated segmental instability, 608
Dynamic moments, in gait, 469

E

Eaton and Littler classification, of trapezio-metacarpal joint osteoarthritis, 606
Effusion
    in facet joint osteoarthritis, 639–640
    in knee osteoarthritis, 564–565
Enthesophytes, ultrasonography of, 509, 513
Environmental factors, in meniscal lesions, 584–585
Erosions, bone, ultrasonography of, 508
Erosive osteoarthritis, of interphalangeal joints, 618–622
European League Against Rheumatism Osteoarthritis Task force, hand osteoarthritis criteria of, 625
External fixation, of tibial osteotomy, 668

F

Facet joint osteoarthritis, 638–640
Femoroacetabular impingement, 470–471, 592–595
Femorotibial angle, in high tibial osteotomy, 668
Fingers, osteoarthritis of, 618–624
    epidemiology of, 605
    ultrasonography for, 509
Fixed-flexion view, for joint space width measurement, 492
Flexor carpi radialis tendinopathy, 609–610
Fluoroscopically-assisted joint space width measurement, 490–491
Foot osteoarthritis, ultrasonography for, 514–515
Force, assessment of, 472
Fracture
    in hip arthroplasty, 664
    in knee arthroplasty, 654

G

Gait
    analysis of, 473
    dynamic moments in, 469

Ganglion cysts, 569, 615–616
Genetic factors
    in hand osteoarthritis, 606
    in meniscal lesions, 584–585
Glenohumeral joint osteoarthritis, ultrasonography for, 511
Granulomatous disease, after hip arthroplasty, 659
Groin pain, in femoroacetabular impingement, 470–471
Guyon canal, ganglion in, 615–616

H

Hamato-lunate joint osteoarthritis, 616–618
Hamstring muscles, impairment of, 454–455
Hand osteoarthritis, 605–626. See also Fingers, osteoarthritis of.
    diagnosis of, 625–626
    epidemiology of, 449–451, 605
    hamato-lunate joint, 616–618
    piso-triquetral joint, 615–616
    radiocarpal joint, 611–613
    radio-ulnar joint, 613
    scapho-trapezial joint, 607–611
    severity of, 625–626
    trapezio-metacarpal joint, 606–607
    ulno-carpal joint, 614–615
    ultrasonography for, 504, 506, 508–509, 512
Heberden nodes, 618–622
High tibial osteotomy, 667–668
Hip osteoarthritis
    arthroplasty for, 656–664
    epidemiology of, 449–450
    in dysplasia, 600
    magnetic resonance imaging for, **591–604**
        biochemically enhanced, 598–601
        in acetabular labrum assessment, 595–596
        in cartilage lesions, 596–598
        in femoroacetabular impingement, 592–595
        semiquantitative assessment in, 537
    mechanics of, 470–471
    ultrasonography for, 506, 512–513

I

Imaging, for osteoarthritis
    before and after joint surgery, **651–673**
    biomechanics role in, **465–483**
    epidemiology and, 448–451
    hand. See Hand osteoarthritis.
    hip. See Hip osteoarthritis.
    in joint space width measurement, **485–502**
    in meniscal damage. See Meniscal lesions.
    knee. See Knee osteoarthritis.

magnetic resonance imaging. *See* Magnetic resonance imaging.
 pathophysiology and, 451–457
 soft tissues, **557–577**
 spine, 626–643
 subchondral bone, **557–577**
 ultrasonography. *See* Ultrasonography.
 wrist. *See* Wrist osteoarthritis.
Impingement test, for femoroacetabular impingement, 592–593
Infections
 in hip arthroplasty, 657
 in knee arthroplasty, 655–656
Infrapatellar bursa, fluid in, 567–568
Infrapatellar fat pad, synovial thickening in, 453–454
Interphalangeal joint osteoarthritis
 distal, 618–622
 epidemiology of, 449
 proximal, 622–623
 ultrasonography for, 512

J

Joint preserving and replacing surgery, **651–673**
 arthroplasty, 653–664
  hip, 656–664
  knee, 653–656
 bone marrow stimulation, 666–667
 cartilage repair, 664–667
 high tibial osteotomy, 667–668
 imaging techniques for, 651–653
Joint reaction force, in patellofemoral joint, 470
Joint space width measurement, **485–502**
 automated methods for, 494–496
 clinical applications of, 497–498
 manual methods for, 493–494
 mean, 496–497
 minimum, 496–497
 protocols for, 488–493
  fixed-flexion view, 492
  fluoroscopically-assisted, 490–491
  Lyon schuss view, 491, 493
  semiflexed AP view, 490–491
  semiflexed metatarsophalangeal view, 491–492
  sensitivity of, 492–493
 semiautomated methods for, 494–496
 tibiofemoral, 493–497
 tibiofemoral joint alignment and, 486–488

K

Kellgren and Lawrence grading system, 448, 625
Kinematics, measurement of, 472–474
Knee images digital analysis, 495–496

Knee osteoarthritis
    arthroplasty for, 653–656
    contact area in, 474
    epidemiology of, 448–451, 465
    gait analysis in, 473
    gender differences in, 466
    high tibial osteotomy for, 667–668
    joint space width measurement in, **485–502**
    kinematics of, 472–474
    magnetic resonance imaging for, **521–555, 557–577**
        mechanical aspects of, 474
        potential of, 522
        quantitative assessment in, 537–545
        semiquantitative assessment in, 523–537
        with effusion, 564–565
        with ligamentous injury, 565–566
        with loose bodies, 570–571
        with meniscal lesions, 580–586
        with periarticular cysts and bursae, 566–569
        with subchondral bone alterations, 558–562
        with synovitis, 562–564
    mechanics of, 466–474
    medial compartment, 654
    meniscal lesions in, **579–590**
    pathophysiology of, 456–457
    progression of, 468–469
    radiography for, 448–449, 473, **485–502**
    risk factors for, 449, 456
    stages of, 457
    symptoms of, 451–456, 469–470
    ultrasonography for, 505–506, 509, 513–514
    whole organ assessment for, 523–537
Knee Osteoarthritis Scoring System (KOSS), 523, 525–528, 530, 535

L

Lateral closing wedge tibial osteotomy, 668
Ligaments
    injury to, 565–566
    ultrasonography of, 509–510
Loading rate, assessment of, 472
Loose bodies, in knee osteoarthritis, 570–571
Lyon schuss view, for joint space width measurement, 491, 493

M

Magnetic resonance arthrography
    for acetabular cartilage loss, 596–598
    for acetabular labrum assessment, 595–596
    for cartilage repair, 666
    for hamato-lunate joint osteoarthritis, 618

for hip osteoarthritis, 592
for joint preserving and replacing surgery, 666
for radiocarpal joint osteoarthritis, 612–613
for scapho-trapezial joint osteoarthritis, 610
Magnetic resonance imaging
for effusion, 453–454
for hamato-lunate joint osteoarthritis, 618
for hand osteoarthritis, 626
for hip osteoarthritis, **591–604**
mechanical aspects of, 471
semiquantitative assessment in, 537
for interphalangeal joint osteoarthritis, 620, 622–623
for joint preserving and replacing surgery
bone marrow stimulation, 666–667
cartilage assessment, 665–666
hip, 657
for knee osteoarthritis. *See* Knee osteoarthritis, magnetic resonance imaging for
for meniscal lesions, 454
for osteoarthritis, epidemiology and, 450–451
for piso-triquetral joint osteoarthritis, 616
for radiocarpal joint osteoarthritis, 612–613
for scapho-trapezial joint osteoarthritis, 610
for spinal osteoarthritis, 628
clinical significance of, 642–643
in bone marrow changes, 634–638
in disc degeneration, 630–634
in posterior element disorders, 638–640
reliability of, 640–642
for subchondral bone lesions, 452
for synovitis, 453–454
for trapezio-metacarpal joint osteoarthritis, 607
for ulno-carpal joint osteoarthritis, 615
pathogenesis and, 456–457
Malalignment, in knee osteoarthritis, 456, 468–469, 544
Mechanics. *See* Biomechanics.
Medial opening wedge tibial osteotomy, 668
Meniscal lesions, in knee osteoarthritis, **579–590**
anatomic considerations in, 579–580
as cause of consequence, 581–584
cartilage loss due to, 544
cysts near, 568–569
environmental factors in, 584–585
genetic factors in, 584–585
imaging evidence of, 456–457
magnetic resonance imaging for, 454
treatment of, 585–586
types of, 580–581
Meniscectomy, 454, 585–586
Metacarpophalangeal joint osteoarthritis, 509, 514–515, 624
Microfracture, in cartilage repair, 666–667
Millette classification, for disc degeneration and herniation, 630–631

Modic classification, of vertebral bone marrow degeneration, 634–638, 643
Mosaicplasty, 667
Motion (gait) analysis, 473
Mucoid cysts, in interphalangeal joint osteoarthritis, 618–622
Muscles, periarticular, impairment of, 454–455
Myelography, for spinal osteoarthritis, 628–629

N

Neuropathic pain, 455–456
Nonsteroidal anti-inflammatory drugs, knee damage related to, 470
North American Spine Society, disc degeneration classification of, 631

O

Obesity, osteoarthritis due to, 455
OMERACT ultrasonography task force, 506–508
Osteoarthritis
    biomechanics of, **465–483**
    classification of, 448
    epidemiology of, 448–451
    for joint preserving and replacing surgery, **651–673**
    hand. See Hand osteoarthritis.
    hip. See Hip osteoarthritis.
    imaging for. See Imaging, for osteoarthritis.
    joint space width measurement in, **485–502**
    knee. See Knee osteoarthritis.
    pathophysiology of, 451–457
    progression of, dynamic moment effects on, 469
    risk factors for, 449
    spine, 626–643
    symptoms of, 451–457
    ultrasonography for. See Ultrasonography.
    wrist. See Wrist osteoarthritis.
Osteoarthritis Research Society International group, hand osteoarthritis guidelines of, 625
Osteochondromatosis, synovial, in knee osteoarthritis, 570–571
Osteolysis
    in hip arthroplasty, 658–659
    in knee arthroplasty, 655
Osteophytes
    in arthritis classification, 448–449
    in knee osteoarthritis, 570–571
    in metacarpophalangeal joints, 624–626
    symptoms related to, 453
    ultrasonography of, 507–509, 511–515
Osteotomy, high tibial, 667–668

P

Pain
    bone, 453

in bone attrition, 562
in femoroacetabular impingement, 470–471
in hamato-lunate joint osteoarthritis, 616–618
in joint effusion, 565
in spinal osteoarthritis, 626
in synovitis, 564
in trapezio-metacarpal joint osteoarthritis, 606
mechanical relationships in, 469–470
neuropathic, 455–456
pathogenesis of, 451–457
versus cartilage loss, 543
Parameniscal cysts, 568–569
Patellar complications, in knee arthroplasty, 654–655
Patellofemoral osteoarthritis, mechanics of, 470, 474
Periarticular muscles, impairment of, 454–455
Periostitis, 453
Peritrapezial osteoarthritis (trapezio-metacarpal joint osteoarthritis), 606–607
Pfirrmann classification, of disc degeneration, 631–633
Piso-triquetral joint osteoarthritis, 615–616
Popliteal cysts, 513, 566
Posterior cruciate ligament, injury to, 566
Posterior tibial slope angle, in high tibial osteotomy, 668
Prosthesis, complications of
    hip, 657–666
    knee, 655

Q

Quadriceps muscles, impairment of, 454–455

R

Radiocarpal joint osteoarthritis, 611–613
Radiography
    epidemiologic information from, 448–451
    for hamato-lunate joint osteoarthritis, 617
    for hand osteoarthritis, 625
    for hip osteoarthritis, 472–473, 592–593
    for interphalangeal joint osteoarthritis, 620–622
    for joint preserving and replacing surgery, 651–652
        cartilage assessment, 665
        high tibial osteotomy, 668
        hip, 657–664
        knee, 654–655
    for knee osteoarthritis
        for joint space width measurement, 486–498
        mechanical aspects of, 466–469
    for meniscal lesions, 454
    for metacarpophalangeal joint osteoarthritis, 624
    for piso-triquetral joint osteoarthritis, 615
    for radiocarpal joint osteoarthritis, 611–612

Radiography (*continued*)
    for radio-ulnar joint osteoarthritis, 613
    for scapho-trapezial joint osteoarthritis, 608
    for spinal osteoarthritis, 628
    for trapezio-metacarpal joint osteoarthritis, 606–607
    for ulno-carpal joint osteoarthritis, 614–615
    pathogenesis information from, 456–457
    symptoms and, 451
Radio-ulnar joint osteoarthritis, 613
Replacement, joint. *See* Joint preserving and replacing surgery.
Resurfacing hip arthroplasty, 658, 660–661, 664
Rhizarthrosis (trapezio-metacarpal joint osteoarthritis), 606–607

S

Scaphoid nonunion advanced collapse (SNAC), 611–612
Scaphoid-lunate advanced collapse (SLAC), 611–612
Scapho-trapezial joint osteoarthritis, 607–611
Scintigraphy, for joint preserving and replacing surgery, 652, 655–656
Scoring systems, for knee MRI, 523–537
Semiflexed AP view, for joint space width measurement, 490–491
Semiflexed metatarsophalangeal view, for joint width measurement, 491–492
Shoulder osteoarthritis, ultrasonography for, 504, 509, 511–512
Software algorithms, for joint space width measurement, 495–496
Spinal osteoarthritis, imaging methods for, 626–643
    clinical relevance of, 642–643
    in bone marrow degeneration, 634–638
    in degenerative disc disease, 630–634
    posterior element stress and, 638–640
    reliability of, 640–642
Spondylolisthesis, degenerative, 638–640
Statistical shape models, for joint space width measurement, 495
Sternoclavicular joint osteoarthritis, 512
Strain, measurement of, 472
Stress, measurement of, 472
Subchondral bone, alterations of, 558–562
SynaFlexer device, 491
Synovial fluid collections, ultrasonography of, 506–507
Synovitis
    in knee osteoarthritis, 562–564
    magnetic resonance imaging of, 506–508, 532–534
    symptoms related to, 453–454, 457
    ultrasonography of, 504–506
Synovium
    hypertrophy of, 513–514
    normal, 504

T

Tendons, ultrasonography of, 509–510
Thromboembolism, in knee arthroplasty, 654

Thumb osteoarthritis, 449–450, 624–626
Tibial osteotomy, 667–668
Tibiofemoral joint
    lesions of, 457
    mechanics of, 470
    osteoarthritis of
        joint space width measurement in, 493–496
        radiography for, 486–488
Tibiofibular synovial cysts, 569
Total hip arthroplasty, 657
Total knee arthroplasty, 654–656
"Trapezial tilt," 606–607
Trapezio-metacarpal joint osteoarthritis, 606–607

U

Ulnar impaction syndrome, 614–615
Ulno-carpal joint osteoarthritis, 614–615
Ultrasonography, **503–519**
    for acromioclavicular joint osteoarthritis, 504, 511–512
    for ankle osteoarthritis, 514
    for bone cortex, 507–509
    for cartilage assessment, 509
    for finger osteoarthritis, 509, 622
    for foot osteoarthritis, 514–515
    for glenohumeral joint osteoarthritis, 511
    for hand osteoarthritis, 504, 506, 508–509, 512, 625–627
    for hip osteoarthritis, 506, 512–513
    for interphalangeal joint osteoarthritis, 512, 618–620
    for joint preserving and replacing surgery, 652–653, 657
    for knee osteoarthritis, 505–506, 509, 513–514
    for ligaments, 509–510
    for metacarpophalangeal joints osteoarthritis, 509, 514–515
    for piso-triquetral joint osteoarthritis, 615
    for scapho-trapezial joint osteoarthritis, 609–610
    for shoulder osteoarthritis, 504, 509, 511–512
    for sternoclavicular joint osteoarthritis, 512
    for synovial fluid, 506–507
    for synovium, 504–506
    for tendons, 509–510
    for wrist osteoarthritis, 506, 509, 512
Unicompartmental knee arthroplasty, 653–654

V

Valgus knee, mechanics of, 466–469
Varus knee, mechanics of, 466–469
Video capture technique, for joint space width measurement, 494–495

W

Whole Organ Magnetic Resonance Imaging Score (WORMS), 523–530, 535
Wrist osteoarthritis, 605–628
    epidemiology of, 605
    hamato-lunate joint, 616–618
    piso-triquetral joint, 615–616
    radiocarpal joint, 611–613
    radio-ulnar joint, 613
    scapho-trapezial joint, 607–611
    trapezio-metacarpal joint, 606–607
    ulno-carpal joint, 614–615
    ultrasonography for, 506, 509, 512

Moving?

Make sure your subscription moves with you!

To notify us of your new address, find your **Clinics Account Number** (located on your mailing label above your name), and contact customer service at:

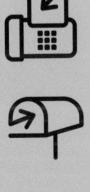

Email: **journalscustomerservice-usa@elsevier.com**

800-654-2452 (subscribers in the U.S. & Canada)
314-447-8871 (subscribers outside of the U.S. & Canada)

Fax number: 314-447-8029

Elsevier Health Sciences Division
Subscription Customer Service
3251 Riverport Lane
Maryland Heights, MO 63043

*To ensure uninterrupted delivery of your subscription, please notify us at least 4 weeks in advance of move.

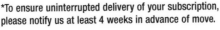

Printed and bound by CPI Group (UK) Ltd, Croydon, CR0 4YY

03/10/2024

01040453-0006